EMPEROR
OF THE NORTH

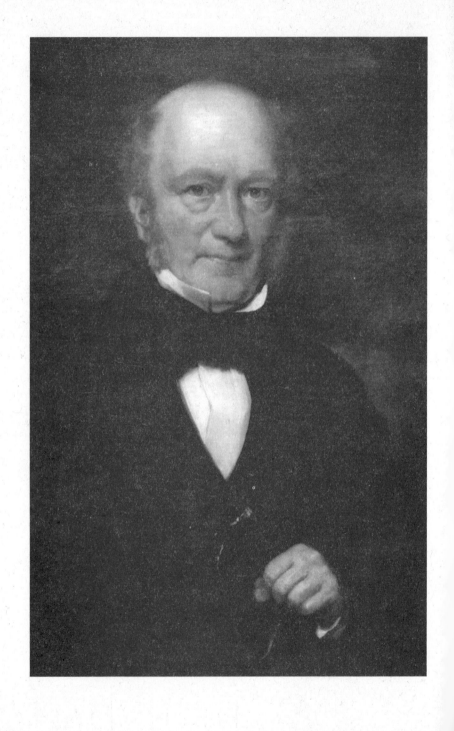

EMPEROR
OF THE NORTH

SIR GEORGE SIMPSON
&
THE REMARKABLE STORY OF
THE HUDSON'S BAY COMPANY

JAMES RAFFAN

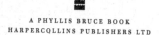

A PHYLLIS BRUCE BOOK
HARPERCOLLINS PUBLISHERS LTD

A Phyllis Bruce Book, published by HarperCollins Publishers Ltd.

Originally published in hardcover by HarperCollins Publishers Ltd: 2007.
This trade paperback edition: 2008.

HarperCollins Publishers Ltd
2 Bloor Street East, 20th Floor
Toronto, Ontario, Canada
M4W 1A8

www.harpercollins.ca

Library and Archives Canada Cataloguing in Publication

Raffan, James
Emperor of the north : Sir George Simpson and the remarkable story
of the Hudson's Bay Company / James Raffan.

"A Phyllis Bruce book".
ISBN 978-0-00-639487-7

1. Simpson, George, Sir, 1792?–1860. 2. Hudson's Bay Company—History—19th
century. 3. Fur trade—Northwest, Canadian—History—19th century. I. Title.

FC3213.1.S5R33 2007   971.201'092   C2007-903560-4

RRD 9 8 7 6 5 4 3 2 1

Printed and bound in the United States
Text design by Sharon Kish

*To Kirk Wipper, who inspired
a new generation of fur traders.*

CONTENTS

———

EMPEROR
OF THE NORTH

———

SIBERIA

Captain Kadnikoff took a long look at the squat dandy in the beaver top hat pacing the foredeck of his Russian-American Company sailing ship, *Alexander*, while it idled in pack ice off the coast of Siberia, waiting for the wind to change. It was June 22, 1842. After forty-three days at sea, the guest from the Hudson's Bay Company was getting more restless by the minute. Being able to see the dilapidated wooden wharves and shanties of the port town of Okhotsk across a cordon of shore-bound ice seemed only to make the fiery little governor more petulant. Above, the red, white and blue stripes of the company flag snapped on the main mast with a stiff breeze that could have easily propelled them the last few miles of the journey, were it not for the spring ice that had preceded them to shore.

Sir George Simpson had been a charming enough passenger in the wardroom as they sailed past the Aleutian Islands and across the rolling waters of the North Pacific to the Sea of Okhotsk. He did have something of an imperious air about him with the stewards, but that might have had more to do with their problems understanding his language. For this Simpson chap was surely a charmer. Many a night his blue eyes had flashed in ship's-lantern light and his freckled little hands had

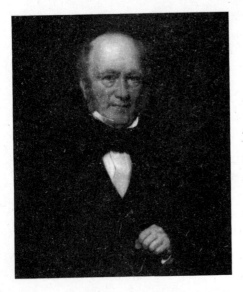

A little known, unsigned portrait of Sir George in the 1850s, in the possession of the Haddon family in Innerleithen, Peebleshire, Scotland. The painter, whose identity is being actively researched, may be Paul Kane or Stephen Pearce.

swept the air as he had told stories of daring canoe exploits and adventures with brave men and beauties in the North American fur country. He ate and drank with the best of the crew, with a seemingly iron constitution. Through foul weather and fair he was last into bed and first up on deck with the dawn watch, pacing like a caged orangutan, wisps of red hair fluttering out from under his hat over clean, pressed collars. Still, the captain liked having such a lively guest aboard. He and the Governor had shared much ribald laughter as they toasted czars, queens, absent wives and lovers—and not necessarily in that order.

With his pinstriped trousers, his spats and his tailored frock coat covered with a blue-lined red tartan cloak, the corner of which he tossed with his cane hand when he turned with a practised aristocratic air on the tar-splattered foredeck, Sir George was a man of style and detail. His manservant had managed to keep him well turned out, no small feat for a man who had bee travelling for more than a year. But now things were not going Sir George's way and, they'd learned, the man had a temper. It was as if, with his affairs out of his immediate control, Simpson had been captured by circumstance and was struggling to contain his frustration.

When he was not below working on correspondence in his suite, he was up on deck pacing. From main hatch to fo'c'sle he would pound, his trim little feet in shiny black leather boots clicking on the *Alexander*'s oaken deck, as if he were vexed with the Almighty himself.

Fifteen months and two hundred degrees of longitude into his around-the-world journey, the newly knighted Sir George Simpson, overseas governor of the venerable Hudson's Bay Company, was frustrated. There was nothing he hated more than inefficiency. Surely, after more than a century of plying the waters of the Bering Sea between Siberia, Kamchatka and the fur posts of the northwest coast of America, the Russian-American Company could have come up with some way to deal with what seemed like such a soluble problem—a bit of ice along the shore. But it was more the circumstance than the problem itself that made him itch. They were not moving. They were stuck. And although the fifty-year-old governor had been caught by ice and weather time and time again across North America during his twenty-two years in the fur trade, George Simpson was never accepting of things he could not control. "If only this tub had steam, we'd be through this ice in an instant," he had muttered more than once to Russian sailors as they went about their business on deck.

The Western world was in the throes of the Industrial Revolution, although word of such developments would not have reached the Russian sailors on a square-rigged ship. George Simpson, who had travelled farther by sailing ship and by canoe than any other contemporary man of business, had experienced personally the dramatic changes that steam had brought to long-distance transportation. Month-long transatlantic crossings that took thirty days on the fastest clipper ships took a quarter to a third of that time with fair seas and plenty of wood to fuel James Watt's amazing, if smelly, invention. And now, with a world view held by few, because they had not had the Governor's drive or opportunity to travel, or his connections with fur traders throughout the northern hemisphere, Simpson was on his way around the world on a route that he had imagined a hundred times. One hundred sixty more degrees of longitude, probably the most difficult seven thousand miles of his entire journey yet to be achieved, and he would be the first person ever to circumnavigate the globe by an overland route—no small feat for an illegitimate child from the north of Scotland. And when his book about this great adventure was published in London by Henry Colburn, who was publishing travel narratives by writers such as Anthony Trollope and Charles Darwin, people would notice—especially those toffs and doubters in London and Inverness. Of that he was sure, or so he told Captain Kadnikoff.

With a wind shift the following day, the *Alexander* was able to poke north through the dissipating pack ice. Eventually the ship was broached by a tender and boarded by a pilot from the Russian-American Company, who guided the ship at high tide into the muddy shallows of Okhotsk harbour. With the pilot came the news that four or five thousand horses carrying supplies for company operations in Kamchatka and Russian America had made it through from Yakutsk. For Simpson, visibly relieved to be moving again, this meant that the treacherous road from Okhotsk on the coast west to Yakutsk on the mighty Lena River, a road that would allow him to continue his around-the-world tour, was open. His plan was to make his way first northwest, then west toward St. Petersburg and, eventually, to London, England, where the journal he had laboured to create would be transformed into a book.

———

For Simpson, halfway through four decades with the Hudson's Bay Company, the epic global circumnavigation that had started in London following his investiture as a knight bachelor by a twenty-one-year-old Queen Victoria on January 25, 1841, was in many respects the zenith of his life and career. Ostensibly, he was knighted for his contribution to northern exploration through his assistance to explorers, including John Franklin and his own cousin Thomas Simpson, but the honour was also a recognition by London society of their respect and his comfort in moving among them, and of his integral role in the politics of

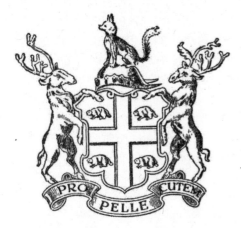

Translated literally from Latin, the HBC motto means "a skin for a skin," which, though variously interpreted, came to mean for men in the trade an exchange of one's hide for employment with the venerable company.

new Britain in North America. But on this journey, moving away from the British–North American axis and onto the international stage, he was travelling more as a statesman or viceroy than as any kind of business leader. He was using his remarkable network of international contacts, but he was also employing his considerable skills of observation, accommodation, negotiation and peregrination. It was a far cry from his apprenticeship as a functionary in a London counting house years earlier, where his business career had begun.

That George Simpson would be drawn to Siberia speaks volumes about his thirst for adventure, his innate curiosity and his broad-minded approach to business. In his earlier dealings with the Russians on the northwest coast of North America, he had been fascinated by their parallel interests. The Hudson's Bay Company had been established in 1670 by royal charter in a more or less monopolistic situation, to conduct the fur trade in North America for Britain; the Russian-American Company had been given a monopoly by Czar Paul I in 1799, to accomplish the same thing for Russia in its corner of North America, in what is now Alaska. Though the RAC, as a corporate entity, was a century younger than the HBC, it was connected through its commercial pedigree to a vast historical fur-trading system in Russia, with markets in China and throughout Europe, a system that was much older and more established than the HBC's in Rupert's Land. There were things the Russians knew about fur and the fur trade that the British did not, and this, as much as the yen to explore new terrain, piqued Simpson's curiosity.

Through discussions with Baron Ferdinand von Wrangel, president of the Russian-American Company, with whom he had negotiated in previous years about company activities on the northwest coast, Sir George discovered that he could use the RAC's established transportation and communication lines to make his way across Asia. In fact, it had been von Wrangel himself—like Simpson, a fiery little man with big dreams—who had suggested that Simpson make the trip. The Russian fur trade was in its denouement by the mid-nineteenth century; Simpson knew that. But he also knew that there were things to be learned from the Russians. He had a sense that what he would experience in a journey across Asia would be similar to what he would see eventually in North America. And he wanted to be prepared.

———

The first moments on shore at Okhotsk were less auspicious than Simpson might have hoped. The governor of Okhotsk, who might otherwise have been at the wharf to meet him, was occupied with his wife who, as the *Alexander* dropped anchor, was giving birth to a baby girl. And the crowd that might have assembled to behold this "governor" from afar were also otherwise occupied. As luck would have it, the following day was the Emperor's birthday, a day of rest and celebration. But because celebratory supplies had yet to arrive on the seven-thousand-mile trek from St. Petersburg, the celebration had been postponed. The eight hundred burghers of Okhotsk stayed in their weathered wooden shacks, avoiding the bugs that infested the coastal marshes surrounding the town and the flies drawn to the corrals of horses waiting for return loads from the docks. And it wasn't as if Okhotsk, at sixty degrees north latitude, caught between the mostly frozen sea and the snow-topped mountains of backcountry Siberia, was expecting visitors from anywhere.

Though he was no stranger to bleak northern landscapes, the harshness of Okhotsk took Sir George by surprise. He knew this had been a penal town for much of its hundred-year history, but he also knew that when the Siberian fur trade had slowed, other economic activities, notably mining, had replaced these revenues. Still, the clutch of weathered wooden buildings on muddy streets would hardly cheer the heart of a visitor. In his account of the journey he wrote,

> A more dreary scene can scarcely be conceived. Not a tree, and hardly even a green blade, is to be seen within miles of the town; and into the midst of the disorderly collection of huts is a stagnant marsh, which, unless when frozen, must be a nursery of all sorts of malaria and pestilence. The climate is at least on a par with the soil. Summer consists of three months of damp and chilly weather, during great part of which the snow still covers the hills, and the ice chokes the harbour; and this is succeeded by nine months of dreary winter, in which the cold, unlike that of more inland spots, is as raw as it is intense ... In summer, in fact, nobody goes out of the house without necessity. If the weather is fine, then the noxious vapours of the stagnant marsh are to be dreaded; and if the weather be not fine, then the rain and wind are to be avoided.[1]

Governor Pavel Nikolaevich Golovin eventually pulled himself away from his wife and new daughter to welcome Simpson and his party to the jurisdiction. Golovin, a former captain of the Imperial Navy, had many questions about North America and the HBC fur trade, and about Governor Simpson's role in it, because—in confusion that would serve Sir George very well during his time in Russia—his British passport listed his occupation as "Governor." Understandably, Golovin, like many people Simpson would encounter in Siberia and across Asia, assumed the title meant Simpson was a man of both politics and business, not just of business. Governor Golovin explained that his jurisdiction, while covering nothing close to the area of Rupert's Land, ran from the

Chinese frontier in the south to the west and north and east. It included all of the Aboriginal people contained therein, as well as about three thousand Russian families. He also explained that though the district was now largely peaceful, its conquest a hundred years earlier had had its moments of conflict between the invading Cossacks and the native Yakuti people. Descendants of these original conquerors, he observed— still proud Cossacks—staffed numerous installations throughout the district and acted as police, as customs and excise constabulary or as a military force, as required.

Perhaps voicing a conclusion Simpson had made in his first few minutes on the docks, that Aboriginal people were clearly second-class citizens, Governor Golovin explained the sometimes strained relationship between the Russians, particularly the Cossacks, and the Aboriginal people of his domain, the Yakuti. Since the conquest, the Yakuti had had to pay a head tax, or *yassack*, levied on each adult male, in addition to bending to Cossack rule, which always brought with it the threat or enactment of force. Though the HBC's relationships with Indians in North America were not as adversarial, these discussions no doubt reminded Simpson of stories to tell the Russian governor about Aboriginal peoples in North America, whose traditional customs were often at odds with HBC policies and ways of doing business. Of course, officially, there was no historical counterpart for Cossacks in the North American fur trade, except perhaps the rough-and-tumble agents of the HBC and its archrival, the North West Company.

The rule of thumb for business or politics in this part of the world, Simpson quickly learned from Golovin, was "God is high and the emperor far off." Translated into the day-to-day reality of life in this isolated Siberian port town, a place dedicated largely to the transshipment of Russian-American Company goods from horse caravans at the end of a supply line reaching all the way west to the Black Sea, this meant that local leaders ruled the day. For example, Sir George learned, freight rates for shipments of goods by sea from Okhotsk to Kamchatka, as set far away in St. Petersburg, were half a ruble[2] per pood (a weight equivalent to thirty-six pounds avoirdupois), but by the time the goods were on the dock in Okhotsk the price had been inflated to fifteen rubles per pood. This, he noted with some amazement in his journal, represented a 2,900 per cent peculation for greedy hinterland shippers.

The immediate order of the day in Okhotsk for Simpson, however, was to negotiate for some of the horses and one or two Yakuti herders, who had brought supplies to the coast. A party was needed to transport Sir George and his entourage over the mountains and several hundred miles inland to the village of Yakutsk, from where they would continue west by boat up the Lena River. Simpson, fancying himself a skilled negotiator with Aboriginal peoples, language barriers notwithstanding, cast around to engage some of the local Aboriginal men who, until they were dragged by enthusiastic Cossacks before Governor Golovin, had no real interest in any kind of contract with Sir George. But, before the governor, a deal was struck with a wily old Yakut called Jacob, who agreed to convey Simpson, his servant and two other companions—an RAC employee who had come across with them from Sitka and a young Gaelic-speaking friend called McIntyre whom Simpson had met on the Atlantic crossing, the first leg of the journey—from Okhotsk to Yakutsk, on the Lena River, eighteen days' journey inland on a track that was a "mere apology for a highway,"[3] at a rental fee of 45 rubles per horse, as long as no single load exceeded 5 poods (180 pounds).

What troubled Sir George in this negotiation was not so much that Jacob and his helpers had to be "encouraged" (with fear of being beaten) into helping them—this was nothing new to a man who knew all the tricks to get voyageurs to shoulder loads when motivation was low—but that a conundrum arose over the pricing of the horses. Simpson had agreed, on advice of Governor Golovin, to rent the horses for forty-five rubles per steed but, having done some comparative shopping on his own, he knew that to purchase a horse outright in Okhotsk cost only thirty to forty rubles. Fortunately for him, he took Golovin's advice, as he noted later in his journal:

Your cheap bargains [for horses] may be unsound from the beginning; even if they are sound, they are seldom able to accomplish the whole journey; and even if they die or break down, they are almost certain to be stolen. In addition to all this, guides and drivers must be separately paid; while from having no interest in your [animals], excepting perhaps an interest adverse to your own, they may prove more troublesome than the brutes themselves. As a general rule, a traveller, whether in Siberia or elsewhere, rarely promotes either comfort or economy by being wise in his own conceit.[4]

So it was that on rented horses, with Jacob, the chief Yakuti herdsman (whom Simpson very soon started calling "the Princeling"), in the lead, the party swung onto the unfamiliar oiled surfaces of overstuffed Cossack-style saddles, with their sweat-burnished figure-eight-shaped leather pads and carved birchwood trees over colourful felted horsehair blankets, and headed upriver and into Siberia. Just as Simpson had felt comfortable with the rocky landscapes throughout much of northern Rupert's Land when he'd first arrived, because they reminded him of his Scottish home, now his journey in twenty-two-hour daylight up narrow craggy paths through thick boreal forests into the snow-covered Stanovoi Mountains north of Okhotsk and onto more sparsely treed steppes must have reminded him of country back in North America. Even the robin-sized mosquitoes that buzzed around his sweating horse's head might have brought for the resilient traveller a minor touch of geographic verisimilitude if not fleeting nostalgia.

Edward Hopkins, Simpson's principal secretary,[5] had left the party prior to the Asian leg, so Simpson was left to do his own journal keeping while he made his way into Siberia, but he was not alone as he continued his round-the-world voyage. On the horse beside him was the young Scot, McIntyre, whom he'd met on the North Atlantic crossing. Because he enjoyed his company, and because the young man spoke fluent Gaelic, Simpson's native tongue, the Governor, as a man with power and means can do on a whim, had invited him along on the rest of the trip. Also travelling with them were an officer of the RAC who had been with Simpson since London (because it would be shorter to go west instead of east to where the officer was going in Siberia) and, of course, a Cossack for discipline, as well as two additional Yakuti herders working with the Princeling. In addition to these seven men on their sturdy little Siberian mounts were twenty-two more horses, loaded principally with Simpson's kit: leather hat boxes, cases of fine wine and port, trunks full of clothing, a handsome wooden toilet kit with polished brass hardware, and what amounted to a dwindling supply of pemmican, taken along in the event that local victuals ran a bit thin. The Governor did not travel light.

The Princeling turned out to have all of the qualities of the most superstitious of the voyageurs with whom Simpson had travelled by canoe in his yearly rambles around Rupert's Land. He had considerable skills as a horseman (and more than enough excuses to travel more slowly than Sir George would have liked), but he was troubled constantly, or so he said, by "spirits of the forest" that required almost constant appeasement with toasts, gifts and other rituals of various kinds. The horse being absolutely central to Yakuti life, the most common gestures to the spirits were symbolic offerings of horsehair, which were tied to trees along the trail. Additionally, impromptu songs, like Norwegian *yoiks*, were sung to the spirits as the horses made their way. As in Rupert's Land, where Indian guides would feed the fire with food or sacred herbs, such as tobacco, as a gesture of thanks to the spirits of the land through which they travelled, Jacob and his crew would always throw the first spoonful or two of their evening trail meal—which usually was a pot of rye flour, butter and sour horse milk—into the fire to "purchase a sound sleep from the genius of the place" and honour "the tutelary divinity of the neighbourhood."[6] As Simpson knew well from his days in canoes, such interruptions, if not dealt with properly and in the necessary amount of time, could delay an expedition indefinitely when the Native guides, as a result, refused to move among angry spirits.

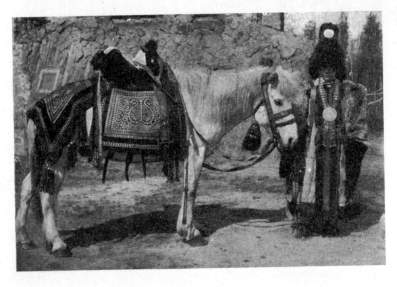

Simpson's Yakuti companions knew their horses.

As in North America, where travelling parties would routinely encounter Native villages and encampments along the way, Simpson and his Yakuti companions passed regularly spaced *ostrogs*, or Cossack encampments, as well as Aboriginal families living in blanket-covered "yourtes" along the trail from Okhotsk to Yakutsk. They even visited Jacob's own family, where they were treated to a tea, more like tobacco than orange pekoe, brewed black in boiling water and made thick by the addition of butter and salt. But these experiences with Jacob, his family and his people, however cordial and welcoming, were never social occasions with equals. There was no doubt that the white Cossacks and the European travellers were of one class of traveller, while the Yakuti were of another. Whatever affections Simpson had for his Princeling, when travel slowed to an unacceptable pace he was not beyond giving the nod to the Cossack to administer lashes with a bullwhip to speed things up. These horsemen, after all, like slaves he had met in his early days in the sugar trade in London, before he joined the HBC, were *not* white-skinned.

Because the trail became more densely overgrown as they moved northwest and away from the ocean, the main hazard was eye damage from bushes and branches that snapped back when an animal passed. As bad luck would have it, one of the party experienced just that. When the expedition stopped to attend to his wound, a vial of an all-purpose opium-based potion called laudanum, from the Governor's personal toilet box, set in motion a cascade of alarming events.

A quantity of this elixir was decanted into a glass and set aside for application to the injured eye, after the wound had been rinsed and was free of irritating debris. While the first aid ministrations were going on, McIntyre noticed the Cossack surreptitiously eyeing the glass on the toilet box. All that was available by way of intoxicants on the expedition, besides Sir George's well-packed personal stock of wine and port, was *kumyss*, a slightly alcoholic brew of mare's milk, fermented by the heat of the sun in a leather skin. The chance to dabble with something stronger was too much for the Cossack. The next time McIntyre turned, the clear colourless liquid was gone and the soldier had a grimace on his face. Knowing that this quantity of medication would surely render the man unconscious, Sir George ordered McIntyre to decant and immediately administer another liquid from the case—a powerful emetic, possibly syrup of ipecac. The vomiting episode that followed may have saved the Cossack's life and left the man astonished at the speed with which liquid justice was delivered, but Simpson's account does not detail the broader scene, which almost certainly included the Princeling and his Yakuti helpers snickering among themselves or madly tying horsehair to the bushes to thank the spirits for their timely intervention.

What most surprised Simpson, as he compared his emerging experience in Siberia with his travels in the hinterland of Rupert's Land, was the amount of other traffic on this busy "apology for a highway." This being spring, they were moving against the traffic, as it were—contrary to the main flow of goods being shipped east on horseback to Okhotsk, for transport to Kamchatka and Russian posts, notably Sitka, in what is now the panhandle of Alaska. Daily they encountered hundreds of horses making their way through the hills to the coast. And as the small group headed the other way, they were often compelled to stop and wait while the bigger herds passed. On one occasion, Jacob sensed that the spirits of the forest were agitated. This premonition was followed by a large herd of jittery horses, guided by even more unnerved herders, who whistled by with news that a she-bear and her cubs had run amok on the trail a little farther inland. They never did see the bears. Mealtime offerings were made, many bunches of horse-hair were tied on bushes at the scene, and the travellers continued on. Bears or no bears, Simpson—ever the businessman—reckoned they had passed not fewer than five thousand loads of goods by the close of their fifth day on the trail.

They encountered a goodly number of other human travellers as well. A judge and his entourage, with their horses, herders and requisite Cossacks, happened into camp for dinner one evening, as they squatted around a buggy campfire. Another day, they met a Mr. Porch, a private businessman who had been travelling east from Moscow for nearly four months. And they made the acquaintance of an RAC clerk, affiliated with another herd of pack horses, who was travelling with coops of chickens and pigeons for the pot. In each of these passings, Simpson must have fairly glowed with embarrassment as his Cossack "supplied the place of a whole regiment of buttons and crosses by the most exaggerated representations of my rank and importance."[7]

On another occasion, proving that the Hudson's Bay Company did not have an exclusive franchise on backcountry bureaucracy, a mail carrier came through alone on horseback, with communications that had been relayed all the way from St. Petersburg. While, through Jacob, he assured Simpson that the mail he was carrying very likely included much-anticipated personal and business mail for the British governor from his family in Lachine, Canada, and from the Hudson's Bay Company governors in London, there was absolutely no way he could unlock the bag: it was against company protocols. He explained that he was seventeen days out of Yakutsk and would have to continue to the end of his journey, at Okhotsk, before the bag could be opened. And in the event that there was mail for Sir George, as there most certainly was, it would be duly sorted and rebound as a load for the next courier headed back up the road. It would be another month before these letters would be read by their intended recipient. But in the world Simpson knew, wherein letters travelled across the Atlantic by ship and then by canoe or snowshoe over vast distances, this delay, however frustrating, would not cause undue harm.

What mattered most to Sir George was the narrative he planned to write on his round-the-world journey, a narrative that would place him among such famed explorer-writers as Samuel Hearne, John Franklin and his own distant relative Alexander Mackenzie, each of whom had made a literary mark in the world and thus secured a place in history. Somehow Simpson had determined that the best way to achieve notice beyond the business community was to write and publish a book. Although this round-the-world journey fed his appetite for adventure and, in some ways, advanced the international cause of the HBC, the trip was really about one thing and one thing only: the book that would one day sit leather-bound in his office library with the narratives of other noted adventurers.

In Sir George's account of the journey, which was finally published in 1847, there are periodic references that reflect his unique knowledge of North American landscapes, technology, First Nations and habits of life. As the trail northwest from Okhotsk threaded its way into the glaciers and mountains of Siberia, Simpson noted an eleven-hundred-foot vertical rock face that reminded him of the famous Thunder Rock on Lake Superior. There were corduroy roads and pack boards for carrying children that also reminded him of home. On the numerous river crossings, too deep to ford on horseback, he was fascinated to see that the Yakuti, like the North American Indians, had sturgeon-nosed canoes made of birchbark—the same peculiar shape, with unusual pointed triangular ends, as those used by the Indians in the Kootenay River region of Rupert's Land. Later on in the journey, he was much impressed with the Russians' efficient use of charcoal and stoves, so much so that he eventually secured the services of a Russian tutor who would travel to HBC posts in North America and teach personnel there how to emulate the technology. And, having seen how well the Yakuti had taken to life as it had evolved for them in concert with the march of progress in Russia—becoming full contractors in the transportation business and various other aspects of the fur trade, workers in the various silver, gold and base metal mines that had been opened by prisoners of the czar, and farmers, of a sort, husbanding horses and cattle on their traditional territories—he wondered, in his journal, if the same might be possible for the First Nations of North America: "How happy, thought I, would it make me to see some of the poor savages of North America thus devoting their lives to peaceful industry, and enjoying all the comforts of pastoral existence!"[8]

When all was said and done, though, Sir George was a man of creature comforts. To get those comforts more quickly than he might have had he stayed with his luggage and travelled at the Princeling's pace, he set his own speed. He and McIntyre left Jacob and the spirits when the trail to Yakutsk was obvious and galloped away on their own, as a pair of couriers might. By now word about this British "governor" had spread up and down the track, so they were able to change horses at RAC depots along the way. They took rough lodging as it came for the last few days of the trip, and arrived well ahead of the main party. Here, as he had been promised by Governor Golovin, he was welcomed with the silver-service hospitality of the head of the Yakutsk District, Governor Roodikoff, and his family. Jacob and his band of Yakuti men—and, of course, the Cossack—plodded up to the south bank of the Lena River with their score of pack horses about three days later, to find the Governor in clean clothes with his belly full of the finest foods the Siberians could offer.

Like Golovin, 880 miles to the southeast, Roodikoff had been a captain in the Russian navy, but he had been taken prisoner by the British in 1806 at the Cape of Good Hope. The result of this incarceration by the ever-so-civilized officers of the British Imperial Navy was that Governor Roodikoff had a soft spot for the British. He made it clear from the outset of the visit that he would do his best to treat the visiting governor royally during his stay in Yakutsk. In addition to providing clean linens and the possible favours of his daughters or other eligible beauties, Roodikoff hosted a soirée that Simpson described at length in his journal.

At the dinner, local dignitaries—the headman of the Cossack detachment, the chief councillor, two doctors and the local merchants—amounted to a table with settings for twenty-five. The food was like nothing Simpson had seen in a long time: "soups, fish, beef, veal, fowls, wild and tame, the former in great variety, with pastry, sweets, and ices, and many other things besides, the whole accompanied by wines in abundance, and graced by a prince of a landlord"[9]—a far cry from fire-singed pots of rye flour stewed in milk or travel-worn pemmican washed down with slops of warm, rancid *kumyss*. Captain Roodikoff restricted his remarks to Russian, at least initially, as formal speeches of welcome were made around the table. In his understated prose, however, Simpson described how the Russian governor relaxed as the night wore on: "[Governor Roodikoff] launched out more and more boldly into such English as he could remember, with every succeeding round of champagne; and, in fact, the glorious old sailor dealt bumper after bumper with such rapidity, that I was fairly driven to rebel against his orders. We accordingly adjourned to the smoking room; but the change was of no avail, for the enemy followed us to our place of refuge, continuing its explosions until all was blue."[10]

And the evening was not done: it continued with a short siesta, followed by dancing with sixty or seventy local ladies brought in especially for the occasion. Simpson describes "waltzing, quadrilling, fallopading &c., till two in the morning."[11] If that led to liaisons of any other kind later on in the evening, he neglected to say. But, given Simpson's generously charged libido, it seems highly unlikely that after months in the company of sailors and other men he did not exercise his carnal urges at this stop in Siberia, given half a chance and a willing woman.

These varied interactions with the people of Siberia allowed Sir George to exercise his ample curiosity about business and customs in this corner of the world so distant from his own. He learned of the Russian equivalent of the luxuriously furred North American marten—the sable—and how, even in the declining trade in this part of the world, these pelts still were sought and had maintained their value in the markets of Europe. And he was captivated by the alloys of silver and copper that the Yakuti had wrought and worked into ornate saddle designs before the arrival of the Russians. But what got him thinking was the trade in mammoth-tusk ivory that was as important as, even more important economically than, either furs or metals.

These tusks, he learned, were found in great abundance all across eastern Siberia, on the skeletons of long-buried woolly mammoths that would be uncovered in glacial till by springtime water movements along the shores of lakes and rivers. Sir George was impressed with the price of ivory on the Yakutsk market, as well as with the fact that Providence seemed to have provided an inexhaustible supply of this organic raw material. Yakutsk, after all, was almost at the Arctic Circle.

After Yakutsk, Simpson and McIntyre boarded a nasty little horse-drawn punt to travel up the mighty Lena River for a distance of more than four thousand miles. The craft had three parts: the fore third had an earthen floor, where a fire for warmth and cooking was tended; the middle third was a cabin (or "crib," as Simpson called it), covered with a kind of canvas canopy, where passengers sat, ate and slept; the aft third was a set of planks on which a helmsman stood with his steering oar to counter the pulling force of the horses being led up the bank by his underlings. Simpson and McIntyre weren't in the boats more than a few hours before the closeness and the clouds of mosquitoes moved Sir George to start referring to the "crib" as a "prison" or a "floating cage." But there were spirits to be dealt with, laconic Yakuti horse tenders to be cajoled by the Cossack, and places to stop, where the Cossack's inflated descriptions of Simpson and company would render townsfolk "more obsequious than words could tell."[12] And, of course, competition between would-be hosts—RAC officials and various governors and district heads—made life at village stops as lively as the boat travel was monotonous.

Simpson amused himself by interrogating people he met along the way and by keeping track of soil and vegetation conditions and what people seemed to be doing for their livelihood. He saw people in birchbark shoes at one point, and at another, where the river narrowed, he compared the Lena to the North Saskatchewan River at Fort Carleton. He went to fairs, watched Cossacks dance, hobnobbed with company and government dignitaries, and ate well on sumptuous local fare—fish patties, sweetbreads, stewed prunes, caviar, radishes, salted fish—switching, as he moved into country more conducive to growing grains, from *kumyss* to gin, rum and *nalifky*, a rye-based spirit flavoured with nuts and berries. And fully a month after he had first crossed paths with them, the letters that had passed him on the trail from Okhotsk to Yakutsk caught up with him, this time in the saddlebags of a special courier, dispatched by Governor Roodikoff, who chased them for nearly a thousand miles up the Lena before making good the delivery.

From the southernmost point of travel on the Lena, Simpson's party travelled on to Irkutsk, where Simpson took a side trip to Lake Baikal and learned much about the interconnected history of Russia and Mongolia. Here, in his narrative, he couldn't resist a bit of blatant self-congratulation:

At the first glance of this the largest body of fresh water on the continent, my thoughts flew back over my still recent footsteps to that parent of many Baikals, the Lake Superior of the new world; and I involuntarily reflected, with some degree of pride, that no preceding traveller of any age or nation had ever stood on the shores of the two greatest of the inland seas of the globe. Even if my previous wanderings through the wildernesses of North America had not given me any personal interest in the matter, I could hardly have refrained from indulging in a comparison between the Baikal, on the one hand, and the Superior, with its great progeny on the other.[13]

The cramped little boat was traded back for travel on horseback and, for the last leg, Simpson and McIntyre settled into a handsome tarantass, a low four-wheeled carriage drawn by five horses, while three telegas with eight horses among them followed with the mountain of luggage. Travelling in a conveyance more fitting a "governor" only increased the obsequiousness of the locals in towns they passed. Although he remarked at one point that he felt disgusted by this show of subservience, which he thought even a sovereign could not accept "without a feeling of degradation,"[14] one gets the sense that Sir George secretly revelled in his celebrity.

Okhotsk, Yakutsk, Irkutsk, Lake Baikal, Krasnoyarsk, Tomsk, Omsk, Tobolsk, Perm, Kazan, Moscow and on to St. Petersburg, with the final five hundred miles on the relative comfort of a macadamized road: Sir George Simpson was the first person to travel overland from one side of the Asian continent to the other, ninety-one days and about seven thousand miles, as part of a circumnavigation of the globe. In St. Petersburg, he and McIntyre boarded the steamer *Nicolai* and headed out into the Gulf of Finland and beyond, through the Baltic Sea, taking on coal at Stitichaun, on the island of Gothland, to Hamburg and, eventually, to Gravesend and up the Thames to London at the end of October 1842. He had travelled around the world in precisely nineteen months and twenty-six days.

That Sir George could make this journey reflected the corporate station he had reached: overseas governor of the Hudson's Bay Company. But this journey had nothing to do with business. It was driven by an agenda buried in a complex and conflicted psyche, by a frenetic drive to make something of himself, to reach an achievement that would not betray his common bastard's birth. And, in completing the trip and eventually publishing his book, he got his wish, as evidenced by one of the shortest entries in Dod's *Peerage* for the year 1854. Surrounded by entries that speak of aristocratic roots and of achievements in business, politics and the affairs of state, Simpson's entry includes nothing about his birth or his wife's pedigree, and little else, beyond his station with the HBC and one other detail—that he had gone around the world and published a book—to position him among the peers, baronets and knights. Why did he take such pride in this journey and its published account, having governed a venerable business enterprise for longer than anyone else and presided over more territory than Queen Victoria? In that there's a story.

PART I

———

THE EDUCATION OF
GEORGE SIMPSON

CHAPTER I

———

DINGWALL

In a 1944 biography, the first on Sir George Simpson, historian Arthur Morton devotes a speculative few pages to Simpson's formative years, placing his birth out of wedlock in the parish of Loch Broom, on the "wild and ... desolate" western coast of Ross-shire, Scotland, and his upbringing in his grandparents' manse in Avoch, on Black Isle, north of Inverness. In a second biography, written sixteen years later, John Chalmers makes no reference at all to the Governor's formative years, nor to his business apprenticeship in London, choosing to begin his story when Sir George joined the Hudson's Bay Company in 1820. The third, most recent—and most thorough—biography, written in 1976 by John S. Galbraith, refers to Simpson's early life as "the unknown years." What is ironic about this is that these years are "unknown" because George Simpson did everything in his considerable power during his lifetime to play down his humble roots, perhaps even altering the historical record.[1]

However, a recent genealogy by Dale Terrence Lahey, Simpson's great-great-great-grandson, has added substantially to an understanding of the Governor's early years. Lahey has shed light on George Simpson Sr., and what he was doing around the time of his son's birth:

Sir George Simpson's father . . . was born and educated in Avoch on the Black Isle, ten miles east of Dingwall. About 1774 [at the age of fifteen] he was sent to Dingwall, where he apprenticed as a lawyer's clerk. He became a writer (the name for a lawyer in Scotland) and practised in the Sheriff's court there, and functioned as a factor and tacksman for local land owners. In 1805, he applied for and was appointed to the position of agent for the British Fisheries Society in Ullapool, a position he held until 1830, when he retired and settled in Redcastle, near Beauly. He died sometime after August 1841. No record for the birth or baptism of Sir George Simpson has been found, but it is almost certain that he was born in or near Dingwall, where his father was living and working during the 1780s and 1790s. There is not a shred of evidence from Simpson's lifetime that he was born in the 1780s; however, there is considerable evidence that he was born in the early 1790s. The best guess at a birth date is represented here as "about 1792."[2]

Sending George Sr. to apprentice in Dingwall was a logical move. Avoch (pronounced "Och") was a small fishing town near the heart of the Clan Mackenzie fiefdom on the Black Isle that could offer little to a bright young man who had finished school and who was not interested in becoming a preacher, a fisherman or a gentleman-in-training with his mother's family. Dingwall Sheriff's Court did more business than any other court in the district, being the Ross-shire county seat and next to the parish of Ferrintosh, which, for many years and for convoluted historical reasons, had the privilege of distilling spirits without paying the King's duties on the proceeds of that labour. This, according to the *Statistical Account of Scotland 1791*, resulted in "a good harvest to Dingwall procurators" to settle the frequent drunken quarrels between and breaches of the peace by Ferrintosh folk. In fact, demographic statistics in that same document indicate a disproportionate number of writers or attorneys (6) for the size of Dingwall town (population 745), who, in addition to dealing with issues of land and property before the Sheriff's Court and dealing with the Ferrintosh

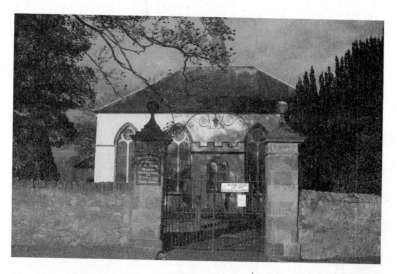

The Dingwall Kirk is where George Simpson would have attended church with his father as a boy. Although both are buried elsewhere, the names of many relatives are etched on stones beneath the chestnut trees in this old churchyard.

thugs, represented people involved in occasional dust-ups at the 19 ale and whisky houses dotted through the Dingwall Parish. But by 1845, temperance had prevailed enough (alongside, presumably, a fall-off in lawyerly business for Dingwall writers) to allow the local preacher, who submitted information to the Scottish statistics books, to report that "the number of habitual drunkards in the place is small, bearing no proportion to the amount of temptation to that vice presented by the great number of public houses. Still the tone of their morality is rather strict than high."[3]

George Sr. either roomed in Dingwall or commuted the ten miles by horse to and from the family home in Avoch as he worked through his legal apprenticeship. He would have been in that position for more than ten years, and presumably by then a journeyman writer making a good living in the Sheriff's Court when his father, Thomas, died in 1786, and the remaining family members—his younger sisters, Jean and Mary, his younger brothers, Geddes, Duncan and possibly Thomas,[4]

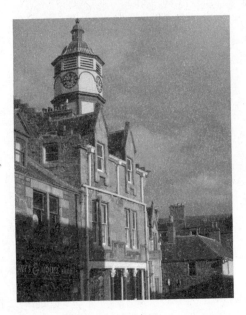

The regular chiming of the bell emanating from the clock tower on the Dingwall Town Hall would have kept young George aware of time and the direction of home.

and his mother, Isobel Mackenzie, moved to Dingwall. At some juncture after this, George Sr. had a non-conjugal relationship that resulted in the birth of his first and possibly only son, George.

To date, not a church or public record, not a birth or death notice, not a letter, a gravestone, an obituary, a medical note, a council minute or a gossip line in any newspaper of the period has yielded even a scrap of information about Sir George's mother. Speculation has led some to wonder if, because of her unusual care and attention to her brother's son, George's aunt Mary might have been his mother through incest, but there is no evidence to support that theory.

What *is* known is that children born out of wedlock were as common in the late eighteenth century as they were at any other time throughout history. Census statistics for 1861, for example—the oldest available—indicate that in northeastern Scotland, fully 15.12 per cent of all births were out of wedlock, with similar values for the cities of Aberdeen and Dundee. And although the Church of Scotland took firm moral stands on all manner of human enterprise, there was not the stigma on illegitimate births—on the parents, at least—at the time of Simpson's arrival that there would be in later years. As for scarceness of records, contemporary research into Scottish illegitimacy[5] points out that it was often leading men in local churches and politics who sired children out of wedlock, men who, with hands on the levers of power, had the wherewithal to keep their indiscretions out of the official record books.

Nevertheless, it was a common occurrence in the Highlands of Scotland for the father to take full responsibility for the child, especially if the mother was young and from a crofting family with too many other mouths to feed. Indeed, Sir George's great-grandmother was born out of wedlock, the product of a liaison between Duncan Forbes of Culloden, a well-to-do lawyer who became head of the Scottish Court of Session, and a woman whose identity he concealed even as he raised the child as his own and made her a legal heir. It was this ancestor who took the family line from Edinburgh north to the wilds of Ross-shire when she married George Mackenzie and moved to his estate on Loch Broom, where George Sr.'s mother, Isobel, was born. And it is this branch of the family that has drawn earlier searchers to the "wilds of Loch Broom" for clues about Simpson's birth.

To whom George Simpson was born, then, is complete mystery. When and where George Simpson was born, however, is much clearer now, thanks to Dale Lahey's genealogical research. And though the "to whom" is incomplete, it is not without impact: George Simpson may have had a plain name, but he became a complex character, combining the discipline and clear-eyed pragmatism of his lowland Saxon Simpson side and the flamboyance and vision of his Highland Mackenzie side, a small bear of a man who had great pride in accomplishment but whose family secrets he himself would never reveal.

———

Born at $57°35'$ north latitude, George Simpson was, to his core, a northerner. Though the weather in the north of Scotland is mild relative to North America's, moderated by the North Atlantic Drift, the town

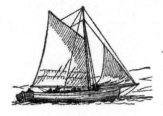

As he grew up on the coast of an island community, small boats, or smacks, would have been an almost daily part of George Simpson's life in Ross-shire.

of Dingwall is at the same latitude as St. Petersburg, southern Siberia, the Alaskan panhandle and the icy middle of Hudson Bay. Hence, Simpson's internal clocks would have been set to the short December days (with only six hours of daylight at the winter solstice). But, like children around the northern hemisphere, he would have longed for those lingering summer days, which, at his latitude, would be eighteen hours long in mid-June. In July and August, the loll of the northern sun would have meant he could play and ramble outdoors to his heart's content, running out of energy most days before running out of daylight.

And what a locale he had in which to venture. Straddling the River Peffery, where it flows toward the north shore of the Cromarty Firth, Dingwall sits in a verdant little valley. When Simpson was born, the town measured a mile and a half by two miles, surrounded by water and by shadowed grey-green hills.[6] To the east, past wheeling gulls that cracked clams over tidal flats, were the gently rolling forests and rich-soiled fields of Black Isle and the town of Avoch, his father's birthplace, and beyond that the distant blue Cairngorm Mountains. To the south, young Simpson's eye would have been drawn by the converging hills along a salt-marsh pasture to the valley of the River Conon, where, in crystalline malt-whisky-making waters, he might have guddled trout or fished for freshwater pearls. To the west was the welcoming southern knoll of the Strathpeffer Ridge, rising past drystone dikes and fat sheep to freshwater Loch Ussie and the Scotch pines, oaks, larches, elms and elephant-legged beech trees in the Woodside of Tollie. And to the north, where he would run and hide on daylong adventures, was the ruin of Tulloch Castle on Tulloch Hill, where he and his friends would look for horse chestnuts on the northern spine of the Strathpeffer Ridge. Beyond that, as he got older and earned the freedom to venture farther, he would have rambled to the twin towns of Dochcairnie and Dochcartie or to the Spoutwell mineral spring. And always, on clear days, would beckon the snow-dusted peak of Ben Wyvis ("Terrible Hill"), six miles to the north and towering 3,430 feet above sea level. Hills to climb, waters and tidal flats to explore—an adventure in every direction, not five minutes from the centre of his own fetching little town.

Farther afield, horse-drawn family affairs would have taken young Simpson to Conon Bridge and across to Avoch or Inverness. And because the waters of Cromarty Firth were never really deep enough, even at high tide, to float a boat of any size, there would have been occasional trips northeast along the north shore of the firth to the port town of Invergordon, where coastal supply boats, called "smacks," which docked every three or four weeks, would give and take passengers and supplies headed for Leith (Edinburgh's port) or London. And, making good the alpine promise of the craggy top of Ben Wyvis, on a road built the year Simpson was born, journeys would most certainly have been made up Strathpeffer Glen to Loch Garve, Blackwater and Loch Glascarnoch and to the heathered highlands of Wester Ross, where the wind tasted of heath and salt air and where the sun walked slowly through clouds, gorse and yellow broom. If there was ever a place to fall in love by proxy with the colour of the North American western prairie or the northern tundra, with the sense of freedom and possibility they imbue, it was the rocky highlands of Ross-shire.

By all accounts, young George's main caregiver was his aunt Mary who, perhaps as a result of close monitoring of his education at the Dingwall school, was courted by the schoolmaster, Alexander Simpson. Alexander Simpson had one "natural" child, Horatio Nelson Simpson, born out of wedlock to another unknown Ross-shire woman, and for whose raising he took responsibility. A second son, Aemilius, arrived in 1792, born to Alexander and his first wife, Emilia MacIntosh, a Dingwall parish farmer's daughter who died soon after his birth. Romance between Alexander and Mary could only have been reinforced and encouraged by the school friendship between Aemilius and young George, both of whom would go into long service with the Hudson's Bay Company, Aemilius as a sea captain and George, eventually, as overseas governor.

What those boys might have done through middle childhood and adolescence, as the century turned and their independence grew, was defined by their imaginations and shaped by the censure of Calvinist parents. But what a rich and adventuresome world it must have been, with perhaps a special bond between Aemilius and George—of similar age, both "motherless," though for different reasons, and both with a yen to venture. Fishing or swimming in the River Peffery, learning horsemanship skills on the Dingwall farms and liveries, digging in the blue clay strata at the edge of Cromarty Firth for ancient seashells, re-enacting the Battle of Culloden, by turns soldiers of the government or of the Young Pretender. Rambling up Tulloch Hill or Strathpeffer Ridge to snare rabbits or perhaps to hunt partridges or deer, or rising early on a long summer's day, perhaps with a dog in tow, to hike the grand circle and scale Ben Wyvis, prattling in Gaelic over a flask of hot tea, with smoked herring, farm cheese and fresh bannock drawn from a handkerchief lumped at the bottom of a hand-sewn rucksack.

And then there were lessons, taught to the strict rule of Aemilius's father, Alexander Simpson, in the schoolhouse (still extant, at the corner of High and Church streets)[7] by the town hall at the centre of Dingwall. Time then, as now, was marked by the quarter-hour chiming of the bells in the clock tower. In the two-room school, several dozen children of mixed grades and ages, all of whom would pay several pence per month as school fees, studied reading, writing, arithmetic and geography. Gaelic was the oral tradition of the common people in Scotland at the time, but there were precious few printed books in that language, so English grammar was taught in conjunction with reading to give students access to written resources, most of which were printed in English, and to the classics of English literature. As a university-educated dominie (school-

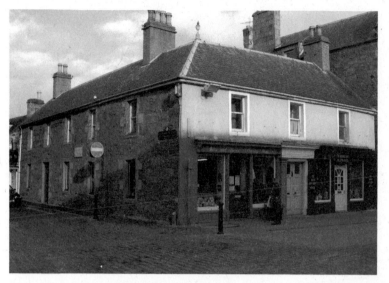

Now a charity shop, the building in which George Simpson went to school, at the corner of Church and High streets, in Dingwall, still stands.

master), Alexander Simpson might have been able to also offer lessons in mathematics to the older children, as well as tutelage in Latin, Greek and possibly French. We know he had facility in Latin because it was in this ancient tongue that he delivered a special oration at the pugilistic festivities on Fasten's Eve, Shrove Tuesday, 1812.[8]

———

The annual cockfight on Fasten's Eve was eagerly awaited by everyone in town. The competition was one on one, individual birds (and their keepers) against all comers in a round-robin fight to the death. It was a very public competition, and among the spectators were some of the parish's most distinguished gentry. In a long-standing tradition that came with the job of schoolmaster, it fell to Alexander Simpson to hold the betting book. There was also money to be made for Mr. Simpson (who supplemented his income with the entry fees and who got to keep "losers" for the pot), but there was also money to be made for the town councillors and others with means to wager on the outcome of the day. The fights involved real money on the floor and a real life-and-death struggle played out before the bettors' eyes. And they were barbaric. Birds that turned tail and ran—called "fugies"—were tied up against a wall and stoned to death by a melee of blood-hungry boys. The owner of the bird that emerged the victor from the bloody day of conflict in the makeshift cockpit in the Dingwall schoolroom would wear the crown and be the toast of the town. And, best of all, there was instant celebrity and privilege for the victor: the right to decide for the dominie, for a period after the fight, who would get strapped and who would not. For boys of a particular character and frame of mind, this must have been a heady day, and particularly so for those with a taste for blood sport and a thirst for power.

The last of these school cockfights took place on Shrove Tuesday in February 1812 and was described in some detail by Alexander Simpson himself.

There was a large entry of birds both from the town and the surrounding Heights, the birds from Dochcairnie and Dochcartie being charged an extra entry fee of 2/6 [two shillings sixpence], the town birds paying 1/- each. The owner of the victor bird, which was crowned the king of cocks, had to pay the schoolmaster a fee of three guineas—the honour was considered cheap at the price, one of the merchants of the town having also to provide the schoolmaster with a new hat. On that occasion the crown for the hero was prepared of a costly velvet, with jewels, the latter being lent for the occasion by ladies of the county. The jewels on this occasion in Dingwall were provided by a sister of Sir Hector Munro, K.B., whose spoils from the East afforded gems and cloth of gold that were worth thousands of pounds. The victor bird was bred and reared at Dochcairnie, then a pleasantly situated hamlet to the west of Dochcartie and east of Dochmaluag, not a stone of which nor trace of the fine garden trees that indicated the spot some sixty years ago now remaining on the site. Assisting the owner was his kinsman who is still remembered in the burgh as "Colin the Laird" of Trinity, whose stalwart figure at these gatherings, as for a generation afterwards at the kirk and market, never failed to excite admiring comment. The cockpit was fitted up in the schoolroom, then at the head of Church Street—the building still remains, but without the quaint stone steps which led from the street outside the north gable, to the Town Hall above the schoolroom—and only a favoured few witnessed the combat. Among them, was "Colin the Laird" with the pure cold water from the Spoutwell and a sponge. In the intervals of the fight he cleaned the bird which had vanquished so many competitors and was now show-ing many marks of the woundings received in the process. When the fight was over, the public ceremonies in connection with the crown-ing were begun. The first of these took place in the Town Hall when the cock was formally crowned, the schoolmaster giving a Latin ora-tion. A procession was then formed which was of considerable length, headed by the Provost, Magistrates and Town Council, with the town officers with their halberds, preceded by the band of the "Locals." The "king of cocks," carried by its owner, occupied a place of honour in the procession, having several equerries in attendance, one of whom was a prominent country gentleman . . . The procession halted at the residences of leading citizens to allow the younger children (if any) to salute the "king." When the procession broke up there was much fun and frolic, the boys in the procession giving themselves an orgy of box-ing in imitation of the birds in combat. The day's proceedings came to a close with a public ball which was attended by the elite of the town and country. "Strange to say"—we are now quoting the words of an eye-witness—"the owner of the king of cocks went to church in state on the following Sunday, with crown and sceptre, attended by his equerries; his reign lasted for six weeks, during which he had the power of sav-ing delinquents from the tawse, but on the expiry of the period he was looked up to with no more respect than his school fellows."[9]

Given the rigours of young life in Dingwall, it is not surprising that George Simpson emerged as a competitive and combative young man.

But he learned more than that. His later inordinate grasp of world geography and of the flow of commerce between Scotland and England and the rest of the world might well have had its roots in a special bond with his well-educated teacher. Alexander Simpson perhaps had a special interest in maps and world affairs that could have seen him presenting the Dingwall classes with "T and O" (*orbis terrae*, or circle of the earth) maps from medieval times, or with the most up-to-date maps of the British Empire and the world.

During Sir George's school years, Napoleon Bonaparte seized power after the French Revolution and was in the process of extending his influence across Europe, in campaigns and coalitions that were covered in the British and Scottish newspapers and that would have been featured current events for senior students in the Dingwall schoolroom. In later life, Sir George idolized Napoleon, for his tactics if not for his dictatorial, anti-monarchist politics. Some have surmised that Simpson identified with both the Corsican's combative nature and his diminutive height of five feet six inches. To most Britons, Napoleon was a despot, and Simpson's eventual adulation of the man speaks to his own somewhat contrarian outlook but, more important, to a schooling in his formative years in which independent thought was nurtured, even encouraged.

Previous biographers have explored this iconoclastic quality of Sir George's character. They have made mention of the fact that his great-grandfather, Duncan Forbes, sided with the government in the Battle of Culloden and, as such, had no sympathy for Bonnie Prince Charlie as heir to the Scottish crown, for the fiercely independent life of the highlanders or for the perpetuation of the Scottish clans as distinct from English society. Their assumption is that through his father and grandfather, Sir George inherited his great-grandfather's Whiggish point of view. Yet Sir George's fascination with the reviled Napoleon Bonaparte would indicate that he had political views of his own. It may have been adulation of an adventuring swashbuckler or feisty Highland pride that led him to name his personal express canoe, in which he crossed and re-crossed North America, *Rob Roy*, after Rob Roy MacGregor, the freebooting rebel who became legendary as a result of his participation in the anti-English Jacobite uprising of 1715.

If one is to believe a nineteenth-century report generalizing the intellectual character of the burghers of Dingwall, it would seem that young George's curiosity, hunger for knowledge and need for independent thought went beyond that of his neighbours and peers. In 1845, Church of Scotland vicar Hector Bethune cast his Dingwall parishioners this way:

> Their intellectual character stands as high as that of most people who labour under the disadvantage of using the Gaelic as their vernacular tongue, in which there existed nothing, at least until recently, deserving of the name literature. Most of them, it is true, were taught to read and write English, but they *think* in Gaelic, which renders these acquisitions of comparatively little use to them. But although thus necessarily, in a great measure, strangers to the intelligence acquired by reading, and consequently a good deal influenced by the narrow prejudices inseparable from ignorance, they are naturally shrewd and observant, sagacious in the management of their affairs, and not altogether destitute of that thoughtful and imaginative cast of mind characteristic to Highlanders.[10]

Good luck, good fortune or, more likely, the blossoming in a fertile learning context of rare natural ability allowed young George Simpson to move and think in both Gaelic and English with acuity and aplomb— and this without formal education beyond parochial school.

With eight or nine years of education in the Dingwall school behind him, George was nearing school leaving time. He did his bit tutoring the younger children—including a lad called Duncan Finlayson, four years his junior, who would follow him into the Hudson's Bay Company and become one of his closest allies to the end—but he was growing up, and his world had undergone some changes toward the end of his school career, some of them profoundly unsettling for a boy in his mid-teens.

In 1805, when Simpson would have been about thirteen years old and going through puberty, his father, now nearly thirty years into his career as a writer and tacksman in Dingwall Parish, sought advancement to a new position as an agent for the Fisheries Society in the newly created model town of Ullapool, on Loch Broom. At a time, arguably, when the son might have most needed a strong male family member to help answer the questions bubbling up out of a young man's changing psyche, his father moved far enough away to be out of day-to-day contact. The relationship they had had up to this point is more or less unknown, but assuming that they lived in the same house, ate at the same table and knew of each other's daily affairs, it seems inconceivable that this separation did not have some overtone of abandonment for young George. Even if the boy had, by dint of circumstance, developed a thick skin and a strong sense of personal autonomy and independence, this new position for George Simpson Sr. must have affected both of them, particularly George the younger, who was motherless.

A second and possibly more unsettling change happened at this time in his life, and may have contributed to the younger George Simpson's leaving the Dingwall family home for good. Aunt Mary, whose near-complete attention he seemed to enjoy, acted upon her long-term courtship with the schoolmaster, and married Alexander Simpson in 1807. Of course, George knew both of these people individually, and he was especially linked to the schoolmaster through his school chum Aemilius, but this betrothal had the potential to change everything. It would make his friend his sort-of stepbrother, which might have been fine. And it would make his teacher his sort-of father, which might have been fine as well, depending on the relationship they'd developed over the years. More significantly, though, it would bring competition into a new household for the attentions of his aunt and de facto mother. His mother had left him at birth. His father had headed to greener pastures on the other side of the county. And now the aunt who had raised him was marrying. We shouldn't wonder when a boy in such circumstances packs his bags and moves on.

How the final days of George Simpson's youth played out we can only surmise. Although his father's youngest brothers, Duncan and Geddes, both went to Aberdeen University and did well, there is no record of talk about this for young George. There might have been some thought of his following his father's footsteps into the legal profession, but that too was never realized. A year after Mary and Alexander were married, a son, Thomas, was born to them—half-brother to Aemilius, first cousin to George. According to Alexander Simpson Jr. (Thomas's younger brother, who wrote much later about their early life together), through Mary's "assiduous entreaty" of her brother Geddes, who was involved in the sugar business in London, young George was offered the chance to board a boat in Invergordon and take up an apprenticeship in his uncle's big-city counting house. Whether the timing of the move was coincidental with or a direct result of the marriage in 1807 and the arrival of Thomas in 1808, we can only guess. What is certain, though, is that in later life, George would have nothing but enmity for his cousin Thomas, to the point where he would deny, at a parliamentary inquiry near the end of his career, being related to him. People even muttered in various places that Sir George might have had something to do with the unexplained death of this cousin. In any case, by about 1807–08, George Simpson's formative years in Ross-shire were over and neither he nor the town of Dingwall would ever look back.

CHAPTER II

LONDON

For a young man with an adventuring spirit, sailing east over the horizon of Cromarty Firth—a journey he had taken a thousand times in his imagination—must have been an exhilarating moment. While we do not know exactly when or how young George Simpson travelled south to start his apprenticeship in his uncle Geddes's London brokerage, best guesses are that he was about sixteen or seventeen years old. With commercial stagecoach travel organized in a hub-and-spoke configuration around bigger population centres, and with sparse muddy, rocky, hilly and at times totally treacherous single-lane tracks to travel, especially in the borderlands between Edinburgh and around the remains of Hadrian's Wall at Newcastle, it seems likely that Simpson would have gone to seek his fortune south by sailing ship, beginning with a trundle down the north shore road to catch the monthly smack from Invergordon to Leith, perhaps changing boats there, and carrying on down the North Sea coast, into the estuary of the fabled Thames River and up to London town.

With his father employed in Ullapool, in Wester Ross, his aunt Mary newly preoccupied both with her husband, Alexander, and now with a baby in the house, with his own fists scarred and his heart hardened by teasing for his small stature, his red-haired temper or his bastard descent, George Simpson probably left Dingwall with more relief than regret, in a new suit of clothes and with his worldly goods neatly packed into one small leather suitcase. In the mix of people on hand to wish him well would have been his grandmother, whom he would likely never see again, perhaps his father, his schoolmate and now half-cousin Aemilius, and his friend Duncan Finlayson who, like Aemilius, would cross paths with him, up to and including the day on which Sir George would die a rich and powerful man in Lachine, Quebec.

Depending on the time of day, the smack would have coasted south around Yarmouth head to Gravesend, at the mouth of the Thames River, to drop passengers, take on a pilot or wait for the twice-daily periods when, since Roman times, ocean-going vessels had, without benefit of sail or power of oar, ridden the tidal bore inland and upstream easily as far as London Bridge. Also in the harbour would have been ships of the Admiralty taking on water or supplies to continue the fracas with France. And at the Gravesend jetty, under the fluttering four-beaver red cross of the St. George ensign of the Hudson's Bay Company, could well have been ships of the HBC fleet, setting sail for Orkney and a North Atlantic crossing. If sight of these ships did not pique the future governor's imagination of what life might be like in North America, perhaps a walk through the grounds of St. George's Church en route to whet his whistle at The Three Daws or The Ship and Lobster—the famous "first and last" pub on the Thames featured in Dickens's *Great Expectations*— might have done so, for it was here, after having been presented to the court of King James and the bishop of London, that the unlucky twenty-two-year-old Algonquian princess Pocahontas had died of white-man's scourge nearly two hundred years before.

The smell of the sea would be replaced by sewage stench as, dodging vessels at anchor, the smack moved upriver past Northfleet, past Grays and eventually past the Royal Greenwich Observatory, on the prime meridian, where the sounds of the City of London would have become audible amid the working calls of bosuns and duty hands working to

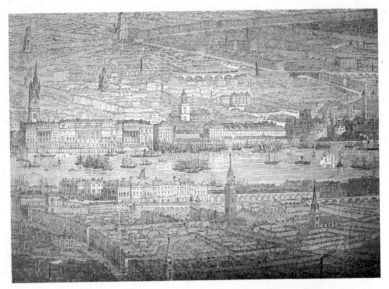

A mid-nineteenth-century etching of Sir George's business neighbourhood in central London, uphill from Custom House on the north side of the Thames. After his start in the sugar brokerage on Great Tower Street, Simpson took employment a few blocks northwest on Fenchurch Street, the London head-quarters of the Hudson's Bay Company, always within reach of the sounds and smells of a bustling Thames River.

keep hundreds of barges, ships, pleasure craft and lighters from running each other down as they made their way up or downriver.

London in the opening years of the nineteenth century was a city about to explode. The seeds of the Industrial Revolution were starting to flower. The making of textiles had been mechanized. "Canal mania" was underway across the United Kingdom, including the recent comple-tion of the Caledonian Canal, south of Dingwall, that allowed ships to cross Scotland through Loch Ness and the Great Glen. Thomas Telford had built his great iron aqueduct over the Dee Valley in Scotland and, in 1807, roughly coincident with Simpson's arrival in London, Robert Fulton launched the first steamship, *Clermont*—a wondrous harbinger of change.

Economically, the promise of fellow Scot Adam Smith's *Inquiry into the Nature and Causes of the Wealth of Nations*, published in 1776, was being realized. Old monopolies like the East India Company and the circumstances that had given rise to the Boston Tea Party and the American Revolution were starting to crumble (though not the single-handed reach of the Hudson's Bay Company in North America, which would only strengthen throughout Simpson's lifetime); they were slowly giving way to individual enterprise and free trade, in spite of the fact that the British government itself, for decades longer, hung onto old ideas of mercantilism. Private business was flourishing, and the "invisible hand" of progress was, as Smith had predicted, starting to control market forces, which, in turn, were spinning off improvements in social welfare. Although far from clean, the state of London sanitation, for example—the quality of the Thames River in particular—was marginally better when Simpson came to town than it had been a century earlier, in spite of the fact that the city's population had grown from 600,000 to 900,000 in that same hundred years.

British trade had doubled and nearly doubled again during that same period. Annual imports were worth about £24 million at the end of the eighteenth century—about £1.2 billion in today's terms—and fully 65 per cent of that business came through London, bringing with it, Adam Smith had argued, certain collateral social benefits, not the least of which was the emergence of a middle class that would be defined by persever-ance and energy, and by individual virtues such as thrift, responsibility and self-reliance.

Technological and social change was accompanied by political tur-moil. Although slavery itself was not officially abolished until 1833, the British parliament passed in 1807 the Abolition of the Slave Trade Act, which enforced a £100 penalty on ship captains for every slave found on a British vessel. The concept of democracy was gaining a notable, if tenu-ous, foothold. The populace was beginning to chafe against upper-class rule. The idea that common people, willing to fight for their individual and collective rights, could participate in the drafting of a constitution under which all could live was being promoted in France and the United States, and similar change was starting to happen in Great Britain.

Simpson's uncle Geddes was a partner in one of the forty London brokerages that handled the most valuable of all imports arriving by ship up the Thames River: sugar. Handy to the docks, coopers and warehouses along Lower Thames Street, most sugar brokerages were based in offices within 250 acres north of the river between London Bridge and the Tower of London, bordered by Fish Street Hill in the west, Fenchurch Street in the north and Tower Hill in the east. Throughout the eighteenth century, rumour was that there was more money in this little plot of Old London than there was upriver in the vaults of King George himself. And it was from the offices of Graham and Simpson, Sugar Brokers, at 73 Great Tower Street, that Uncle Geddes would have walked or called for his double-bodied carriage to transport him to a public wharf on the bustling nearby Thames to meet his wide-eyed nephew and—though neither had an inkling of it at the time—future son-in-law.

Fourteen years younger than George Simpson Sr., Geddes Simpson was in his early thirties when his apprentice came to town. Geddes had attended Aberdeen University, after parochial school in Avoch, and moved to London to seek his fortune after graduating in 1794 with a master of arts degree from Aberdeen's King's College. He had married, and in scarcely a dozen years of buying and selling cane sugar and sugar derivatives like rum and molasses, he had learned the business, gone into partnership and formed his own brokerage. He had done exceptionally well. By the time young George arrived, Geddes Simpson had built a very comfortable life for himself and his family, commuting two and a half miles to Great Tower Street each day from New Grove House in Bromley-on-Bow, east of the city centre.

The apprenticeship the Dingwall lad would undergo in his uncle's firm in the following decade, and to which he would take so naturally, would be in the skills of accounting and business management but, perhaps as important, it would also be in culturing the look, habits and politics of a merchant gentleman. However progressive George's Dingwall upbringing might have been, one must remember that it was built on a spartan Church of Scotland foundation. In spite of the young man's fearless efforts to present a suave and worldly impression to his uncle and his uncle's London colleagues, the relative simplicity of a world view cast in a little Scottish town must have left him looking occasionally like a bumpkin in a city a thousand times bigger, the political and commercial hub of the British Empire.

Sugar was king of commodities. In the three hundred years since European contact in North America, what had once been a condiment used only by nobility and royalty had, on the backs of African slaves working in the cane fields of the West Indies, come down in price to the point that, when Simpson entered the trade, middle- and even working-class Britons were developing a serious sweet tooth. High on the list of ways in which sugar was ingested were molasses for cooking, granular sugar in tea and coffee, and fermented sugar—rum—which, like gin, was in some circles almost a food group unto itself. Indicative of the significance of sugar in the economic scheme of things in London at the turn of the nineteenth century was the fact that the plantation owners and brokers who grew, processed and traded it were able to essentially rework and transform the totally congested London docking system with the creation of the first walled loading and unloading facility in the city's history. Opened in 1802 on land circumscribed by a huge oxbow in the Thames called the Isle of Dogs, the West India Docks enclosed a thirty-acre excavated import basin and a twenty-four-acre artificial export basin. At either end, opening to the tidal basins of the river, were locks that could be opened before and after high tide to allow six hundred large ships to be hauled by horses and loaded or unloaded at half-mile-long rows of five-storey warehouses. For some traders, this reduced the waiting time for unloading from four weeks to four days. Equally important, the twenty-foot-high brick wall that surrounded the whole facility reduced the piracy and pilfering that had been cutting into business profits for years. It was the sugar trade and the construction of the

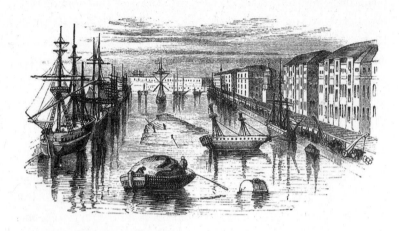

The West India Docks surrounded a basin that was kept full at low tide by wooden locks. It was here during his early days in business that George Simpson paced back and forth checking shipments of Jamaican raw sugar and rum on behalf of his uncle's brokerage.

West India Docks that allowed nineteenth-century London to surpass Amsterdam as the richest city in the Western world.

The West India Docks fascinated Simpson. At one level they were about the imposition of a plan that would produce economy of effort, minimization of cost and maximization of profit. But at another level, they would have been full of people and stories that could scratch his curiosity and extend the young man's reach. There would have been walks through the West India Docks where he could stop working men, their two-wheeled trucks or barrows loaded with sagging sugar sacks, to ask what they were doing, where they were from, noticing all the while—and remembering—their routes and motions on the pier, noting how things might be done more smoothly. As well he could stride up gangplanks, dodging loads going the other way, to speak with the ships' officers supervising the unloading about sea conditions, where the cargo originated, trouble with pirates en route.

Knowing little of business beyond what he might have gleaned about property and the law from his father or from Dingwall retailers and marketeers, Simpson would have begun his apprenticeship as a clerk, at the very bottom of the counting house Graham and Simpson. However, as his later performance as a shrewd operative for the HBC would indicate, George Simpson would have been no desk-bound Bob Cratchit, following the boss's bidding for some paltry wage. Simpson hungered to experience all aspects of the business: totting up sacks or barrels of product in or product out, making trips to the wharf or the warehouse to see the shipment for himself, speaking with ship's captains about spoilage, meeting sellers or buyers face to face at auction.

In his early years at least, someone—perhaps his uncle Geddes—set before Simpson a systematic course of study, an unofficial curriculum that guided his education in all aspects of the sugar trade. He would have learned about accounting, record keeping, insurance and office management; about the seasonality and production rhythms of the commodity itself, the triangular trade routes of the Atlantic, and the vagaries of West Indian weather and an increasingly fractious slave labour force. And there would have been points to glean about markets and pricing, excise and exchange strategies, cash flow and leveraging, customer relations—countless issues at both micro and macro levels of business administration. It is clear from his later expertise inside the Hudson's Bay Company that he had a gift for observing and processing the minutiae of trade while simultaneously conducting business in a larger national and international marketplace.

And George Simpson's London apprenticeship would have extended to venues beyond the private offices of Graham and Simpson and the West India Docks, to the Royal Exchange off Cornhill, the Custom House on the banks of the Thames just below his office and, perhaps most influential of all, the various London coffee houses. These "seats of English liberty" were becoming more and more popular in the shifting winds of the late Georgian period.

Long since dubbed "penny universities," coffee houses were places where men from different walks of life would congregate and discuss

matters of mutual interest and concern. King Charles II, who granted
the Hudson's Bay Company its royal charter, was suspicious enough
about the very earliest of these democratic gathering places that he made
a half-hearted attempt to outlaw them. But by the turn of the nineteenth
century, there were several hundred thriving coffee houses in the City
of London where patrons could discuss issues of the day, do business
deals on the fly and read newspapers both for and against the government. Garraway's Coffee House in Change Alley was where the founding
partners in the Hudson's Bay Company had their first little fur auction
in 1671. Given his secret passion for Napoleon's antics, Simpson would
have also enjoyed a visit to a place like Lloyd's Coffee House, located
inside the Royal Exchange, knowing that both the American and the
French revolutions were tied to early discussions in similar insurrec-
tionist establishments in Boston and Paris.

Lloyd's Coffee House, founded by Edward Lloyd in 1688 at a bow-
windowed storefront shop[1] a few doors down Great Tower Street from
the offices of Graham and Simpson, had become a meeting place for
merchants, ship owners, sailors and ship's masters, and had experienced
such success that in 1774 the proprietor had moved his business into
rooms at the Royal Exchange. Here, perhaps after participating in the
sale or purchase of some sugar-related product for his uncle, Simpson
could retire to read, in Lloyd's spacious subscription room, up-to-date
newspapers from around the world. He could share bone china cups
of steaming white coffee with people who had first-hand experience in
the places named on the mastheads of those periodicals. At the time
Simpson would have been frequenting Lloyd's Coffee House, what had
begun a century before as gentleman's agreements on how to share the
risks and perils of putting their ships to sea around the world were slowly
changing into more formal agreements to ensure the well-being of each
business. Lloyd's was being transformed into an insurance company for
the expanding business world. And George Simpson would have been
on the margin of all that, watching with rapt attention.

Simpson would also have spent time in the Jamaica Coffee House, at 1 St. Michael's Alley in Cornhill, between his office and the Royal Exchange, whose main patrons were merchants trading with Madeira and the West Indies. If there was any place to glean intelligence or listen to scuttlebutt about shipping or sugar business concerns in the West Indies, it was the Jamaica Coffee House. This was also the place to pick up occasional correspondence from the mail packets carried by the merchant ships that were travelling back and forth across the Atlantic—those that were not delivered personally by courier to Graham and Simpson directly on the ship's arrival at the West India Docks.

Given the public nature of these coffee houses, there were unwritten rules about how and with whom to be seen to make an advantageous impression. A young man of Simpson's status took pains with his appearance: cutaway jacket with silk waistcoat, watch and chain; tailored fine cotton shirt with starched and studded high-pointed collar and detachable French cuffs; outlandishly coloured cravat; tight trousers covering high-topped Wellington boots; beaver hat and burnished brass-trimmed hickory cane to finish the effect. George Simpson may have been a clerk to start, but he was not a clerk for long, especially in his own imagination.

For some of his early time in London, Simpson may have stayed with his uncle at New Grove House, but more likely he would have taken rooms nearer the centre of the city where, in the manner of the day, given an ample income, he would have hired help to do the cooking and cleaning. Every day of his working life with the Hudson's Bay Company, George Simpson was on the job before everyone else, worked as hard as or harder than they did when on duty, and was often the last to retire. It is safe to assume that this drive to work, to advance the cause of business—to succeed in making something of himself—was a habit forged in Dingwall and shaped and polished during his time in London. Staying within walking distance or a short omnibus or coach ride of 73 Great Tower Street would have allowed him to exercise his passion for business without the complication of domestic details. A centrally located residence would also have put him in the midst of the London dandies, thereby furnishing him with a reason to dress smartly, or even beyond his means, to make the right impression, and it would have placed him within the range and purview of Britain's best haberdashers, tailors, milliners and boot makers, who could, for a fee, dress him impeccably as a gentleman of business.

And of course, London then, as now, was alive with music, theatre and dance. He would have visited the homes of his business friends and associates, including attending Sunday dinners and important family anniversaries at New Grove House with Uncle Geddes and his family. There would, no doubt, have been some kind of celebration at Bromley-on-Bow, at St. Leonard's Church, perhaps, in August 1812, when Geddes's wife, Frances, gave birth to a winsome baby girl they christened Frances Ramsay Simpson. And, as a still eligible bachelor and a bright and engaging guest, Simpson would have had no shortage of invitations to dine in or out with friends, some of whom, no doubt, would have introduced him to their daughters, nieces and female neighbours, whose attentions they hoped might catch the eye of the handsome, if short, up-and-comer. And, as friends and associates inquired into his Scottish roots, Simpson may have begun the process of either telling diversionary tales—perhaps regaling them with stories of cockfights in the Dingwall school—or being coy about his out-of-wedlock birth.

We do not know with whom Simpson had liaisons during his time in the sugar business, but we do know that he sired two daughters with two different women during this period of his life. Maria Louisa was born on October 25, 1815, to a woman called Maria, about whom nothing else is known; two years later, a second daughter, Isabella, was born to an unknown mother. Like his father before him, Simpson appears to have taken responsibility for these children; they may have been cared for in infancy by his London housekeeper, or perhaps even by their mothers for a short time. Both Maria and Isabella ended up in Scotland when Simpson joined the HBC, where they were looked after by Simpson's uncle Duncan and his wife, or possibly, for a time, by his father, in Ullapool. And both went on to marry lawyers from Inverness, though, for reasons that may have had something to do with the younger daughter's choice of mate, their dowries from their father were dramatically different.

The most significant turning point in Simpson's life and career came as his uncle Geddes strategized with his partner, Mr. Graham, about how to continue growing their business in a bullish sugar market. In 1812, roughly four years into Simpson's apprenticeship, Graham and Simpson merged with another brokerage, Wedderburn and Company, bringing the artful and influential Andrew Wedderburn into the firm. Wedderburn, who changed his surname to Colvile (sometimes spelled Colville) two years later, intrigued and inspired George Simpson and, in time, would change the course of his life.

———

Wedderburn was a Scot, like Simpson, with dark roots reaching back to the '45, except that his ancestors, unlike George's great-grandfather, Duncan Forbes, were on the side of Bonnie Prince Charlie, the Great Pretender. Wedderburn's father, James, was sixteen years old in 1746 when his father was hanged, drawn and quartered for his support of the Jacobites. The Wedderburn family estate, near Inveresk (just east of Edinburgh), was confiscated by the king, and the rest of the family, out of necessity, joined a Scottish exodus to Jamaica, where young James set himself up as a doctor without qualification.

For a white person in the sugar plantation culture of Westmoreland County in Jamaica, it was only a matter of time before doctoring gave way to the purchase of land holdings and slave labour. And after twenty-eight years of "rapacious" slave ownership, during which the family regained title to the original Scottish estate, James moved back to Inveresk in 1773 and married Isabella Blackburn, the winsome daughter of a west-coast steel magnate. Andrew was their first child, born in 1779; Jean, a sister, was born sometime after that. Both Andrew and Jean would play roles that in some respects shaped, coloured and ultimately darkened George Simpson's life.

The main problem was that Andrew Wedderburn, who had inherited significant Jamaican sugar plantation holdings from his father, connected Graham and Simpson directly to sugar production in the West Indies. While this was good for business, the partnership also exposed George Simpson to the culture, attitudes and racist assumptions of the slave trade. Coming from the north of Scotland, Simpson undoubtedly came to London with xenophobic fears and racial biases of his own, but the connection to Wedderburn may well have helped those flower, as he watched his new mentor respond to a mulatto half-brother who had turned up in England from Jamaica.

Robert Wedderburn—who was a colourful character in his own right, and a supporting player in the abolitionist movement—was the last thing his father, James, wanted while he was in the process of moving back onto the family estate and trying to re-establish the Wedderburn name in the social hierarchy of post-Culloden Scotland. Having arrived on his father's doorstep and been given short shrift there, Robert moved to London and began a very public campaign to tell his story to anyone who would listen. He eventually published an important book about abolitionist times, but before that he wrote to newspapers to try to gain credence and momentum for his case. In a London weekly called *Bell's Life*, he described his situation this way:

> I was born in the island of Jamaica, about the year 1762, on the estate of a Lady Douglas, a distant relation of the Duke of Queen'sbury. My mother was a woman of colour, by name Rosanna, and at the time of my birth a slave to the above Lady Douglas. My father's name was James Wedderburn, Esq. of Inveresk, in Scotland, an extensive proprietor, of sugar estates in Jamaica, which are now in the possession of a younger brother of mine, by name, A[ndrew] Colvile, Esq. of No. 35, Leadenhall Street.
>
> I must explain at the outset of this history—what will appear unnatural to some—the reason of my abhorrence and indignation

at the conduct of my father. From him I have received no benefit in the world. By him my mother was made the object of his brutal lust, then insulted, abused and abandoned; and, within a few weeks from the present time, a younger and more fortunate brother of mine, the aforesaid A. Colvile, Esq. has had the insolence to revile her memory in the most abusive language, and to stigmatize her for that which was owing to the deep and dark iniquity of my father. Can I contain myself at this? . . .

My father's name, as I said before, was James Wedderburn, of Inveresk, in Scotland, near Musselborough, where, if my information is correct, the Wedderburn family have been seated for a long time. My grandfather was a staunch Jacobite, and exerted himself strenuously in the cause of the Pretender, in the rebellion of the year 1745 . . . When I first came to England, in the year 1779, I remember seeing the remains of a rebel's skull which had been affixed over Temple Bar; but I never yet could fully ascertain whether it was my dear grandfather's skull, or not. Perhaps my dear brother, A. Colvile, can lend me some assistance in this affair. For this act of high treason, our family estates were confiscated to the King, and my dear father found himself destitute in the world, or with no resource but his own industry. He adopted the medical profession; and in Jamaica he was Doctor and Man-Midwife, and turned an honest penny by drugging and physicking the poor blacks, where those that were cured, he had the credit for, and for those he killed, the fault was laid to their own obstinacy. In the course of time, by dint of his *booing* and *booing*, my father was restored to his father's property, and he became the proprietor of one of the most extensive sugar estates in Jamaica. While my dear and honoured father was poor, he was chaste as any Scotchman whose poverty made him virtuous but the moment he became rich, he gave loose to his carnal appetites, and indulged himself without moderation, but as parsimonious as a weaver. My father's mental powers were not of the brightest which may account for his libidinous excess.[2]

With this kind of scandal brewing, Andrew Wedderburn had to distance himself from public unseemliness. Arguing that it was a move taken to honour his mother's family, from whom he had received a substantial inheritance about the time Wedderburn and Company merged with Graham and Simpson, Andrew Wedderburn changed his surname to Colvile and from then on went by that name or by Wedderburn-Colvile. Whatever honour it brought to his mother's family's memory, the name change also separated him from his vociferous half-brother. Yet this was not enough to create that distance, and Colvile eventually found himself forced into responding publicly to Robert's accusations:

Sir—Your Paper of the 29th ult. containing a Letter signed by Robert Wedderburn, was put in my hand only yesterday, otherwise I should have felt it to be my duty to take earlier notice of it.

In answer to this most slanderous publication, I have to state, that the person calling himself Robert Wedderburn is NOT a son of the late Mr. James Wedderburn, of Inveresk, who never had any child by, or any connection of *that kind* with the mother of this man. The pretence of his using the name of Wedderburn at all, arises out of the following circumstances:—The late Mr. James Wedderburn, of Inveresk, had, when he resided in the parish of Westmoreland, in the Island of Jamaica, a negro woman-slave, whom he employed as a cook; this woman had so violent a temper that she was continually quarrelling with the other servants, and occasioning a disturbance in the house. He happened to make some observation of her trublesome temper, when a gentleman in company said, he would be very glad to purchase her if she was a good cook. The sale accordingly took place, and the woman was removed to the residence of the gentleman, in the parish of Hanover. Several years afterwards, this woman was delivered of a mulatto child, and as she could not tell who was the father, her master, in a foolish joke, named the child Wedderburn. About twenty-two or twenty-three years ago, this man applied to me for money upon the strength of his name, claiming to be a son of

Mr. James Wedderburn of Inveresk, which occasioned me to write to my father, when he gave me the above explanation respecting this person; adding that a few years after he returned to this country, and married, this same person importuned him with the same story that he now tells, and as he persisted in annoying him after the above explanation was given to him, that he found it necessary to have him brought before the Sheriff of the county of Edinburgh. But whether the man was punished or only discharged upon promising not to repeat the annoyance, I do not now recollect.[3]

Colvile then threatened to sue the paper if it published any further slander upon the character of his father. The paper published a long editorial that concluded, "After all, the intelligence we have obtained by the above letter, is but a 'contradiction' of an assertion, *without one single* proof that the assertion is untrue."[4]

Other evidence points convincingly to the veracity of Robert Wedderburn's version of events. This was the sordid underbelly of the British sugar industry, an enterprise through which more than a million black Africans were transported into slavery. On these transatlantic voyages—the Middle Passage—"successful" captains lost only a quarter of their human cargo to disease. White men on plantations in America and the West Indies had free access not only to slave labour in the fields but to other young black women. One plantation owner who recorded all his sexual conquests in a diary documented 3,853 acts of sexual intercourse with 138 women in his 37 years in Jamaica. That this particular planter saw himself as "a harbinger, in a modest way, of the Enlightenment in the Tropics; a scholar and perhaps a gentleman; loyal friend and respectable Imperial subject; a man of principle and integrity,"[5] indicates the presence in the sugar business of a systemic double standard predicated on racism of the worst kind.

George Simpson was connected to this double standard, however tangentially. He heard about it from Andrew Colvile, likely talked about it in coffee-house conversations, and may even have experienced the situation at first hand on trips across the Atlantic to survey the West Indian end of the sugar business, long before he entered the largely Aboriginal population of Rupert's Land. For some sugar brokers, the assumption was that black people were not actually human or that they somehow benefited when white people dominated their lives. Simpson would have taken with him into the fur trade and into the rest of his life disturbing notions about the relative power and authority vested in skin colour. Possible evidence of this is in how Simpson dealt with the marriages of his first two daughters. To Maria's husband-to-be, Donald Mactavish of Inverness, he gave £500 "in consideration of the marriage."[6] To Isabella's betrothed he gave nothing, making it known that he did not approve of the union to Mr. John Cook Gordon of Jamaica. Was John Cook Gordon of mixed race? Could it be that, like Andrew Colvile, Simpson had no interest in willingly admitting into his family the half-caste progeny of planter and slave?

Andrew Wedderburn's sister Jean also shaped George Simpson's future, through her choice of spouse. On November 24, 1807, coincident with the time Simpson arrived in London, Jean Wedderburn married Thomas Douglas, the 5th earl of Selkirk. Selkirk was a young man of means and privilege who had a special sympathy for people, especially for Scottish highlanders displaced by late-seventeenth-century "progress." He had already taken one group of settlers to Prince Edward Island, and had written a book, *Observations on the Present State of the Highlands in Scotland, with a view to the causes and probable consequences of emigration*, which had given him a measure of celebrity.[7] Selkirk's convictions about the need for settlement were strong, and this, along with his experience in Canada and his research for this book, left him convinced that the organization with which to mount a new North American agricultural settlement initiative was the Hudson's Bay Company. It was Selkirk's dream of a new life in Canada for displaced Scottish highlanders that eventually connected Simpson to the Hudson's Bay Company, in a cascade of events that began the day Andrew Wedderburn's and George Simpson's worlds collided at 73 Great Tower Street.

At the time of the 1812 merger between Graham and Simpson and Wedderburn and Company, Andrew Wedderburn had for some years been on the Board of Governors of the Hudson's Bay Company, because of his brother-in-law, the earl of Selkirk. Following his marriage to Jean, Selkirk had put his plan into action by starting to purchase HBC stock, in the hope that this might help leverage his settlement dream. In May 1809, he purchased a substantial block of HBC shares, valued at £4,087 10s.

Always the businessman, Andrew Wedderburn heard about this purchase, liked what he was hearing from his brother-in-law and gambled that this stock was undervalued. He purchased some a month later. Indeed, through the 1790s the HBC had been having a very public struggle with the fledgling North West Company for supremacy in the North American fur trade and this, combined with the fact that European fur markets had more or less collapsed as a result of the Napoleonic Wars, made the stock an attractive investment. HBC dividends had fallen off for a number of years, and its £100 share, which at one time sold for £260, could be purchased in the £60 range. So Andrew Wedderburn joined the family action with a purchase of £2,166 13s 4d in June of the same year, and a further £507 10s purchase in July. Strengthening Selkirk's position with the Hudson's Bay Company even further, Andrew Wedderburn's sister's husband (and his first cousin), John Halkett, a lawyer who was commissioner of the King's West Indian Accounts, joined the initiative, adding £3,717 10s worth of HBC stock to the family position. The upshot of these purchases was predictable: Halkett and Wedderburn were invited to take seats on the HBC Board of Governors in London (also called the London Committee) in the spring of 1810, where Wedderburn proposed and had approved by the board a retrenching system, to restructure and reorganize the antiquated North American trading and accounting practices of the venerable, if moribund and nearly bankrupt, Hudson's Bay Company. In due course, aided by his brothers-in-law and by the wish of the HBC to confound the North West Company, Selkirk was able to secure a land grant from the Hudson's Bay Company of 116,000 square miles

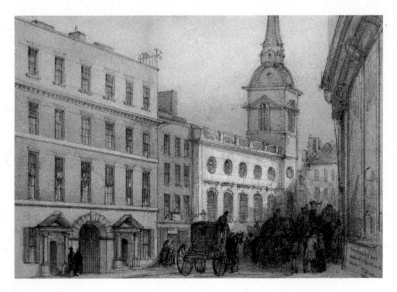

Hudson's Bay House at 3/4 Fenchurch Street was where the governors of the company met to control an empire half a world away. In the main boardroom hung a massive set of moose antlers weighing fifty-six pounds and a life-sized painting of a trophy elk in Rocky Mountain splendour.

of arable land at the junction of the Red and Assiniboine rivers, in the heart of fur country.

By the time the Selkirk settlement plan was being enacted, Andrew Wedderburn had joined the firm, and there would have been no avoiding a scheme of this scope around the Great Tower Street office. While Simpson went about his business in the sugar trade, he no doubt would have also been getting daily updates on the fortunes of the Hudson's Bay Company and its protracted competition with the Nor'Westers, as well as news from Selkirk, also filtered through Wedderburn, of the imminent departure of settlers for York Factory and then south to the new land grant, called Assiniboia.

Almost from the moment King Charles II signed the charter for the Hudson's Bay Company on May 2, 1670, people—possible competitors in the British Isles—had voiced concerns about the propriety of a monopoly over 480,370 square miles—a tract of land covering more than half of what is now Canada. Most of the dissenters contested the HBC's right to exclusive trade and commerce in Rupert's Land, and the right to property (that is, settlement) within the granted lands. For many years, settlement was the last thing on the minds of HBC's London-based governors, but as the eighteenth century wore on—and especially when the North West Company, out of Montreal, started to grow strong—the idea of broadening the scope of activities in Rupert's Land through settlement had more appeal. Hence, when Lord Selkirk floated the idea of creating a settlement in HBC lands below Lake Winnipeg, there were those on the HBC's London Committee who thought this an ideal opportunity to vindicate the company's royal charter, even though there were many in the rank and file, those who had direct experience of life in Rupert's Land, who thought the idea was ludicrous.

The problem with situating an agricultural settlement in the middle of North America was that it interrupted a main transportation route between Montreal and the west. Eastern Canada had been trapped so heavily that the North West Company and, to a lesser extent, the HBC were now concentrating their efforts in the west, around Lake Athabasca. The HBC's supply line began at York Factory on Hudson Bay, but the NWC's main depot was at Lachine, near Montreal. For the Nor'Westers to reach the fur riches of the Athabasca Country now, they had to pass right through Assiniboia.

Notwithstanding problems of weather and logistics, the Selkirk settlers got a modest start in Assiniboia, just as the earl had dreamed, in the summer of 1812. But from the outset, the Nor'Westers, in conjunction with their Métis allies in the west, made life difficult for the new arrivals. A full-scale attack was mounted in 1815. The settlers were driven from the land, only to be led back by an optimist called Colin Robertson, another character who would wend his way in and out of Simpson's life for the next couple of decades.

Selkirk himself, angered by the nasty reception his settlers had received, travelled to Montreal that same year and petitioned the King's

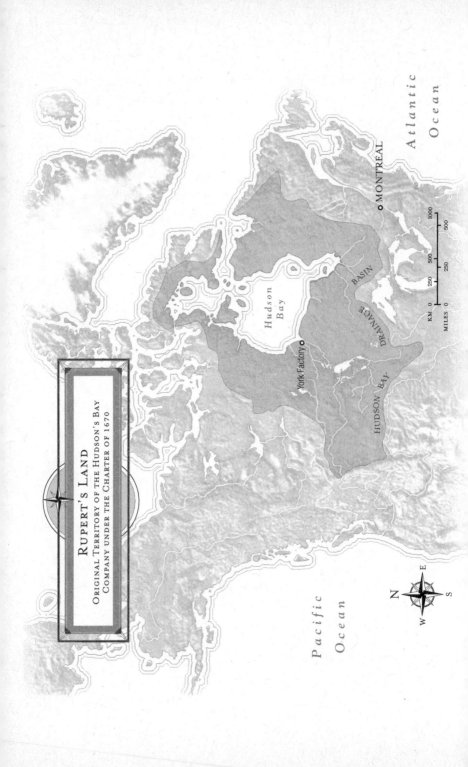

RUPERT'S LAND
ORIGINAL TERRITORY OF THE HUDSON'S BAY
COMPANY UNDER THE CHARTER OF 1670

Pacific
Ocean

Atlantic
Ocean

Hudson
Bay

York Factory

HUDSON BAY DRAINAGE BASIN

MONTREAL

KM 0   250   500   1000
MILES 0   250   500

N
W   E
S

representative in Canada, Lord Bathurst, for soldiers to protect the settlers. Bathurst considered the problem an instance of corporate bickering
and lent Selkirk only a handful of soldiers—six privates and a sergeant.
Selkirk was able to purchase the services of a hundred or so additional
Swiss militiamen, but it was not until the following summer that he was
able to move his unit westward. By then it was too late. Along the way,
Selkirk learned that Governor Robert Semple and nineteen other settlers had been killed in a skirmish with Cuthbert Grant and a band of
Métis sympathetic to the Nor'Westers, on June 19, 1816, at a location
called Seven Oaks, inside the bounds of Selkirk's land grant.

The Massacre of Seven Oaks turned the tide. The Selkirk settlement
struggled on, but it never realized the young earl's dream. Selkirk himself died a few years later. But Lord Bathurst, the colonial minister, saw
that there was more to this situation than a few fur traders fighting in
the hinterland and urged the government to get involved. The partners
in the North West Company and the governors of the Hudson's Bay
Company realized that if there was any money left to be made in the
North American fur trade, it had better be done without the level of
competition that had brought both companies to the brink of bankruptcy and too many of their employees to their graves. Various fur trade
and government officials were travelling around Rupert's Land arresting
and locking up competitors for crimes both real and imagined. Selkirk
himself, on hearing of the death of his settlers, detoured to Fort William
and summarily arrested most of the North West Company partners who
were there for their summer rendezvous. Selkirk would be reprimanded
for that, and most of the accused were set free in due course, but there
was a need for stability in the fur trade.

The Hudson's Bay Company sent William Williams, an experienced East India Company sea captain, to get company affairs sorted
out, but he too was dragged into the fighting and infighting. Worried
about Williams's imminent arrest in Rupert's Land, and knowing that
his removal might result in the collapse into total anarchy of company
fortunes in North America, the HBC governors wrung their hands

around the table at Fenchurch Street, pondering what they might do. Whom could they send to smooth the situation during this time of crisis? Andrew Colvile (formerly Wedderburn) had an idea: Why not recruit a bright young broker from his office on Great Tower Street? Might George Simpson take up the challenge?

In one of the very first letters from a rich, varied and voluminous collected correspondence, Simpson wrote excitedly to an associate, Mr. Pooler, in Reigate, forty miles south of London, to let him know about this astonishing turn of events:

London 23d. Feby 1820

My Dear Sir:

Since I last had the pleasure of seeing You an unexpected circumstance has occurred which renders it necessary for me to leave Old England for a time, and at the short notice of 5 Days.—I was most anxious to shake hands with You and my highly valued Friends at Nutley Lane previous to my departure but my time is so much occupied in winding up publick & private affairs that I have not one hour to spare and a visit to Reigate is utterly impracticable.—

On Sunday afternoon I leave Town for Liverpool, embark in the Packet for New York on Tuesday, from thence I proceed directly for Montreal and afterwards take an inland Route by the St. Lawrence, Lakes Ontario, Huron, Superior, and Winnipeg to Hudsons Bay and afterwards thro Athapascow to Slave Lake and Copper Mine River.— The Journey is rather a serious undertaking and with the Mission is important business connected with the affairs of Lord Selkirk, the Hudsons Bay & North West Compys.—Travellers you know meet with extraordinary adventures I shall therefore have some wonderful Tales to relate when I again have the pleasure of visiting You.—

I expect to return by the Hudsons Bay Compys Ships in November but if they are gone before I arrive at the Bay I must just take up my quarters for the Winter in the Northern Regions.—

London

The short notice I have had and the multiplicity of my arrangements have so completely occupied my attention that I have scarcely
had an opportunity of thinking seriously about the task I am about
to undertake and the difficulties I am likely to encounter; Yet in
the midst of all my hurry & bustle I must admit that as the time
of my departure approaches I begin to feel a certain depression at
the idea of leaving my Native Land and so many near relations and
sincere Friends amongst the latter Your good Self and Family stand
prominent.—

Pray offer my affectionate regard to Mrs. and Miss Pooler Dick
& the Children as also to Mrs. Palmer and with unfeigned esteem
believe me always to be

> My Dear Sir
> Yours Most truly
> Geo. Simpson
> 73 Tower Street

—

CHAPTER III

ABOARD THE
JAMES MONROE

The clatter of spoked wooden wheels and hackney hoofs on cobblestone outside Simpson's central London lodging would not have come a moment too soon on Sunday, February 25, 1820. Notice of this new appointment with the Hudson's Bay Company had been short, and the days prior to departure had been a blur of activity as Simpson made arrangements to ship four-year-old Maria and two-year-old Isabella to Scotland, to close down his rooms and to assemble his travelling kit. Unlike his arrival in London twelve years before, as a wide-eyed novice with a wish and a carpet bag containing a mackintosh, clean socks, a crust of bread and a letter from his uncle Geddes, his exit was auspicious. It was a gentleman's departure, complete with manservant (a trusted black man he called Sample), a brand-new portable brass-detailed leather armoire with compartments for studs, hats, collars, cuffs and shoes, and a pull-together of hand-tailored garments made of fine cotton and wool to clothe a girth that had grown in proportion to his station since Dingwall days. But Simpson was ready precisely when he said he would be ready, and Andrew Colvile's personal landau was late. "Sample, check the street, and if there is nothing to be seen, send a boy to Tower Street to hurry the horses." The footman, however, was finally at the door. Simpson sat in the carriage, his rosewood cane between his knees, and stared straight ahead while the luggage was loaded. And they were off.

Motion soothed his restless soul. The run to Liverpool, he knew, would be a chance to collect his thoughts on this move he was making. From sugar to fur. From slaves to Indians. From a family firm that had been incorporated for decades to a venerable company, founded by royal charter a century and a half ago. About all of this he knew very little, but he did know—he knew, as he had known when he left Dingwall twelve years earlier—that he would show them that George Simpson was up to the job. More than that, he would do the job as no one had done the job before because, without privilege of title or university education, he had had to pull himself up by his bootstraps and learn twice, thrice, ten times more than others. But Simpson stock was good stock. He was a fighter—that was what his uncles had always told him. "Look them in the eye, son," they would say. "Cuff them if you must." And there would be nothing that would get in his way. He would show them, or so he might have promised to himself as he rolled northwest to the rhythm of a six-horse hitch, his pink head beneath thinning red hair bobbling between narrow shoulders, his darting blue eyes scanning the sombre winter fields of Buckinghamshire, Northamptonshire and on up to the coast.

It was a good time to be leaving England. The ailing king had finally died on January 29, and the Prince Regent had become King George IV. The British Regency period was officially over, and anarchy was breaking loose across the land. The Luddite riots of 1811–15, largely confined to the textile industry, had given way to more broadly based and better-organized discontent calling for government reform. At St. Peter's Field in Manchester, not far from where he was headed on this overcast day, a cavalry unit had charged into a large public gathering organized by the Patriotic Union Society, killing eleven and injuring four hundred more, including many women and children, an incident that would be

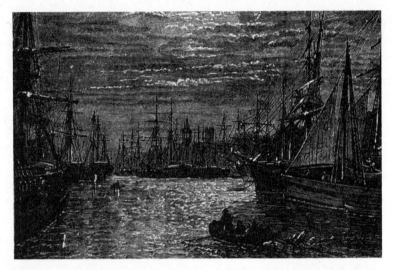

Although the HBC's outbound shipments of men and supplies and inbound loads of furs moved through docks in London and Gravesend, Simpson's transatlantic travel was most often on the more comfortable commercial packet ships of the Black Ball Line and other carriers that sailed from Liverpool (above) to New York.

known as Peterloo. Just two days before his departure, *The Times* had announced more deaths in London, as the government foiled an attempt to assassinate several members of the British cabinet.

At a public house on Cato Street in central London, west of Great Tower Street, near Westminster, a group of conspirators, enraged by Peterloo and by new laws—the so-called Six Acts, which made any meeting for radical reform an "overt act of treasonable conspiracy"—had put in place a plan to overthrow the government by killing a goodly portion of the cabinet. Government forces had uncovered and put down the uprising, but not without bloodshed. Editorials noted that it was only a matter of time before the conspirators who had not been killed in the apprehension would be tried, convicted and hanged.

Once, George Simpson had secretly sided with the revolutionaries in the American Revolution and had admired the insurrectionary tactics of

Napoleon. He may even have lauded the motives of ordinary folk who were demanding change in these changing times. But there was another side to his politics, that of the increasingly hard-headed businessman who knew that political discord and social unrest were just plain bad for business. Whatever sympathies a man might have for the intelligence and tactics of the young Corsican who was flexing his muscles across Europe, the Napoleonic Wars had knocked the bottom out of the sugar market and, he'd learned over the last couple of years from his mentor Andrew Colvile, from the fur market as well. First and foremost, Simpson was a champion of business, and anything that needed to be done to maximize profits would be done.

Change was very much on Simpson's mind as his carriage crested Everton Brow to reveal a bustling vista of downtown Liverpool and the Merseyside quays. This was the port that had grown busy and fat on the proceeds of the slave trade. The quality of the roads had improved, the skyline of Birkenhead across the river was busier and the aging Georgian facades along the Strand were darkened by industrial soot in the maritime air. And among the forest of masts of ships made fast lest they be drawn upriver or back out to sea on the riptides of the Mersey Estuary were to be found Cheshire salt, Lancaster coal and textiles, Staffordshire pottery and Birmingham metal.

Under less pressing circumstances, a position with the Hudson's Bay Company would have secured a man passage to Rupert's Land on one of the company's small fleet of sturdy little supply vessels, but these sailed only in spring, when there was some hope that Hudson Bay would be ice-free or would have leads of open water sufficient to see a supply ship into Five Fathom anchorage off York Factory. But, as the Committee had explained, the company was in something of a perilous position at this juncture in its history, making it imperative to put a new manager—or governor *locum tenens*, as they were calling him—into the field immediately. To achieve that end, passage had been arranged on a relatively new packet service that now sailed year-round between Liverpool and New York: the Black Ball Line.

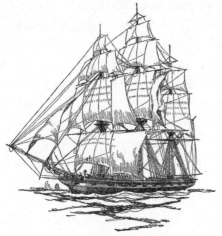

Packet ships of the Black Ball Line were the best and sleekest of Yankee clippers that could make transatlantic crossings in a fraction of the time it took stumpy British trade ships to make their way on similar routes.

The idea of a packet ship was not new. Government-owned vessels often carried mail, important passengers and valuable cargo between Britain and the ports of Europe. Although these ran, in theory at least, full or not full, the European packets were notoriously late or unpredictable. The new Black Ball Line headed the other way, west across the Atlantic. Even after American independence, there was much business to be done with the former colonies, and that business was growing year by year. Fortunately, the five associated merchants who had founded the Black Ball Line in 1797 had built something of a reputation for reliability and punctuality.

What made this possible was their choice of ships. Instead of the sluggish oaken East Indiamen, since the beginning synonymous with British maritime exploits, the Black Ball Line took advantage of American innovations in naval architecture—the faster and more manoeuvrable designs that had allowed American craft to run circles around British ships during the War of Independence and in the Great Lakes during the War of 1812. The Black Ball Line, so named for the unimaginative but memorable black disk on its distinctive house flag (the first in vexillological history—the firm named for the flag instead of vice versa), had purchased one of these early Yankee clippers—the

Pacific—and had started sailing between Liverpool and New York. So popular was this service that the firm soon commissioned three more in close succession: the *Amity*, the *Courier* and the largest, at 424 tons, the *James Monroe*, named for the fifth president of the new United States. The *James Monroe* was launched and christened in 1817, coincident with Monroe's election to the White House. And it was this ship that would provide the new governor's passage to Rupert's Land.

Simpson's sharp eye spied the flag that matched his ticket and, as the tired horses picked up their feet to avoid being jigged from behind by another carriage, he followed shrouds to deck and beheld the most handsome vessel he had ever seen. The *James Monroe* was a raked three-masted full-rigger with the classic concave bow and long, low-sweeping sheer of a clipper. Replacing the bulwark of a chunky British man-o'-war was a balustrade of delicate turned stanchions and a stem-to-stern hand-rail along the spar deck, white-painted like the hull, that emphasized the ship's sleek commercial lines. Before Simpson's coachmen could pull down his luggage, the *Monroe*'s bosun had called down a coterie of ruddy-faced sailors from the rigging to see to the settling aboard of Mr. Simpson and his things.

It would be a few days before the *James Monroe* would sail from Liverpool, but there was some acclimatizing of the passengers and crew to be done in the intervening days. Because these transatlantic pack-ets were a premium service, every appointment, every service offered on these early "Blackballers" was first class. Although records of the *Monroe*'s actual interior layout and decor are lost, subsequent vessels in the Black Ball Line, made by Donald McKay of East Boston, had a score of cabins abaft with mahogany wainscotting, recessed sofas, ottomans, marble-covered tables, mirrors and elliptical panels ornamented with pictures, all arranged around a spacious main salon, with a fine library for use of the passengers and crew and a galley with silver, linen and china service that rivalled the best hotels in Europe. Simpson mused on this elegance in his topcoat and muddy shoes, stretched out on a clean bedspread like Lord Byron himself, while Sample put away his things.

With the trappings of a gentleman and the confidence of a new and very senior (for his age and experience) corporate position, Simpson stepped into the salon to meet the other passengers. Originally there were a dozen: General Vevas, the Spanish ambassador, and his entourage; a number of businessmen; and two women who were on their way to America to reunite with husbands who, for reasons of their "treasonable proceedings," had found it necessary to seek asylum in the United States to avoid the Six Acts and their consequences in England.

Also aboard, as Simpson later described to his friends the Poolers in a letter, were "two Vile Radicals," vociferous political reformers—anti-government types who may also have been seeking asylum in the United States. Whatever the case, it was not long before Simpson (and presumably some of the others) got into conversation with these chaps, as he had with strangers countless times in Lloyd's Coffee House or elsewhere in his London rounds. Whatever it was that they said, and however measured and restrained was Simpson's initial response, eventually his temper flared. As he had before and would in the future, he persuaded the malcontents to see things his way, with tongue first and, when that did not have the desired instant effect, with his fists. "[These two] would have kept us in continual discord during the Voyage," he explained to the Poolers, "had we not sent them to Coventry . . . not only by threats but actual hard lumps."[1] The *James Monroe* sailed on March 4, 1820, with only eleven passengers, including the young governor and another, much more experienced fur trader—a dreaded Nor'Wester, as it happened—who would become a central figure in Simpson's life from that moment on.

———

As one of the conditions of the Treaty of Paris—signed in 1763, about thirty years before Simpson was born—France ceded Canada and all lands east of the Mississippi River to the British, but this did not end the role of the French and the Métis in the North American fur trade. Since the very beginning of the fur industry in North America, the French,

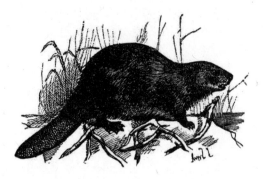

By the time Sir George arrived in North America, the beaver had been all but trapped out in eastern and central North America, forcing the HBC to find markets for other types of fur and to push farther north and west.

through strategic alliances with Canada's First Nations, had taken to canoes and snowshoes and moved across and through the land in search of peltry for European markets. Fur as a textile would become fashionable during Simpson's tenure with the HBC, but the early demand for fur, especially the thick underpelt of the beaver[2] with its fine barbed hairs, was as fibre to be used to make felt, particularly for the construction of fine hats. The European beaver, *Castor fiber*, which was indigenous to Britain and large portions of Europe, had been trapped to extinction in the sixteenth century, largely because of its rich and valuable fur. So when French traders first came back across the Atlantic with pelts from the European beaver's North American cousin, *Castor canadensis*, a whole new industry was born.

Unlike the French, who paddled into the country to trade, the Hudson's Bay Company, since its inception in 1670, had set up shop in tidewater forts and factories and waited for the furs to come to them. Slowly, however, especially after the Treaty of Paris, competition with savvy Canadian traders, who flourished in the absence of French rule, forced the British traders with the HBC to rethink its operation and move inland. Cumberland House, their first inland post, was built in 1774, and dozens of other posts were constructed after that. From that moment on, rivalry between the HBC and everyone else involved in the fur trade dominated events in the North American wild.

The HBC presented a formidable obstacle to its competitors, to some extent because its main resupply point, York Factory, was strategically located at the mouth of the Nelson and Hayes rivers on the shores of Hudson Bay. Independent traders, who by now included a variety of enterprising Scotsmen, concentrated on Montreal as their point of sale and resupply. They quickly saw that alliances of independent brokers, coureurs de bois and merchants were valuable means of building economies of scale that would enable them to compete against the HBC.

Although there might have been a quasi-official alliance as early as 1776, it was not until 1779 that a group of Montreal fur merchants, under the leadership of Simon McTavish, Benjamin Frobisher and Peter Pond, formally created a sixteen-share corporation they called the North West Company, which, in a scant few years, would compete with—and indeed nearly topple—the venerable Hudson's Bay Company. Yet throughout the growth of the new organization, as it built its own posts to rival every major HBC installation and went head to head with the HBC for the allegiances of First Nations people across the land, the problem of supply remained.

It was actually the problem of distance to Montreal that led Nor'Wester (and distant cousin of George Simpson) Alexander Mackenzie to seek other routes back to England, including the great river that still bears his name. Ironically, because this long river the Dene Indians call Dehcho didn't reach the Pacific Ocean, Mackenzie considered the 1789 expedition a failure—he named it Disappointment River. But when he did actually make it across North America by land in 1793, he fundamentally changed the fur trade and, in some respects, intensified the competition between rival companies. Stories about this distant relative on Simpson's grandmother's side, told around the dinner table in Dingwall, may have led George Simpson to follow in his North American footsteps. As it was, while Simpson was aboard the *James Monroe*, Alexander Mackenzie died and was buried in the churchyard in Avoch, where George's grandfather had preached before the family had scattered and George had moved to Dingwall. No doubt in his conversations with the older Nor'Wester, Simpson might have mentioned his connection to Mackenzie by way of giving some credence to his new position in the trade.

On the strength of his explorations north and west and his awareness of the damaging competition between the NWC and the HBC, Alexander Mackenzie had become convinced that the only way to make the fur trade work as a continuing business enterprise was to use York Factory as a depot and to merge the two companies. So convinced was Mackenzie of the rightness of this plan (though he was unable to convince senior wintering NWC partner Simon McTavish) that for a time he joined a splinter interest called the New North West Company (later dubbed the XY Company, for the mnemonic mark used on its cargo bales), established in 1798, as a step toward eventual amalgamation of the two companies. It would take until 1821, a year after George Simpson entered the fray, for amalgamation to occur, but it was Alexander Mackenzie who had put those wheels in motion, and there was much internecine fighting between the archrival companies to be done before the young governor from Dingwall would arrive on the scene.

There were other problems as well. A murder in the valley of the Saskatchewan River at the turn of the century, on top of miscellaneous pillaging, looting, intimidation and other unnecessary deaths—all perpetrated by officers of the NWC or the HBC—gave the British parliament no choice in 1803 but to pass the Canada Jurisdiction Act, designed specifically to deal with lawlessness in the fur trade. This new law provided for various alternative strategies to bring offenders to justice, including the designation of justices of the peace in "Indian Territory," with the power to arrest malefactors and bring them to trial in the courts of Canada. Still, the struggle between the two companies continued as they saw their markets and territories increasingly overlapping.

As a result of the Jay Treaty of 1794, written to clear up lingering problems of separation between the United States and Great Britain, the

NWC was forced to move its main inland depot at Grand Portage, which was now American territory. On land acquired from the Ojibwa who controlled the land on the west end of Lake Superior, the Nor'Westers shifted north and built a big new depot at the mouth of the Kaministiquia River: Fort William, named after wintering partner William McGillivray. Fort William did not give them the resupply benefits of York Factory, but it was a place to stockpile goods and much-needed staples, which substantially bolstered the strength and efficacy of their brigades further west. Fort William effectively divided NWC operations. Crews in much more efficient thirty-six-foot *canots du maître* could run freight between Montreal and Grand Portage. Smaller crews in twenty-five-foot birchbark *canots du nord* could work the rivers west of the Great Lakes, giving the NWC something of a chance against the HBC, which had the two-thousand-mile advantage of bringing freight in and shipping furs out from York Factory. Like York Factory, Fort William became the scene of great revelry during summer rendezvous for the glorious first two decades of the nineteenth century. It was also a place where plots were hatched to disrupt the HBC.

Great quantities of liquor and trade goods were expended for diminishing amounts of furs during the opening years of the nineteenth century as the rival companies tried to out-compete each other for the attentions and allegiances of the First Nations people. It is very likely that a goodly quantity of the Jamaican rum that was used in this trade by the HBC was in fact purchased from Graham, Simpson and Wedderburn back in London, perhaps even with one George Simpson as broker. This petty bickering kept up until Lord Selkirk's settlers began arriving in Assiniboia in the summer of 1812, a move seen by every Nor'Wester as a threat to the fur trade because the huge land grant at the forks of the Red and Assiniboine rivers effectively bisected the main trade route from Montreal to the west. There was even a considerable constituency of Hudson's Baymen who were against settlement, arguing that every available company resource should be going to the fur trade and to the battle against the Nor'Westers.

The situation went from bad to worse when the first governor of the Red River settlement, Miles Macdonell—a Canadian Glengarry high-lander and former sheriff of the Home District in Upper Canada—worried that his people would starve, issued an edict in 1814 forbidding the export of provisions of any kind from Assiniboia, including the thirty-five tons per year of that delicate and long-lasting blend of dried pulverized buffalo meat (or moose, elk or deer), dried Saskatoon berries (or cherries, currants, chokeberries or blueberries) and rendered marrow fat that was called pemmican. The Métis, who prepared and traded this commodity, and the Nor'Westers, for whom this was the key supply that allowed them to extend their operations into the far west and northwest, took Macdonell's so-called Pemmican Proclamation as an act of war.

There were raids on the Red River settlement throughout the spring of 1815. In June, under threat of imminent attack, Governor Macdonell surrendered to representatives of the NWC in return for a promise from the Nor'Westers that no settlers would be harmed. Fort Douglas, the stronghold of the settlement, and the hard-won few houses that had been built to date were burned to the ground. The "charge" against Macdonell, and the justification for what amounted to a citizen's arrest under the by now somewhat fuzzy auspices of the Canada Jurisdiction Act, was illegal confiscation of pemmican. An HBC surveyor and vet-eran of much hurtful struggle between the NWC and the HBC, Peter Fidler, who had escorted a second wave of settlers to Assiniboia, was given temporary command of the settlement, and Macdonell was taken off to Montreal for a trial (which never happened).

The harassment of the Red River settlers by the Métis and the NWC continued. Only a couple of weeks after Macdonell had been removed, Fidler surrendered the colony and took the settlers north to Jack River House, a staging point on the way to York Factory. It was there that a col-ourful ex-Nor'Wester-cum-HBC-officer called Colin Robertson, himself on an expedition to mount renewed opposition to the NWC in Athabasca Country, gave over command of his group to second-in-command John Clarke. (Both Robertson and Clarke would figure largely in Simpson's early years in the trade.) Clarke continued on to Athabasca, where he established a rival post to Fort Chipewyan (which had been established by Alexander Mackenzie), on an island in Lake Athabasca. Clarke called the new post Fort Wedderburn, after the new HBC London governor.

Meanwhile, Robertson led a band of the most determined, if beleaguered, settlers back to Red River. In November 1815, Macdonell's replacement, the unfortunate Robert Semple, arrived with another coterie of settlers, from Sutherlandshire, Scotland, joining Robertson and the others, but it would be less than a year before continuing skirmishing would come to a nasty climax at Seven Oaks, when the young Cuthbert Grant, "captain general" of the Métis, and his men killed Semple and a score of unwitting settlers, setting the stage for amalgamation and Simpson's arrival on the scene. It was Canada's wild west.

———

How did all of this connect with the *James Monroe*? Among those who came in the second generation of Scots adventurers to join the fray for the NWC was a distant relative of founding partner Simon McTavish who would eventually shepherd Simpson's entry into the fur trade. John George McTavish was born in Dunardy, Argyll, Scotland, in 1778, the year before the official founding of the North West Company. Fourteen years older than Simpson, he came to North America at age twenty, worked his first five years for the NWC at its headquarters in Montreal then went with the NWC to James Bay to challenge the HBC presence there. From there he worked his way west, spending time at Fort Dunvegan on the Peace River and eventually heading over the mountains, where he stickhandled the "purchase" from John Jacob Astor of the overstretched and isolated Pacific Fur Company's installation on the Columbia River. J.G. McTavish was there when Fort Astoria became Fort George, named for the ailing king. By 1816–17, McTavish was in Athabasca Country, where Peter Pond and Alexander Mackenzie had been before him, running affairs at Fort Chipewyan on the west end of Lake Athabasca. But while heading out from there in the spring

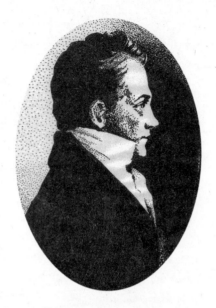

Young London businessman George Simpson, as he would have looked when he entered the trade, in robust health with a full head of hair.

of 1818 with the post's winter bounty of furs, bound for Fort William, the NWC's inland depot on Lake Superior, McTavish was ambushed, arrested and shipped back to England by an HBC officer vested (or so the officer thought, incorrectly, as time and subsequent court action would reveal) with powers afforded him as a magistrate of Rupert's Land, under the Canada Jurisdiction Act.

The charges against John George McTavish didn't stick, but they did take him out of play in fur country, which pleased the HBC no end, and which may have brought him a period of respite and modest material comfort after years of privation. When legal matters were finally sorted out and he was free to return to the fray, early in 1820, he was a Nor'Wester hungry for retaliation against any and all operatives of the HBC. His packet of choice? The only passenger transportation game available in the damp middle of the British winter, the pride of the Black Ball Line—the *James Monroe*, slated for a March 1 departure from Liverpool. On embarking, he found a quick-tongued, fellow Gaelic-speaking Scot who had just thumped and sent packing two English radicals twice his size.

The long-standing enmity of their employers notwithstanding, McTavish immediately took to Simpson, and the brand-new Bayman found good company in the older Nor'Wester. In the course of thirty-one days at sea from Liverpool to New York, in the sumptuous if occasionally wave-tossed salon of the *James Monroe*, McTavish decanted story after story about the fur trade for the novice, including the tale of his most recent arrest and acquittal. By degrees, Simpson was able to put it all together.

The HBC officer who had arrested McTavish was one William Williams, the former East India Company sea captain who had been sent to North America in 1818 by the HBC as a "fighting governor" to oversee the end of hostilities with the NWC—or the end of the NWC, whichever he could engineer more expeditiously. As head HBC man in Rupert's Land, Williams had made arrests on bench warrants from Montreal and on bills of indictment found by Montreal grand juries, as well as on his own initiative. Over quantities of brandy and sumptuous food, often in his native Gaelic tongue, McTavish took to imitating Williams when he was in his cups. In his own voice, he would re-enact the bellowing he himself did at Grand Portage, in the name of his rights as a true Nor'Wester to travel freely wherever he pleased, and then he would mince his words and feign a slight limp to play the part of Williams, who, he said, bellowed in reply, "I care not a curse for the Prince Regent's proclamation or for Lord Bathurst [the colonial minister] or Sir John Sherbrooke [the governor general], by whom it was framed. They are damned rascals. I act upon the charter of the Hudson's Bay Company, and as governor and magistrate of these territories. I will do as I think proper!" And with that, McTavish would, in the best plummy English accent an inebriated Argyll tongue could muster, say again, "I will do as I think proper. Proper!" and collapse on the slide bars at the edge of the ship's table, slapping his hand on the polished surface as if it were the funniest thing he had ever heard.

When it came time for Simpson to tell his story, he was able to spin it out for Captain Baines, the Spanish ambassador and the rest of the passengers, emphasizing new connections he had made as a result of characters and events he had learned from McTavish's tales as the ship worked its way west across the wind-whipped winter North Atlantic. And what a delicious irony he had uncovered in this chance meeting. He was heading to Rupert's Land as governor *locum tenens* (meaning "in place of") in case the HBC's head man in the country was arrested. That head man had already taken powers into his own hands, or so the Committee (and its legal counsel) thought, and he had arrested people he should not have arrested, not because they didn't deserve it—in the NWC-HBC fight between 1780 and 1820 there were very few innocents—but because he had acted beyond his jurisdiction. And that man was William Williams. And now here they sat, Williams's former fugitive and Williams's future replacement, on a frigid March night in the middle of the broad Atlantic with ice a foot thick on the decks and the rigging. Two would-be enemies, in the lantern-lit cloister of a coal-heated packet salon, laughing until their sides ached.

CHAPTER IV

———

TO RUPERT'S LAND

S impson was in a decidedly mixed frame of mind during his first few hours in North America. After a nasty storm off Newfoundland, the *James Monroe*—decks, sails, rigging and all—had been entirely coated with ice, making the decks off limits for passengers. The restless Simpson was effectively locked in his berth. But somewhere off the Boston coast, they sailed through a warm front and the sun shone. Land on the south shore of Long Island looked low and uninviting, dressed in drab March colours, but as the snow-covered forested hills of New Jersey hove into view against an Appalachian blue sky, the place looked almost inviting. Captain Baines's explanation that in spite of the unsettled weather they had made the crossing a week ahead of the thirty-eight-day average added to the sense of arrival. Travelling with speed felt good. Time was too precious to be wasted travelling slowly.

Sailing through the narrows of New York harbour, past the fortifications of Governor's Island and into the bustle of vessels of steam and sail against a skyline of handsome wooden steeples, Simpson compared the city to London or Liverpool. But here everything looked new. Spring was in the air, and he was filled with hope and promise of intensity equal to that he felt only on leaving Dingwall, twelve years—or another lifetime—before. Still, it was all a bit confusing. His leaving Graham, Simpson and Wedderburn with almost no notice; the hurried departure from London; meeting McTavish, who scurried away moments after the *Monroe* docked to make his way to Montreal, hell bent to find and punish his nemesis, the man who had sent him back to England: Simpson's new boss, William Williams.

Here, in New York, Simpson was on his own as an agent of the Hudson's Bay Company, and that, with the anticipation of new adventures in business, might have brought more than a tinge of dread to a lesser man. But doubters were weak. Simpson was a man of position. He had paid his dues in the counting house. And no one was more conscious of his arrival than the man himself. In the satchel cocked under his arm, as he made his way up the carpeted stairs of Mechanics Hall, were dispatches for important men of the trade, two in particular: one from the colonial minister, Lord Bathurst, to deliver to the partners of the North West Company to tell them to toe the line; the other very likely a reprimand and an introduction to his eventual replacement to be delivered, by hand, from the London Committee to Governor Williams. These Simpson would deliver in due course. Meantime, here in New York, he had letters of introduction to the houses of some of America's most prominent businessmen, and these he had to oblige, if only to try out his new corporate identity and to promote contacts for later dealings on behalf of the HBC.

It is not known exactly on whom Simpson called during his several days in New York City, but it is reasonable to assume that these meetings were calculated to achieve maximum personal and corporate benefit. HBC governor Nicholas Garry, who came across the Atlantic with similar letters of introduction the following year, met J. J. Astor, head of the American Fur Company (and erstwhile head of the Pacific Fur Company, which McTavish had relieved of its assets on the west coast during the War of 1812). Simpson may well have called on him as well: Astor's rise from labourer to chief executive officer would have appealed no end to the striving Scot. The politically connected Astor would be another of the players in the game of international politics in which Simpson would dabble later on in his career.

A second possible call would have been to another principal in the Pacific fur trade, the colourful and flamboyant "merchant prince" Colonel Thomas Handasyd Perkins, who owned, among other significant assets, a fleet of ships that served the needs of a tripartite business strategy: "short speculations in the West Indies, longer ones in Europe, and major investments in the growing China market."[1] Simpson, when he eventually reached the west coast of North America, seemed to have remarkable fluency in the geography of the China trade, and this may well have come from an early association with Colonel Perkins. Marking steps that Nicholas Garry would following the next spring, with letters of introduction from the London Committee of the HBC, Simpson may have connected with Perkins, who, through his firms Perkins and Company in America and J. & T.H. Perkins in Canton, had been shipping furs to China on behalf of the North West Company in the late eighteenth and early nineteenth centuries—Perkins may have been an influence for Simpson as a role model in the more flamboyant American tradition of entrepreneurship.

Simpson may also have crossed paths with a Mr. Robert Lenox, whom Nicholas Garry later described as "one of the most opulent men in the United States." Lenox was involved in a scheme hatched in 1819 by then governor of New York State DeWitt Clinton to build a canal from Troy, on the Hudson River, through to Oswego, on the south shore of Lake Ontario. Simpson would have been drawn to Lenox and the Erie Canal scheme because it was all about improving the efficiency of transportation and lowering costs to business of moving people and resources between the Atlantic seaboard and the middle of the continent.

After his New York City visiting was done, Simpson boarded the eighty-horsepower steam vessel *Chancellor Livingstone* and sailed 170 miles up the North (Hudson) River to the town of Albany, which was near the point at which Lenox's proposed seven-million-dollar, 40-foot-

wide, 4-foot-deep shipping canal was to link existing New York waterways west to Lake Ontario. Churning north on the turbid spring waters
of the Hudson River, he was quite taken by the "bold and romantick"
landscapes of the Catskill Mountains. But, as he dined and danced on a
ship that was larger and more sumptuous in its appointments than the
James Monroe, admiring the snow hanging in the verdant, steep-sided
Adirondack valleys, he had no idea that fate had handed him the absolute worst time to travel through upstate New York.

Had it been summer, when a narrowing river would have precluded
travel by steamboat, he would have transferred to horse and cart for a
short jaunt to Whitehall, where he could have reboarded a vessel and
continued sailing north 120 miles up Lake Champlain and the Richelieu
River toward Montreal. But Simpson left New York in mid-April, and the
waterways above Albany were still icebound. Demonstrating the toughness and irrepressible spirit that he would exhibit travelling around
North America throughout his career with the HBC, Simpson hired an
open four-horse hitch and literally crashed, bounced and dragged himself north to La Prairie, on the south shore of the St. Lawrence, where
after the insult of the rickety cart ride he took a dunking in cocktail ice
on the way across to Montreal.

Where an ordinary gentleman, softened by title or privilege or too
many lazy Sundays punting on the Cam, might have called it quits after
a few spills from an open cart into snow-slurried mud, Simpson seemed
untroubled. One pictures the man, long since bereft of creases, starch
and boot polish, staggering in the dark "19 out of 24 hours," following
four knackered horses and a driver who would sooner have stopped two
inns earlier, down some rutted cart track in the Adirondack Mountains.
Then there was a seven-mile push—and a swim, apparently—across the
St. Lawrence River in rising spring floodwaters. The Governor was no
ordinary gentleman.

With each stop on his way into the country—Liverpool, New York,
now Montreal—Simpson seems to have settled more and more comfortably into the persona of his new executive role with the HBC. And

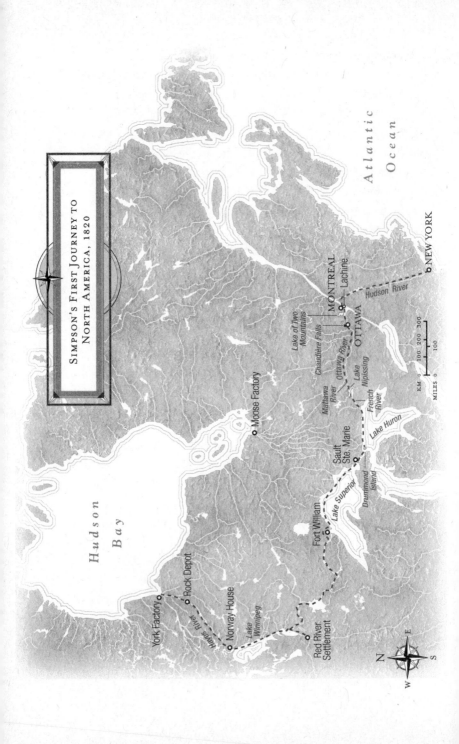

SIMPSON'S FIRST JOURNEY TO
NORTH AMERICA, 1820

Atlantic Ocean

NEW YORK

Hudson River

MONTREAL
Lachine
OTTAWA

Lake of Two Mountains
Chaudière Falls
Ottawa River
Mattawa River
Lake Nipissing
French River

KM 0   100   200 300
MILES 0   100   200

Moose Factory

Sault Ste. Marie

Drummond Island

Lake Huron

Lake Superior

Fort William

Hudson Bay

York Factory
Rock Depot
Hayes River
Norway House
Lake Winnipeg

Red River Settlement

N
W   E
S

although the Hudson's Bay Company had yet to establish a base in Montreal—in 1820, this was, after all, the home court of the Nor'Westers, with whom the HBC was for all intents and purposes at war—as a man of business, with letters of introduction from the London aristocracy, and no doubt with remarks in the right ears from J.G. McTavish on his way through town a week or so earlier, Simpson settled into Montreal life like Phileas Fogg settling with a long cognac and a fat cigar at the Reform Club back in London.

To get some idea of the Montreal Simpson entered in the spring of 1820, we can again turn to Nicholas Garry's account, written the following year. Besieged as he was by bugs, Garry liked the location but was not terribly impressed by much else in the bustling centre of Canada. He wrote:

> Montreal is very pleasantly situated on the St. Lawrence in Lon. 73.13 in Lat. 45.33 The Houses are built of Stone and with some exceptions are old fashioned and ill built—the stone has a gloomy dirty Appearance. This Town has been so often visited by Fires that the Inhabitants have hit upon an Expedient which renders the Town very uncomfortable—the Heat being almost insupportable. The Roofs of the Houses and Churches are covered with Tin Plates and the Shutters are of Iron. On my first Arrival we were dreadfully annoyed by an innumerable number of Flies which took possession of the town. They pay the Town an annual Visit and come with the Shad Fish. In walking it was necessary to keep the mouth shut. Montreal contains about 15,000 Inhabitants, three-fourths Canadian-French. The Island on which Montreal is built is about 30 miles in Length and belongs almost entirely to the Priests (St. Sulpice). Their Income would be immense but they do not exact their Rights and all they receive is given away in charity.[2]

In correspondence, Simpson described being in excellent quarters and "quite at home" with many of the "First Families" of Montreal, dividing his time between business and pleasure. At the suggestion of one of these acquaintances, he took advantage of a steamer service offered by the Molson Line and sailed on the *Accommodation* down-river to Quebec City and back, just to acquaint himself with the lay of the land and to get a sense of where the North American fur trade had begun. Back in Montreal, he was busy attending dinners, tea squalls, card parties, balls, theatre evenings and masquerades, as if these were completely within the normal range of things he might have done in London in his previous life. His warm welcome in a town ruled by his employer's arch-enemy might well have had something to do with a certain constituency in Montreal to whom he was connected through his benefactor and mentor on the London Committee, Andrew Colvile. Samuel Gale Jr. was a close friend of Colvile's sister, who was married to Lord Selkirk, and was seriously agitating for union of the two compa-nies. He had a strong interest in connecting with the HBC "new broom" in North America. Simpson carried with him a very complimentary let-ter of introduction from Colvile to Gale. Getting to know an executive for the company you would like to take over or merge with seemed an advantageous thing to do.

Simpson's descriptions of his time in Montreal have almost an over-tone of incredulity. To the Poolers, he wrote, "I assure you the repre-sentative of the Hudsons Bay Coy [Company] & Lord Selkirk is looked upon as no inconsiderable personage in this part of the world."

The social power of Simpson's new position was extended and reconfirmed as he embarked on his very first North American journey by canoe, heading west with his letters into the *pays d'en haut*. His rank was reinforced by his means of travel: the voyageurs, the lowest of the low in the fur trade hierarchy, the most hard-working and colourful con-stituency within the trade, the paddlers of the big canoes, men—many of them Mohawks from the St. Lawrence community of Caughnawaga (today's Kahnawake)—who would become some of Simpson's most loyal followers in Rupert's Land.

Simpson's affinity for these iconic characters of the fur trade appears to have been almost instant. Most were of mixed blood, some pure French Canadian, some pure Aboriginal, many Mohawks of the Iroquois Confederacy. Closer to five feet than six in height (like Simpson), known for their incredible toughness, their willingness to endure pain and privation, their ability to work in rain and snow and sleet and to carry more than twice their body weight on a leather tump strap affixed by gravity alone to their tanned foreheads, the voyageurs were by all accounts men who took the utmost pride in the hallmarks of their trade. It mattered who could sing the most beautifully, who had loved the most women, who had consumed the most alcohol, who carried the heaviest load, who paddled the wildest rapid, who jogged the fastest on portages and who, at the end of a run, could carouse until he dropped, get up, and do it all over again. These were strong-backed, quick-tongued men of motion, afraid of nothing but le diable himself, men defined by what they did as much as who they were.

In his time with the HBC, Simpson had almost nothing good to say about the stolid Orcadian oarsmen who rowed the York boats up and down the rivers of the west, but for the Canadian voyageurs he seemed to have a soft spot. In his heart, George Simpson was more voyageur than viscount, and that may have been one of the reasons why the voyageurs would do almost anything for him.

From the moment Simpson disembarked from a carriage, having driven the nine-mile road from Montreal to the village of Lachine on Lake St. Francis, where the thirty-six-foot freight canoes were loaded and the brigades began, the engagés, as the paddlers were called, would have met his every need, in the hope that this might curry an extra moment of sleep or a supplemental tot of rum somewhere down the trail. But in those days, the road from Montreal to Lachine continued along the north shore of the river to the Church of Ste. Anne, and, delaying the inevitable discomforts of canoe travel, dignitaries often went by road to the church on the upstream end of Lake of Two Mountains, where the voyageurs typically encamped on the first night of a trip to sleep off the excesses of departure and pray for safe passage

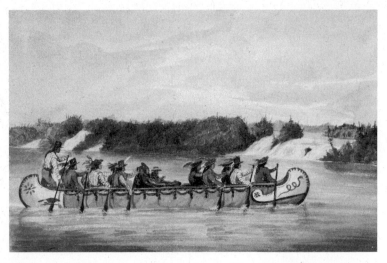

A painting by British Army officer and artist Henry James Warre of George Simpson in his express canoe passing Chats Falls en route up the Ottawa River.

to the interior. It was customary, then, for passengers to enter the big canoes as passengers on day two. Even if Simpson did just that, his natural curiosity and his intuition that transportation was at the core of finding economy in the fur trade would have seen him inspecting every aspect of the loading, noting how and with what the canoes were being filled, and how they were ingeniously packed with their four and a half tons of supplies.

First, long wooden tent poles, likely made of balsam fir, would be placed carefully along the longitudinal axis of the bottom of the craft to protect the fragile hull—birchbark with seams waterproofed with a special mix of tallow, ash and pine pitch on the outside, hand-hewn cedar ribs and wafer-thin planks on the inside, all sewn up tight with wattup, split spruce root. In the front of the canoe would be a large roll of spare bark as well as a pot of pitch and a rolled length of spruce root for repairs on the trail. The heavier items would then be placed on the poles in the bottom of the canoe. Lighter items like cassettes of provisions and cooking utensils and regularly used items like liquor barrels would be placed on the top of the load. Everything would be covered to keep out rain and spray with canvas tarps, or even tents, if someone of consequence was riding in the canoe. In all there would be about sixty individual loads to be carried in a thirty-six-foot *canot de maître*.

Simpson's first canoe, which may have carried supplies heading inland for the Selkirk settlement, would have also carried about a dozen voyageurs, including a specially trained *gouvernail* in the stern to steer and an *avant* in the bow to help navigate in fast water, perhaps also one of the *mileaux*, or middle paddlers, getting an extra shilling or two of pay for agreeing to lead songs to keep rhythm and good spirits along the way. Also in the canoe, besides Simpson and Sample (who would have headed back to England from York Factory at the end of the summer), was an interpreter who spoke French and a smattering of Aboriginal languages, and a young HBC clerk, who was heading west to Red River. It is likely that this special governor's brigade was organized by Montreal agent and entrepreneur George Moffatt, with his partners George and Robert Gillespie, of Gillespie, Moffatt and Company, one of the biggest independent import-export houses in Montreal at the time.

———

Simpson took to canoe travel like a boy to a Strathpeffer raft or a skiff on Cromarty Firth. Passengers were typically offered "seats" in the middle of the canoe, which were boards suspended on wattup or rope from the gunwales or thwarts so as to avoid damaging the integrity of the sides of the canoe with the constant motion and friction. Voyageurs perched right on the thwarts or sat on the cargo. Neither pew was comfortable until and unless its occupant learned to pulse with the shifting balance of the canoe and to the changing rhythms of the paddling. Comfort in a canoe was and is possible, but it takes some learning and accommodation, and there are, as one might then expect, two types of people in the world: those who can get comfortable in a canoe and those who can't.

In his long career, Simpson demonstrated annually, when the rivers would thaw and the furs would move again, that he was in the first

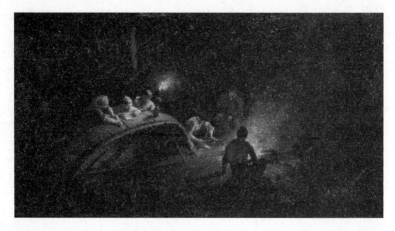

Often setting up camp after dark, even on the long days of June at northern latitudes, Simpson would eat and retire, but his voyageurs would still have chores to do before they could settle in for a four-hour sleep.

category. When, in early mid-life, his health started to fail, he said, "It is strange that all my ailments vanish as soon as I seat myself in a canoe." In fact, after some years of experience with canoe travel, after dictating letter after letter in the canoe to his corresponding secretary, Simpson would nap, but he would let one hand dangle over the gunwale in the water as a sort of motion-meter that would allow him to know if his crew was slacking off when his eyes were closed.

Camping was slightly more involved than he described to the Poolers. As romantic as it may have sounded in a letter, Simpson's cloak very likely didn't "answer the purposes of a bed," nor did the canoe's upturned bottom become his chamber. Simpson's travelling habit was likely very similar to that of Nicholas Garry when the latter came upriver the following year:

> The ceremony of encamping is, that the moment we land a fire is
> made, the tent raised, the kettle put on the fire and in the short space
> of a quarter of an hour your inn is prepared. Our tent is about 30 feet
> by 15, of canvas, handsomely striped in paint on the top. An oil cloth

is placed as a carpet at the bottom, this forms the covering of the tent [when packed up]. Our boxes and our cassettes become our chairs and tables. After supper all this is cleared and our beds are spread. First, canvas which forms the cover of the bed and our seat in the canoe. Then a bed of blankets sewn together which form an article of trade in the interior; on these two fine blankets as sheets and above this a coloured blanket as a coverlet. The fire is kept up all night for the purpose of boiling the men's dinner which consists of Indian corn and pork, from which they are called Pork Eaters.[3]

As he did the travel routines, Simpson learned the routes by rote. This was a major part of his modus operandi as a manager. And, perhaps from some land sense inherited from his ancestors in the days of the clans, Simpson seemed to know in his bones that particular pieces of land had attached to them particular people with particular points of view. From the moment he paddled onto the North America landscape, he employed a keen eye and an open ear to learn the lore and legends, the people and politics, the fur yields and the social patterns across Rupert's Land and beyond.

From the Church of Ste. Anne and the Lake of Two Mountains, they continued up the Ottawa River to Long Sault and the village of the seminary of St. Sulpice, where Miles Macdonell, the first Red River governor, would live after fleeing the Selkirk settlement in the coming months. Simpson would have taken note of the canal-building activities going on at this location, adding this to his knowledge of the Erie and Lachine canals. A canal would enable loaded boats to move more quickly, with less effort and less cost, around the rapids of Long Sault. Little did he know at this juncture in his life that investment in canal building would make him a very rich man.

Farther upriver, the little brigade may have smelled the smoke and the sweet vapours of the last of the maple syrup being candied and pressed to maple sugar to sweeten the root vegetable stews, pies and preserves of another winter. Before Chaudière Falls, where in 1805 Philemon Wright had set up the Ottawa Valley's first sawmill, at the present site of the city of Gatineau, Quebec, Simpson would have been awed by the full width of the Rideau River, falling sixty feet like a ribbon of light cascading over undercut limestone into a knifeline of effervescent foam.

And in the mornings, when the *gouvernail* would awaken the brigade with calls of *"lève, lève"* or *"embarquez!"* the *engagés* would rise in the only clothes they owned and whip out the tent poles to load them first, hoping to drop the tent on the boss. But with Simpson there was never any fun to be had on that front because he was usually up before them, having a skinny dip and raring to go. All that was left to do was tease him gently about his fancy luggage, or about having to carry him, piggyback style, when sharp rocks made it impossible to land the canoe right on shore.

From Chaudière Falls it was on to Lac des Chats, so named, the interpreter would have told them, for the unusually large population of raccoons that lived in the nearby falls. And on upriver, paddle and portage, past Calumet Island and around the rapids of Portage du Fort. Along the way, they would pass Algonquin Indians who, if they wanted to talk, would whoop and fire a rifle, although sometimes they fired their rifles as sport on a sultry spring afternoon. Then Lac des Allumettes, Allumette Island, Rivière Creuse, Portage des Joachims—many of these rapids and portages now drowned by power dams—and on past Rivière du Moine on the right and upriver to the turnoff at Petite Rivière where they would veer west to Lake Nipissing.

Along the way, in addition to meeting Indian families and other brigades bringing furs down to Montreal, they would encounter the campsites of those who had gone ahead long before them. Where voyageurs had died of strangulated hernias on portages or of drowning or in fights, small crosses marked the spots, and Simpson's voyageurs would fill in the details before they crossed themselves or sprinkled tobacco as an offering on the nearby water. And from those who were just a few days ahead, occasionally there would be a strategically placed egg, balanced on a rock beside or on a portage, on which a note for someone they knew was following would be written in pencil.

Up the Petite Rivière (now the Mattawa), moments of frenzied upriver paddling were punctuated by short, steep carries up worn trails in the thin soils covering old granitic rocks of the Canadian Shield. Portage du Prairie, 287 paces; Portage de la Cave, 100 paces; Portage de Talon, 300 paces—each one with a story, if there was anyone in a mood to tell it. Near Talon Portage, for example, there was a dramatic waterfall where, so the story goes, a brigade was making its way one day during a storm when lightning struck a tree, which exploded and fell, wrecking the canoe and killing every person but one. Simpson would have wanted to know the name of the one.

And on they would go, to Turtle Portage, which would take them into a series of nasty swamps, where, in May, after the scourge of blackflies that had dogged them on the river, they would have been greeted by legions of bloodthirsty mosquitoes. The mud and insects of the headwaters of the Mattawa River would have been almost forgotten as they crossed the height of land and slid down into Lake Nipissing and toward the Rivière des Français (today's French River). A year later, Nicholas Garry wrote of this transition, "At once the Lake Nipissing came to our view and a change from misery to the greatest pleasure and comfort. Not the poor wanderer in the desert could be more delighted with the sight of a well after being parched with thirst than we were on entering the lake."[4]

On they continued, down the French River, across the north shore of Lake Huron, past Manitoulin Island and on for respite and minor resupply at Drummond Island before heading up to the Falls of St. Mary at Sault Ste. Marie for a breakfast of the succulent whitefish for which that post was well known. Three separate carries along the St. Mary's River would have taken them to the misty maw of Lake Superior, the largest freshwater lake in the world and, in May, possibly the coldest as well.

As his canoe headed out onto the swells of Superior, setting aside thoughts of home and the Cromarty Firth brought on by the rocky hills and rolling blue horizon, Simpson may have opened his correspondence satchel and fingered the letter from Lord Bathurst, perhaps even knowing something of the portent for change that this dispatch would bring to the bristly Nor'Westers at the end of the lake. Fort William was a couple of hundred miles and still several days' paddle away, depending on the weather.

Notwithstanding the fast friendship he had made with J.G. McTavish during their passage on the *James Monroe*, Simpson had a pretty good idea that he was moving into something of a hornet's nest in the fur trade. He knew the risks, and he was coming as well prepared as he could be, given the short time frame within which his move into the fur trade was being made. He mentioned something of his apprehensions and preparations in a letter to the Poolers, written dramatically in Montreal before embarking by canoe: "There is a possibility that I may be obstructed in my route as the N.W. Coy [Company] a band of unprincipled Lawless Marauders stick at nothing however desperate to gain their ends; I am however armed to the teeth, will sell my life if in danger as dear as possible and never allow a North Wester to come within reach of my riffle if flint steel an bullet can keep him off."[5]

The letter he was delivering was the same one the HBC had received from Secretary of State for War and Colonies Lord Bathurst, which stated in no uncertain terms that if the NWC and the HBC did not curb the escalating violence and obey the governor general's proclamation to that effect, the government would step in. Bathurst had been indifferent in the early days of the fighting, but with very public debacles like the Massacre of Seven Oaks and other incidents, word of which had travelled like wildfire through the "moccasin telegraph" in North America and around the United Kingdom, lack of peace in the fur trade was becoming a political issue that could no longer be ignored.

After paddling up the mouth of the Kaministiquia River, Simpson would have disembarked at the Nor'Wester stronghold's dock for a stretch and then walked with his motley band of voyageurs up to the double gates in the palisade wall of Fort William. Difficult as it is to walk with dignity after sitting in a canoe for a month, Simpson must have done his best to make a good impression, wondering if he would be greeted with hostility, or perhaps with musket fire. But nothing like that happened.

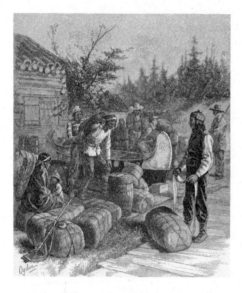

Once his express canoes were loaded at a dock or landing, Simpson would embark under his own power. If the canoe had to be loaded some distance from shore to avoid shallow water, the last item for loading would be the Governor, on the back of a willing canoeman.

On arrival, over cordial cups of tea, Simpson learned that his new friend McTavish had arrived a couple of weeks earlier and had just departed with other NWC partners and a force of sixty men en route to Grand Rapids, to avenge his own capture by William Williams, to rectify the wrongs inflicted on the NWC by Lord Selkirk and to generally continue their campaign of interruption and inconvenience against the HBC. When Simpson opened his still new leather correspondence satchel and delivered Bathurst's letter to whoever was left to mind Fort William, the moment came and went without notice. By 1820, although there was still fight in some of the hardiest Nor'Westers, everyone in the trade knew that something had to give. Bathurst's letter may not have come as much of a surprise, and, indeed, its arrival may even have brought a measure of relief.

But there was still one letter left to deliver, which, along with the results of McTavish's raid at Grand Rapids, would set the ink on Simpson's future trajectory with the HBC.

To continue inland, the Governor's brigade traded its 36-foot *canot de maître* for two 25-foot *canots du nord*. The voyageurs were redeployed, with perhaps another couple being added to the complement of paddlers, depending on available resources at Fort William. One officer and the interpreter would have travelled in one canoe, Simpson and Sample in the other for the next leg of the journey, 470 miles and 78 portages over the height of land to Lake Winnipeg and the Red River settlement, and another long, rough paddle up Lake Winnipeg to Norway House and eventually to Rock Depot, on the Hayes River. Here he might catch up with the infamous William Williams, about whom he had heard so much—that was, of course, if McTavish and his crew of hungry Nor'Westers had not captured him and spirited him off to Canada for trial.

If that were the case, Simpson knew what he had to do. He knew what his own letter of commission said—knew the full meaning and significance of the phrase *locum tenens*. Andrew Colvile had shown him the accusatory contents of the long letter in his satchel from the London Committee. He knew that it would fall to him to pick up the pieces of HBC operations in Rupert's Land and somehow figure out how to fit them all back together again before the NWC crushed the HBC once and for all.

Williams, as circumstances transpired, evaded the dragnet at Grand Rapids on his way east from Cumberland House, where he had spent the winter. But Colin Robertson, the leader of the Hudson's Bay Company campaign against the Nor'Westers in Athabasca, was not so lucky. He was arrested a second time. So when Simpson finally caught up with William Williams at Rock Depot in early July 1820, he delivered the letter to a man who was his superior, a man who, in turn, assigned Simpson to lead the charge in Athabasca in Robertson's stead. This, as it turned out, would be where the final winter skirmish between the two fur companies would transpire. And this was where Simpson would cut his teeth in the fur trade, as head man for the HBC at Fort Wedderburn on Lake Athabasca.

The Committee's letter to Williams provides an illuminating view on this juncture in history, and on the start of Simpson's fledgling career.

Williams was in trouble with the law, and in trouble with his London bosses, and the new man had just arrived in a white birchbark canoe with the following orders:

Hudsons Bayhouse
William Williams Esqr
London the 26th. feb^y 1820

Sir

 This will be delivered by Mr. George Simpson to whom we shall have given a Commission to act as Governor in Chief locum tenens in the event of your absence from the Country—. We have been enduced to grant this Commission in Consequence of the Indictments found against you in Canada, under which we are apprehensive some attempt may be made to drag you from the Country.

 2. We have perfect Confidence in Mr. Simpson's honor and integrity and from his general knowledge of Business and the information which he has been able to acquire here of the Company's affairs, we think he will not find much difficulty in making the general arrangements for the trade, provided he receives the candid and ready assistance of our Chief factors and other traders, which from their experience and local knowledge they are qualified to afford him.

 3^d. If your apprehensions of your being seized and carried down to Canada should prove unfounded, it is our wish that Mr. Simpson shall return by the Ships of this Season and you will besides writing fully, confidentially communicate with him on any points relating to the Company's affairs which it may be difficult to explain thoroughly by letter—. If however you should be of opinion that Mr. Simpson's Services in the Country would be of essential importance, we leave it to your discretion to employ him in the Superintendance of any part of the Business which may be considered to require a person of his abilities.

 (4) We have Stated a case to Counsel upon your transactions at the Grand Rapids and have obtained the opinion of Mr. Tyndall upon

it, and you will receive the Case & Opinion herewith. Mr. Tyndall is a Lawyer of considerable eminence but we cannot admit without further investigation and discussion, that his opinion of the Canada Courts having a concurrent jurisdiction over the Company's territory is a sound one. Since it differs from the Opinions formerly given by Lawyers of the first eminence at the Bar and of which you have Copies—. It is not possible however to have this further investigation in time to write by this Conveyance and we must leave it to your own discretion to act according to the best of your Judgement in the situation and Circumstances under which you may be placed—. We think it right however to add, that we understand that some other Lawyers entertain the same Opinion of the 43 Geo. 3 Chap 138 with Mr. Tyndall, and as there are doubts on the Subject it would be imprudent to resist the Execution of the Warrant, where from the Circumstances you have reason to fear Serious Consequences may ensue.

5. With regard to your transaction at the Grand Rapids we think you have in some points exceeded your authority and have not acted according to proper legal forms. You have no right to issue a Warrant to apprehend a person accused of having committed a Crime at any place not within the Limits of the Company's territories, nor to take a Recognizance to appear at any place out of the territory.

You ought also to sign your name to all official papers as "Governor in Chief" and not as "Magistrate." You will perceive Mr. Tyndall's Opinion touches on these points, and there can be no doubt of his correctness upon this point.

In similarly condemnatory language, the Committee's letter goes on to set William Williams straight on a number of other oversights and transgressions with which the Committee had had to cope. Evident in every aspect of the now famous letter, even as it collapses in the end into minutiae about damaged skins, skins not prepared properly and the proper marking of goods for export, is the fundamental tension in the running of the whole HBC—namely, the problem of having the administrative nerve centre of a corporation located several thousand miles and a cultural ocean away from the day-to-day affairs of its core concerns. In the same letter in which arrives a stern rebuke from Williams's directors and an introduction to his likely successor, delivered by that selfsame new man, there is administrative flotsam and instructions that would have taken weeks, if not months to digest:

10. From the altercations which have taken place in the Customs duties on furs it is requisite that the very damaged or staged bearskins (known here by the name of Drawback Bears) and the very common Wolve skins should not be sent to this Country, if they cannot be advantageously made use of in the Bay they should be destroyed, as they will not produce on Sale even the Amount of the Import duty and no Drawback is now allowed on exportation.

11. More attention should be paid in preparing the Swan skins and although we have formerly written upon this Subject, requesting that the Skins should not be scraped so much as generally had been the practice, it continues to be done; it would be better to suffer the fat to remain on the pelt and to dry them thoroughly, than to scrape them into holes which injures the down and lessens the value of them—.

12. We have again to call your attention to the packing and marking of the Goods, and regret that we have to mention that the marks and numbers on many of the Bales of Cargoe 1819 were completely obliterated; to remedy this inconvenience, a piece of parchment or leather with the number and contents written upon it should be enclosed in every bale, and we desire that in future each description of Fur be packed separately using nothing but Wolf skins as Wrappers (Beaver skins should on no account be used). By the Ship a correct Copy of last year's Invoice will be handed to you, which will demonstrate the irregularity with which this part of the Business is conducted.

13. We request you will send home a Sample of the different sorts of Canadian Belts and Silver works which were last Season indented for

from Montreal, it is probable that the latter article may be procured cheaper in England than in Canada, and we desire that you will in future put the Indent which is sent by that route under cover sealed with the official Seal, and give directions to the agents to forward it to England by the first means of communication.

14. Since writing the above we have Received a Letter from Lord Bathurst of which we enclose a Copy. The enclosure which it contained has been delivered to Mr. Simpson, that it may be delivered according to its address in case he meet with "the wintering proprietors of the North West Company" in his way to Jack River House—. If he does not meet them he will deliver it over to you, and you will take the earliest opportunity of delivering it according to its address—.

15. Should the Evidence on the trial to which we have alluded in the 6 Par. and the Verdict of the Jury be such that the prisoners are found guilty of a capital offence, and that you are consequently under the necessity of passing the Sentence of Death you will make an accurate Report of all the proceedings at the trial, the Evidence, the Verdicts of the Jury and the Sentence of the Court and Sign the Report as Governor that the same may be laid before the Secretary of State for the purpose of taking His Majesty's pleasure as to the execution. We are

> Your affectionate friends
> J.B. G^r
> J.H. Pelly DG^r
> B.H.
> A.C.
> N.G.
> W.S.[6]

But William Williams had no head for detail in comparison to George Simpson. From Simpson's first moments in Rupert's Land, it is clear that the new man had an amazing—possibly eidetic—memory, a complex and very effective internal filing system and a keen sense of how every scrap of information fitted into the bigger picture. He would have remembered every detail, every nuance, every character, every situation, and filed it away in the back of his head for future reference. Still, the old sea captain had not been arrested. He remained in charge of HBC operations in North America, and he had given young George Simpson a job. It was on to Fort Wedderburn.

CHAPTER V

FORT WEDDERBURN

Accompanying Simpson was the bright and talkative British clerk Robert Miles, twenty-five years of age, who had already spent two seasons in Athabasca Country. Miles had entered HBC service in 1818 as an accountant and writer, but with those qualifications came a keen mind and direct experience with the world Simpson was entering, including with the illustrious Colin Robertson, who had led the HBC charge into Athabasca. Simpson, always one to make the best of time with people who knew things that he did not, would have prodded Robert Miles for as much detail as he could provide about the history and context of HBC operations in Athabasca, especially at Fort Wedderburn.

As two of sixty-eight men (and at least one Indian woman) in one of twelve big bark canoes that were part of the Athabasca brigade that summer, heading west from York Factory with a winter's worth of supplies and trade goods, Miles and Simpson would have sat amidships, kipped up among canvas bales against hand-hewn spruce thwarts and gunwales. And over the course of the fifty-two days it took them to travel to Fort Wedderburn on Lake Athabasca, as he had done with John George McTavish on the *James Monroe*, Simpson would have taken advantage of the captive audience to pepper Miles with questions. In return, through hours, days and weeks of joint occupancy of a canoe-office that was in motion for eighteen to twenty hours each day, Miles would have had all the time he needed to curry favour by apprising his new boss of every nuance of events contributing to the situation at Fort Wedderburn in the fall and winter of 1820–21.

Miles would have told Simpson details of the messy story of the fight for fur in Athabasca between the NWC and the HBC and how, sooner or later, everything and everyone in the trade is connected to everything and everyone else. There was Nor'Wester John Clarke, who was with them on this journey as well, heading to take charge of the HBC post at Isle à La Crosse. When Clarke was out of earshot within the brigade, his ears might well have been burning as stories about him flowed back in the Governor's canoe. Miles would have been explaining that Clarke had fallen out of favour with many of his peers in the trade because of his huge ego.

Seeking better personal fortunes, Clarke had changed sides to the HBC about 1815. He and fellow former Nor'Wester Colin Robertson had been charged with the task of building HBC capacity in Athabasca. As they made their way west, they had come across the defeated rump of the Selkirk settlers who had been driven by the Nor'Westers from their homes at Red River. Robertson had made the choice to lead these settlers back to Red River. This left Clarke to carry on alone with the rest of his men north to Athabasca, where he built Fort Wedderburn on Coal Island just offshore from Fort Chipewyan. The goal, of course, was to vie for the trade in the area, but also to keep an eye on the Nor'Westers' main post on Lake Athabasca. But Clarke had bungled the fight and, as a result of bad decisions or bad luck (he would claim the latter), the Nor'Westers were able to cut off Clarke's connection to his Aboriginal provisioners. Clarke ended up having to barter trade goods, not with the Indians for furs, but with the NWC for food—and, still, he lost men from starvation that winter.

Clarke had had a rough go of it. He'd been imprisoned by the Nor'Westers at Great Slave Lake after this disastrous winter, but he'd found his way back into the trade. He'd even been given a promotion. In 1818, he had extended the HBC's reach in the northwest by establishing Fort St. Mary in Peace River country. As luck would have it, Clarke, with his returns from Fort St. Mary that spring, met up with HBC governor William Williams at Cumberland House and was with him, on their way out to York Factory in 1819, when Williams ambushed, arrested and sent packing back to England one John George McTavish. It was a small world. But no one liked Clarke. In one way or another, Miles would have been able to tell Simpson that it was the view of several HBC officers who knew Clarke that "his inordinate vanity is such that the management of John Clarke is as arduous a task as that of opposing the NWC."[1]

Robertson, on the other hand, Miles would have continued, went back to Red River with a mission to rectify the wrongs perpetrated by his former colleagues and allies in the North West Company. But things he did there that summer to avenge the ousting of the settlers eventually led to his arrest and shipment east to Canada. He was acquitted and scampered back to Athabasca, but no sooner had he settled in there, replacing John Clarke and the remainder of his men, than he was arrested and confined by Nor'Westers at Fort Chipewyan, where he spent the winter in the brig. The Nor'Westers, coming out that spring under the leadership of Samuel Black, thoroughly fed up with Robertson's antics in captivity, loaded their turncoat prisoner in a canoe at Portage des Epingles on the English River (now the Churchill) and, while they portaged around the raging waters, sent Robertson and a skeleton crew of hapless voyageurs into the frothing water. Robertson would later contend that this was meant to kill the lot of them. He survived and later escaped, but two of the voyageurs did not. Back Robertson went to Athabasca, or so the story went, and, on his way out in the spring of 1820, he was one of a group of Baymen arrested by . . . John George McTavish, in a well organized ambush at Grand Rapids portage at the north end of Lake Winnipeg. Of course, McTavish (as he'd told Simpson on the *James Monroe*) was actually looking for William Williams, but any senior HBC man would do, including the illustrious Colin Robertson. This event had set in motion the circumstances that had created the "vacancy" in the post manager's position at Fort Wedderburn that William Williams had asked Simpson to occupy.

Robert Miles had been there, in Athabasca, for two years, long enough to experience some of what went on. Some of the news, like the gory details of McTavish's arrest of Robertson, was absolutely fresh and might well have come from people they met at Norway House or on the water as they made their way west. But of the many people with whom Simpson travelled in the early years and from whom he would have heard stories that he salted away in his remarkable memory, perhaps none of these informants was more influential than Robert Miles.

Simpson developed very quickly during his first winter a surprising command of the way the trade worked. It was Miles who was at his side during this pivotal time in his career. It might well have been Miles who helped Simpson understand that there were large-scale patterns of fur out, trade goods in on which HBC commerce with local trappers was based, but that at each of the posts were smaller patterns as well—unique circumstances and idiosyncratic politics involving the history and sentiments of the local Aboriginal people, the background and temperaments of the officers and men conducting the HBC's business, and distinctive geographic and climatological issues that had to be understood in order to effectively comprehend how business worked at each node in the HBC's vast network of posts.

And so began the partnership that produced the *Journal of Occurrences in the Athabasca Department, 1820 and 1821*, dictated by Simpson and penned by Robert Miles in a moving freight canoe, the first lines of what would turn into shelves of journals, reports, ledgers and correspondence produced by one governor and his clerks in the course of forty years with the Hudson's Bay Company. Even in this very first journal, George Simpson seems to have had an uncanny grasp of the workings of the trade. In truth, although he would come to his own comprehensive understandings and never really acknowledge in any meaningful way those who helped build it, the grasp reflected in this document was likely not so much Simpson's as that of his willing clerk and scribe, Robert Miles.

Having heard about all the action at Grand Rapids and being worried about another ambush on his first trip into the country, Simpson issued each man in the brigade a musket, bayonet and ten rounds of ball cartridge. No ambush came to pass, however, which is probably just as well because, as Simpson's journal recounts, he was travelling with a band of incorrigible drunks. They revelled at Oxford House, Norway House and every chance they got as they made their way west, some voyageurs even trading their blankets to the Baymen for their share of rum and spirits. But they were sobering up by the time the brigade reached the bottom of Grand Rapids, at the north end of Lake Winnipeg, when they insisted that the threat of a Nor'Wester attack demanded a hearty dram to calm nerves sufficient for loads to be carried into possible danger up the trail.

Luckily, the threat had moved on. They learned from a free trader named Martin, who was camped in a cabin near Grand Rapids, that James Leith, Simon McGillivray (twenty-year-old son of the "Godfather" of the Nor'Westers, William McGillivray) and a large contingent of clerks, interpreters, Métis and voyageurs had passed through a few days before, amid much public rumination and clattering of arms about the imminent destruction of the HBC in Athabasca. They also learned that the illustrious Samuel Black had shimmied west, up the Peace River and over the Rockies, to avoid arrest for his part in the cruelty to Clarke, Robertson and the others at Fort Wedderburn, with a promise that he would be back to Athabasca the minute he heard they needed help to confound the HBC's best efforts to compete. In due course, Simpson would meet all of these characters, and he would not have to wait long to begin the introductions.

Two days beyond Grand Rapids, as a result of Simpson's waking his men at one and two o'clock in dark of the early morning, they overtook the NWC's Athabasca brigade. Simpson's first observation was that this whole outfit was of superior quality: their canoes were newer and in much better shape, their crews were happier and better disciplined, and their kit, including their brand-new company flag fluttering on a short standard from the stern of the lead canoe, looked to be fresher and in much better repair than his. In a show of bravado that had characterized the often lethal posturing between operatives of the two companies, young Simon McGillivray took leave of his brigade to silently circle the HBC brigade in his light canoe and have a good look at what they were carrying.

By now, thanks to Miles, Simpson knew that McGillivray was well known for his low cunning and that he had something to do with "every nefarious transaction" that had taken place in Athabasca. Next to Samuel Black, Miles had explained, McGillivray was "more to be dreaded than any member of the N.W. Co." But Simpson seems not to have been intimidated by McGillivray in the slightest way, saying simply, in his journal, "a day of retribution I trust is at hand for this worthy." His chance would come.

A few days later, making their way up the Sturgeon-Weir River to the English River, Simpson's canoes caught up to John Clarke's portion of the brigade, which had gotten a little bit ahead. Simpson was irked to see that Clarke, whom he had liked well enough until he'd learned something of the man's chequered history, had left behind some of his cargo and two of his men so that he could accommodate his Indian wife in his canoe. Clarke's lot in Simpson's eyes dropped even further when he let on to the new governor that one of his men had found a bag of ball shot, left behind on a portage, and that for a gallon of rum for his men, he would gladly return it to its rightful owner. Ruminating on these low tactics by an officer of his own company, as well as on the trouble he'd had with drunken men up to that point and the overall poor turnout of his brigade in comparison to the Nor'Westers, Simpson wondered if he was not travelling with the "very dross and outcast of the human species."

By the time they left Clarke and his portion of the brigade behind at La Loche post and continued northward to Athabasca, over the

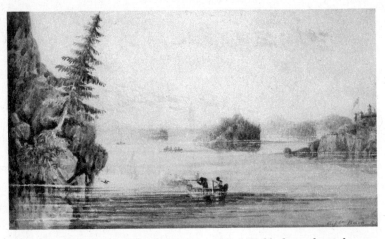

Simpson's first charge in the fur trade was Fort Wedderburn, located on an island in Lake Athabasca within sight of the original North West Company outpost, Fort Chipewyan, on the north shore. In a watercolour by Franklin midshipman George Back, painted when he passed through in 1820, an Aboriginal hunting party is seen with Fort Chipewyan in the background.

thirteen-mile Portage La Loche (Methye Portage) and into the Little Athabasca (Clearwater) River, Simpson's view of the man had completely changed. "One of the Company's worst bargains," as Simpson later wrote, would have his comeuppance, but not until the Governor was good and ready to mete out appropriate punishment. He would start, in due course, by billing Clarke, against his salary, for costs associated with reclaiming the goods and personnel he left behind.

After a canoe-based six-week crash course in the workings of the fur trade under the tutelage of Robert Miles, immersed in the experience of travelling with a working HBC brigade in all its tattered drunken glory, Simpson arrived on September 20, 1820, at Fort Wedderburn on Coal Island at the west end of Lake Athabasca. Clearly visible on the bluffs of the northern shore of the lake, a mile and a half away, were the magnificent wooden palisades, peaked roofs, watch tower and opposing flag of the rival Nor'Westers' long-standing Fort Chipewyan. Wedderburn, by contrast, was more or less as John Clarke and his men had laid it out in 1815, a "scarcely habitable" north-facing assemblage of damp and smelly low-doored, sparsely windowed, hand-hewn, moss-chinked log buildings with its own approximation of a pointed log palisade surrounding the installation. Behind the "fort" was a huge cliff—good for defence, bad for keeping direct sunlight out of the buildings for six months of the year. And in front, off to the right, barely ten paces from Fort Wedderburn itself, was a most vexatious watch house built by the Nor'Westers, "an army of murderers, robbers, bullies and villains," in the summer of 1819 to intimidate the enemy.

There at the ramshackle gate to meet their new boss were William Brown, master of the post, and four other officers of the district, including Simpson's old chum from his Dingwall school days, Duncan Finlayson, who had entered HBC service in 1815 in the capacity of a clerk, latterly at Fort St. Mary in the Peace River District. According to Simpson's journal, there was no time for idle chit-chat, even with boyhood friends, for there was much work to be done to distribute the supplies he had brought from Rock Depot.

Considering that Simpson had been in transit by this time for nearly seven months, having left London in February, and that the only business he had known up to this point in his career was the London-based sugar trade, the speed and vigour with which the twenty-eight-year-old governor *locum tenens* took up his duties at Fort Wedderburn speaks to his astonishing tenacity and his remarkable intelligence. In a few short weeks, he seemed to have absorbed the macro picture of the fur trade across North America as well as the micro picture in the various districts of the Hudson's Bay Company's purview from York Factory southeast into Canada, south into Assiniboia and west into Athabasca and beyond. His mind was in constant motion. From the outset, the key to his success seems to have been an ability to see and assess his world through the eyes of his officers and underlings and to make snap judgments on the veracity of the information received based on his assessment of the character traits of the individuals from whom the information had come.

As the HBC's head man in the northwest, Simpson had charge of the Athabasca District, which included 6 officers and 44 men at Fort Wedderburn, 2 officers and 6 men at Berens House, south of them at Pierre au Calumet on the Athabasca River, and 2 officers and 7 men at Harrison's House at the east end of Lake Athabasca. Also in his charge was the Peace River District, which included three installations up the mighty river west of Lake Athabasca: 4 officers and 21 men at Fort St. Mary, 2 officers and 10 men at Fort Colvile and 2 officers and 10 men at Fort de Pinnette. And, to the north, Simpson oversaw operations in the Great Slave Lake District, which, at the time, had only one post, Fort Resolution, at the mouth of the Slave River, housing 2 officers and 17 men. In total, in an area equivalent to that of Canada's four Maritime provinces, Simpson had immediate responsibility for 115 men, not including cooks, guides, interpreters and voyageurs, most of whom, he quickly decided, were underworked, overpaid and lacking respect for discipline and authority.

And whatever the inventory of goods might have been that he had routinely handled or tallied in his daily round in the sugar business, the fur trade was a much more complex proposition. In the alphabetically organized list of goods included in the Athabasca outfit his brigade had brought west were hundreds of individual items, from augers to anvils, borax to buttons, hooks to hatchets, needles to nails, pistols (fourteen) to plough shears (one), rasps to razors, beeswax to binding wire and everything in between—beads, bells, belts and blankets—along with a surprisingly short list of comestibles: butter, coffee, chocolate, flour, mustard, pimento, pepper, raisins, Jamaican rum, sugar, black tea, green tea, wine, brandy and shrub (fruit cordial). All had to be unpacked, inventoried, repacked and sent to destination before the onset of winter in the northwest.

In letters of self-introduction, he wasted no time in letting his district managers know that life as they knew it was about to change. He entreated everyone to eschew waste: "Economy must now be the order of the day, indeed our means are this season so limited, that we cannot follow up the extravagant system which has hitherto been adopted, and your influence with the Indians will I have no doubt soon reconcile them to the change."[2] But he also moved deftly and with precision to tighten things up on the basis of what he had learned from the people around him.

He had heard from reliable sources (perhaps Duncan Finlayson) that Joseph Greill at Berens House was a hopeless alcoholic. He met that situation head on, writing, "It has been hinted that you are rather addicted to the Bottle, this report I cannot believe until it is substantiated on conclusive evidence, and I trust your conduct will be so perfectly correct as to challenge the strictest examination; a Drunkard you are aware is an object of contempt even in the eyes of the Savage race with whom we have to deal in this country."[3]

To Charles Thomas at Fort St. Mary in the Peace River District, about whom he had heard nothing good from Robert Miles or from other officers during his first few days on Coal Island, he handed a summary demotion:

Fort Wedderburn, 26th Septr., 1820
Mr. Charles Thomas
St. Mary's

Sir

I beg leave to inform you that in the consequence of Mr. Robertson's unexpected visit to Canada, the Govr. in Chief has appointed me to the charge of the Athabasca Department.—This will be handed to you by Mr. Finlayson, to whom you will be please to deliver up the charge of the Peace River District; he is a stranger to your part of the country, and I trust you will render him every assistance by your council and advice in the management of the business, which from your judgement and experience cannot fail to be of the essential importance to him. I intend visiting St. Mary's in the course of the Winter when I shall have the pleasure of introducing myself personally to your acquaintance, meantime, I remain, Sir,

Your Obedt. Servt.

(signed) Geo. Simpson[4]

This one-two delivery—giving Thomas's job to a stranger followed by flattery of Thomas's judgment and experience—is an early and classic example of what was later called "Simpsonian smoothing."[5] Thomas had not done a stellar job at St. Mary's River, and likely no one knew that better than the man himself, but he was not beyond acquiescing to Simpson in his lowered position in favour of jockeying for higher wages. Simpson, who now had the person he wanted in the post, decided to spar with Thomas in an almost playful correspondence, eventually giving him a portion of an expected annual raise in pay with the tongue-in-cheek admonishment, "Pray do not give the censorious an opportunity of saying that you drove a hard bargain with me."

To Duncan Finlayson, whom he appointed to replace Thomas at Fort St. Mary, Simpson expressed concern about the possible effects of the change on top of damage already caused or exacerbated by Thomas in the social hierarchy at the main post in the Peace River District. Simpson cautioned, "I beg to call your attention to the following observations. Jealousies and private misunderstandings amongst the Officers have hitherto been most prejudicial to the general service; you will therefore no doubt see the propriety of keeping on friendly terms with all the Gentlemen in your District, using every exertion to reconcile any little differences that may exist between them."[6]

In his letter of charge to Finlayson, it is clear that Simpson had an ulterior motive for setting him up as head operative in the Peace River District. In fact, Finlayson had been on his way west to set up an HBC presence in New Caledonia (the region of the Stuart and Upper Fraser rivers between the Coast Range and the Rockies) when the season had closed in on him and he was forced to retreat for the winter to Fort

Wedderburn. Simpson seems to have had a very clear sense about the good fur prospects of Athabasca and the west, which stood in stark contrast in the ledgers to the mid-parts of North America, now effectively bereft of beaver. This knowledge is evident in his instructions to Finlayson on departure to Fort St. Mary: "It is of the utmost importance that New Caledonia should be established next year, the delay that has already taken place in settling this rich and valuable country is deeply to be regretted."[7] He felt that Duncan Finlayson was the man to make sure that this move happened.

In the middle of these early letters, Simpson's attention was also drawn north, toward Great Slave Lake and to John Franklin's Northern Discovery Expedition, which had had a terrible time trying to ship inland what supplies it had brought to York Factory late the previous year. Nominally the transport of five extra pieces had been in the care of the NWC, but the expedition had left them at Grand Rapids, and Clarke, who was supposed to be helping on behalf of the HBC, had refused to carry them as well—another black mark against the man and his ego. The same day Simpson wrote to Duncan Finlayson about New Caledonia, he wrote a conciliatory letter to Lieutenant Franklin. He knew the five errant pieces were somewhere between Grand Rapids and Great Slave Lake, but he was not sure exactly where. But he wrote to Franklin anyway, saying that he would do everything in his power to assist. He apologized also for not being able to send Franklin a newspaper, saying that the last news he had was on March 4, the day he left Liverpool. But he took a moment to summarize major political events: "The most important recent occurrences are in the decease of our late much beloved Monarch, and His Royal Highness the Duke of Kent in the Month of January; the proclamation of his Majesty King Geo. the IVth; the dissolution of parliament, and the fortunate discovery of a horrible plot to assassinate the whole of the Cabinet Ministers."[8]

No sooner had Simpson sent off brigades to the outlying HBC posts (along with his orders) than serious trouble began anew with the Nor'Westers. James Leith and Simon McGillivray made sure there were one or two NWC personnel manning the watch house outside Fort Wedderburn at all times. The Nor'Westers would paddle the mile and a half of open water from Fort Chipewyan to Coal Island and march back and forth outside the Wedderburn gate from time to time with muskets shouldered and cutlasses at the ready, trying to look as menacing as possible. They would watch as HBC men from each district would parade by, reload their canoes and head out, noting who was there, what they appeared to have by way of supplies, and any other useful intelligence. The engine of the trade was fur: no fur, no trade; no trade, no London sales; no London sales, no cash for new outfits, no dividends for shareholders—for either company.

By mid-October, Simpson was intrigued by the fact that the back windows of the NWC watch house commanded a full prospect of proceedings at Fort Wedderburn, and so he instructed his men to go out and build a high fence. Before making this provocative move, Simpson called his officers together and ordered them to load their guns. It was only a matter of time before the Nor'Westers took umbrage at this and, in due course, out came Simon McGillivray with two of his larger men, loaded pistols in hand. Simpson had already learned that there were mutually agreed upon lines of demarcation drawn around both installations on Coal Island. Now he knew his bargaining position.

With his men leaning on their shovels beside the partially completed stockade fence, Simpson and McGillivray (who, it should be remembered, did not speak when McGillivray circled the HBC brigade a month or so earlier) stood face to face, guns at the ready. In his journal, Simpson recounts what happened next ("in case it may be of importance at any future period"):

When standing close to McGillivray on the bank of the Trench I remarked, "My name is Simpson, I presume yours is McGillivray", he replied: "it is."—I then said, "I intend erecting these Stockades from the corner of the Bastion in a direct line to that stump" (point to the stump of a Tree, about five feet within another stump which is understood to be the boundary of the two establishments) "pray Sir, what are your objections?" He answered: "I understand from Mr. Oxley that he intended to run them beyond the boundary line which I shall not permit." I rejoined: "we have no intention to encroach on what is understood to be the line of demarkation, nor shall we tamely submit to any encroachment on our rights, we are inclined to be quiet orderly neighbours if permitted to be so, but are determined to maintain our privileges with firmness, and shall promptly resent any injury or insult that may be offered." . . . Here ended the conversation; McGillivray and his bullies retired somewhat crestfallen, and in the course of two hours afterwards, the fence was completed and an annoyance removed which has been a source of great vexation to the inmates of Fort Wedderburn since it has been established.[9]

McGillivray was not to be intimidated so easily. He immediately commanded his men to start gathering mainland timber on the island to see about some additional building of their own. The following Sunday, October 22, 1820, one of Simpson's men was beaten up as he returned to Wedderburn with a load of firewood. The NWC bullies kept the wood and the man's hat as victory spoils, knowing someone would be back for both. Simpson demanded an explanation but was given only the cap. His temper piqued, he strode out of the fort with his armed officers, who had been given an order to shoot anyone who came between them and return of the firewood. The wood was returned, and all was quiet until the following day when William Brown reported to Simpson that the Nor'Westers were now digging the foundation of a new bastion within two feet of Fort Wedderburn.

Meanwhile, Simpson had hatched a nefarious plan of his own. On October 18, an HBC employee, Mr. Grignon, had arrived at Fort Wedderburn in a canoe with additional supplies and, in conversation with this French-speaking *engagé* who could neither read nor write, Simpson learned (through various officers who translated for him) that under powers of the Canada Jurisdiction Act, or something similar, he was a sometime constable for the District of Montreal. He had in his kit a King's warrant for the arrest of one Simon McGillivray, for previous alleged offences committed in the war for fur trade supremacy. Simpson knew just by looking at him that Grignon was no match for the strength and cunning of the wily McGillivray, so he announced to his men that in the event that an officer of the law called for help in the execution of a warrant, any law-abiding citizen was obliged to assist in the King's name, if necessary. With his band of pistol-toting conspirators behind him, Simpson stumped out to the new hole in the ground demanding to speak to McGillivray on the subject of the boundary line. When McGillivray appeared, Grignon collared him and escorted him promptly into locked quarters inside Fort Wedderburn.

In this strange enclave in the far-flung reaches of the North American wilderness, Simpson seemed right at home. Bickering with the Nor'Westers added spice to life. Having a man of equal cunning and pluck, like McGillivray, at his disposal for dinner conversation or to while away the lengthening nights was an unexpected pleasure. To a point, the prisoner capitulated to this hospitality. And when everyone was where they were supposed to be for the winter and the lake began to freeze, the pace of life at the Fort Wedderburn post dropped, or at least that is the impression one gets from Simpson's journal. Best kept in mind, however, is the knowledge that this journal was an official document, written by Simpson as an HBC employee for the London governors. Simpson seemed well aware of the possibility that any point committed to paper could well come back to haunt him. The pace of post life, then, may not have been quite as humdrum as the written record would have us believe, although their diet, which consisted largely of unspiced Lake Athabasca whitefish, would have indeed been a trifle monotonous, even to a pragmatist like Simpson.

When winter came in early November, canoes were replaced by snowshoes, and hand-hauled toboggans and dog carrioles—three-dog sided toboggans called "trains"—were used to transport people and goods, mostly fish and firewood, from place to place. Simpson seems to have had something of a soft spot for dogs. It's not known how a dog called Boxer came into his life, or how long the dog stayed, but on November 5, the eve of dogs being called into requisition, Simpson wrote in his journal, "From the beginning of November until the latter end of May they are daily in Harness, hard wrought and sparingly fed; if in tolerable condition at the end of the season, many of them are eaten by their masters, and those who have the good fortune of being so lean as to escape the Kettle are allowed to starve the rest of the year. They are a great article of traffic amongst the Canadians who value a dog according to his points as we estimate a Horse in the civilized world. Three active dogs have been known to run ten miles within the hour drawing a carriole and passenger with the driver standing behind and fifty pounds of luggage."[10]

Simpson, ever the businessman, was thinking about how the HBC could profit from this aspect of the business by creating a monopoly of female sled dogs. He wrote, "By proper attention to the breeding of dogs the Company may make a very profitable trade of them and in spring I intend to issue an Order that none shall keep bitches except the Compy., by this arrangement we shall always have a good stock of dogs, and can supply the people at fair prices." He speculated about increased use of horses at the most-travelled posts, and also about the possible use of another northern transportation resource: "I see no reason why Rein Deer should not be employed in this country as in the North of Europe, and intend giving orders that the experiment be tried next season."[11]

As the days got shorter and the stars got brighter, the temperature dropped, and not once did Simpson complain. The pace of life did not entirely drop, though. At a dance on December 4, McGillivray (who was eightsome reeling on the floor with his wife) managed to escape. And Simpson suspected a Mr. Knipe, a Swiss De Meuron Regiment[12] soldier who had joined the HBC after helping Colin Robertson capture Fort Gibraltar and restart the Red River settlement, of bribery and collusion with the enemy. But the interrogation ended without success when Knipe made it known that he would discuss the matter only in German, even though the alleged collusion was supposed to have happened in English.

Christmas Day meant an extra dram and a "holyday" from regular duties. The gentlemen at Fort Wedderburn were treated to the most English meal the cooks could muster: a roast of buffalo with bannock and gravy, followed by plum pudding and a "temperate kettle of punch." That meal was interrupted by news that Simon McGillivray was in the watch house, so Simpson had to muster a guard detail for the night. They also celebrated on Hogmanay (Scottish New Year); the festivities began at 4 a.m. with a salute of firearms followed by an all-day regale with a "few flagons of rum, some cakes, a full allowance of buffalo meat, and a pint of spirits for each man." Simpson added in his journal that "the women [all of whom were Aboriginal] were also entertained to the utmost of our ability." During this celebration, in came news of an impending Nor'Wester attack, but no one seems to have done much about it, perhaps because Simpson was otherwise occupied, with activities not recorded in any official document. Two women, part of the help contingent at Fort Wedderburn, would eventually bear children by George Simpson. In his chambers this Hogmanay may well have been Betsy Sinclair, the young daughter of Chief Factor William Sinclair and his Cree wife, Margaret (or Nahovway) Norton.[13] Betsy was originally from Oxford House, but either was already at Fort Wedderburn (which is unlikely) or went west with Simpson. Young Betsy Sinclair conceived a child with George Simpson in April or May of 1821. As in England, evidence suggests that when the nights turned cold, he was not quite as alone as his journals might indicate.

On January 2, 1821, while most of the fort was still drunk or hungover to the point of incapacity, George Back, one of Lieutenant Franklin's officers, turned up looking for the Northern Expedition's lost supplies. Simpson, by this time, knew that Franklin had gear farther back in the supply line, and that it was his shifty manager, John Clarke, who was withholding it (along with much-needed food and supplies for Fort Wedderburn). But Simpson also knew that Robert McVicar at Fort Resolution had already given the expedition all that he could possibly give them, to the point that Simpson was worried that his most northerly post would be unable to conduct effective trade in the spring. Yet George Back persisted, and through a series of strong letters back and forth between Fort Chipewyan and Fort Wedderburn, with occasional visits with Simpson in between, eventually retrieved some of the lost supplies. But he had to suffer the brunt of Simpson's temper as well.

There is an especially lively exchange of letters from February 5, 1821. From Fort Chipewyan, Back wrote, "Sir, I have been anxiously expecting for several days past an intimation on your part of fulfilling your promise—I mean 'the additional supply.' If you do not intend further assistance, you will oblige me by mentioning it in direct terms, as I shall consider any deviation as mere equivocation and quite foreign to my request."

Simpson replied immediately: "Sir . . . The expected supplies from Isle à La Crosse alluded to in my Letter of the 4th Ulto. [from the Latin *ultimo*, meaning "last month"] have not come to hand nor have I received any communication from that establishment of a later date than the 15th Octr. so that it is quite uncertain whether Mr. Clarke can furnish them or not, and if you will take the trouble of referring to my correspondence I think you will find that any promise made of further assistance is qualified with the proviso of my receiving the expected supplies from Isle à La Crosse . . . If you would be pleased to refer to my former remarks on this subject I think you will find that I have not in any instance amused you with 'equivocation' but that my observations have been directly to the point."

The response came back across the frozen lake within the hour: "Sir . . . I must inform you that I need no prompting as to references or any former correspondence. This I know—that you have had several arrivals during my residence here and I imagine they were not all empty."

To which Simpson replied curtly, "Sir, The object of my referring you to former correspondence was to correct an error into which you appear to have fallen in regard to my promises of additional supplies. The arrivals you allude to have no connection with the Goods expected from Isle à La Crosse and your conjecture that 'they were not empty' is perfectly just."

A few supplies did, in fact, arrive from Isle à La Crosse in the nick of time, and Back was sent packing with at least some small portion of the goods Lieutenant Franklin had requested. Still, the Northern Discovery Expedition was woefully undersupplied and undermanned, in significant measure because of the internecine bickering between the HBC and the NWC. Franklin and Back, whatever their own shortcomings in planning and execution, got caught in the middle. And in what history would show was a portentous statement written well before Franklin's well-publicized disaster—in which nine men died of starvation or exposure and a tenth, who was suspected of cannibalism and possibly murder in the death of midshipman Robert Hood, was executed by expedition doctor John Richardson—Simpson had this to say about their prospects for success:

> February 8th, 1821 Mr. Back paid me a visit preparatory to his departure; from his remarks I infer there is little probability of the objects of the expedition being accomplished, not so much on account of any serious difficulties to be apprehended, but from a want of unanimity amongst themselves; indeed it appears to me that the mission was projected and entered into without mature consideration and the necessary previous arrangements totally neglected; moreover Lieut. Franklin, the Officer who commands the party has not the physical powers required for the labor of moderate Voyaging in this country; he must have three meals p[er] diem, Tea is indispensable, and with the utmost exertion he cannot walk above *Eight* miles in one day, so that it does not follow if those Gentlemen are unsuccessful that the difficulties are insurmountable.[14]

Simpson had problems of his own as the winter wore on. The fort's fishery, which was located at Big Island, several miles down the lake, became less and less productive. People were hungry and fractious. Constant preparedness in the face of imminent Nor'Wester attack wore everyone down. The would-be constable, who had enjoyed more favour than he should have on the strength of his arrest of McGillivray, turned up at the fort with a load of buffalo meat in early March, but Simpson reckoned that during the journey, which had taken sixteen days instead of the expected nine, they ate more meat than they brought home. He complained in his journal: "Grignon is quite useless about the Fort and it is really vexatious to be saddled with the expense and have the name of so many Clerks when we derive no benefit from their services, I would gladly exchange half a dozen of our present officers for two good English Halfbreeds. Grignon talks of breaking his Engagement, I shall however save him that trouble as he consumes more provisions and tobacco than his services are worth."[15]

With the first whiff of spring in late March 1821, Simpson sent several trains to Harrison's House, at the other end of the lake, for supplies, but they returned with news that officers were trading the clothes off their backs for furs lest the Indians go away with nothing and trade with the enemy.

———

Breakup in early May swept away three nets from the fishery, and from then until departure from the fort on May 26, they were at near starvation rations. On May 21, for example, Simpson noted that the working men in the fort had had nothing to eat for three days, the women and gentlemen nothing for half that time.

But in this dismal context, his mind was sharp as ever in its assessments of the Athabasca Department's business performance. The good news, he reported to the Committee in his year-end report, was that he was convinced that the Nor'Westers were in even more desperate straits than the HBC and would not, he reckoned, be able to sustain their activity in Athabasca for another winter, two at the most. However, he reported, the bad news was that as a result of previous mismanagement, the Athabasca Department—Fort Wedderburn in particular—was in a total shambles. The Native trappers, who had been lavished with gifts and credit for several years running, had learned that they could

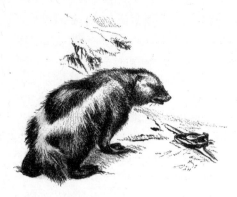

Although beaver was the prized pelt, the HBC traded many other skins as well. Fur from the elusive wolverine, however, was often kept by the Aboriginal people, because oil on the fur made it less likely to frost up in cold weather when used as a ruff around a hood.

get everything they would ever require in trade goods, and then some, for fewer and fewer furs. He had worked hard, he told the Committee, to reduce expenses, but even with those austerity measures added to his constant "encouragement" of the Indians in the area, the district had incurred two more years of loss in a row. The returns for the district in 1819/20 had been £1,165 14s 3d, with expenditures of £7,623 15s. The returns for 1820/21 had been better, but still disastrous, at £1,892 6s 7d on expenses of £6,569 5s 1d.

What Simpson may have under-appreciated as he prepared to paddle east with the 1820/21 returns, but would better come to understand through correspondence with the London Committee, was that this protracted internecine fighting with the NWC not only had made both companies unprofitable but had driven them deeply into debt—specifically, the HBC. Despite overall fur sales in London that had realized £95,000 in 1818, £86,000 in 1819, and £69,000 in 1820, the firm's overdraft with the Bank of England had risen from £23,500 in 1814 to £75,000 in 1820, and the value of unpaid bills languishing on the HBC treasurer's desk in London had risen over the same six years from £4,734 to £30,502.

Finances aside, Simpson laid a large proportion of the blame for the company's lack of performance on mismanagement, saving most of his scorn and sarcasm in his report of 1820 for his predecessor in charge at Fort Wedderburn, fellow Scotsman Neil McDonald. Simpson wrote:

The important services of Mr. McDonald who had charge of this District last year are not unworthy of remark . . . One would conceive him to be a *rara avis*, possessing the abilities more fit to govern an Empire than [an] Athabasca trading Post, but if he did possess those luminous talents, he must have kept them entirely to himself, one thing is clear, that the Honble. Compy. reaped little advantage from them. This phenomenon at a Saly. of £265 p annum last Year never took the trouble of putting Pen to Paper, looking after his people, or into the state of officers of the District, speaking to an Indian, keeping either Books or accounts or even crossing the threshold of his chamber (except to answer the calls of Nature) but actually passed the whole of his time inland Eight Months in eating and Drinking the Compy's property, smoking their Tobacco, and Sleeping their time away: if the responsible Man thus deports himself it is but natural that his officers and Men should follow his example; the result may be anticipated, the business got deranged and was left in a chaos of confusion.[16]

Perhaps warmed by his ire (although his stomach might have also been grumbling), George Simpson's spirit and constitution were as strong as his business acumen as he headed east, hiking the thirteen miles of the Methye Portage, hoping to have a feed of pemmican his old nemesis John Clarke was to have left on the ice at the edge of Lac La Loche. But there was no pemmican to be found, and Clarke had gone on ahead with his own returns. When they finally did get food in early June, the Wedderburn brigade was "nearly worn out with hunger and fatigue . . . having had little or no sustenance for eleven days." Simpson called a day of rest, but even still the following day he encountered something of a minor mutiny when the call was put out to load the canoes. If any one of these unhappy *engagés* was thinking that the fire had gone from the Governor's emaciated belly, he was wrong. Simpson described his little tantrum this way: "When embarking this morning at six o' clock several of the people were extremely insolent and refused to ship a small Box, one in particular (Jaudoins) was so mutinous that I found it necessary to

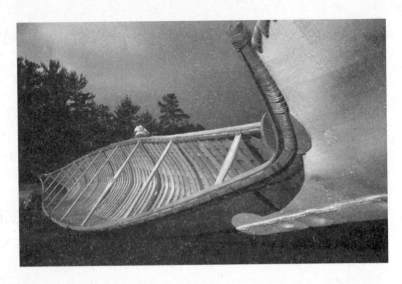

Construction details, showing birchbark sewn together with spruce root seams, waterproofed with pine pitch on a frame of hand-split cedar gunwales, ribs and planking, seen here on a modern replica of a thirty-six-foot canot du maître, fabricated at the Canadian Canoe Museum in Peterborough, Ontario. The canoes used by Simpson to travel into Athabasca Country were twenty-five-foot versions of more or less the same thing—strong, light and able to carry prodigious loads, but not indestructible.

plunge into the Water, and drag him ashore for the purpose of compelling him to embark the box; he was back and encouraged by eleven of his comrades who it will be requisite for the sake of example to punish severely by fine."

With the recalcitrant crew back at their posts, the Athabasca brigade made its way down the Sturgeon-Weir River, into the North Saskatchewan and on toward Lake Winnipeg. Their muskets were loaded before they approached Grand Rapids, and a contingent of men was sent ahead in the bushes to make sure that the half-loaded canoes landed safely in the upper basin. Simpson shot the upper rapid—two miles in six minutes—and was totally exhilarated by the experience: "the finest run in North America," he called it in his journal. (It is now submerged behind a power dam.) But they all recoiled as they swept around the final bend and saw an NWC canoe suspiciously beached on a small island in the river. It looked like a trap. Another trap.

But it was not a trap. A clerk of the North West Company stepped onto the beach as the Athabasca brigade approached and called Simpson by name, with news that they were now working for the same outfit—that the NWC and the HBC had merged. He produced copies of letters from various officials on both sides, including William Williams, to prove that this was indeed the case. At first Simpson thought that this might be a hoax but, having talked at length with Andrew Colvile and so many others in his travels both in the United Kingdom and now in North America, he knew that there was a ring of truth, an inevitability even, to it. The clerk asked him to address a number of NWC officers, camped farther down the portage, on the subject, but he declined. Guard was still required. And in the end, he was disappointed that the war was over. He wrote, "The information seems to disconcert both Officers & Men, and I must confess my own disappointment that . . . our Opponents have not been beaten out of the Field, which with one or two years of good management I am certain might have effected."[17]

This year in the trenches of Athabasca, on the last front line of the greatest rivalry the fur trade had ever seen, was a pivotal time in George Simpson's life. On top of a dozen years of business apprenticeship in London, he could now add a fifteen-month internship under battlefield conditions in the fur trade. The last words of his first trade journal are these: "As the contest is now terminated I beg to conclude this apology of a Journal after presenting my most respectful congratulations to the Honble. Committee on what appears to me a very advantageous and satisfactory arrangement of the serious differences which have for a length of time kept the country in a state of Warfare."

——

CHAPTER VI

NORTHERN GOVERNOR

On the water highway from Norway House, just off the northeast end of Lake Winnipeg, to York Factory, at the Hayes River estuary on Hudson Bay, there were thirty well-trodden portages. Even after receiving news of the merger of the NWC and the HBC at Grand Rapids, Simpson knew that regardless of what had happened at head office, as a field manager his first duty was to see the year's returns from Athabasca over every bug-infested, mud-sodden step of those trails around impassable sections of river before he could in good conscience pass on his precious cargo to the men in York boats below Rock Depot on the Hayes River. They would row the furs on flat water over the last 120 miles of the journey to the HBC depot at York Factory.

There, at Rock Depot in early June 1821, Simpson had turned to retrace his steps, thirty portages and days of upstream travel 265 miles back to Norway House, where post managers had been summoned for the first meeting of the newly amalgamated companies. Senior managers from both the NWC and the HBC had been summoned to Norway House to hear explained the terms of the merger, to hear pronouncements on appointments as required by the new arrangement and to hear the details of a carefully engineered corporate plan to stop rough and ready traders and fur operatives from killing each other.

Back he had gone, with his trusty clerk, Robert Miles; his personal assistant, Tom Taylor; and his "washerwoman," Betsy Sinclair. And there, at Norway House, he had shaken hands with his acquaintance, London Committee member Nicholas Garry, to whom had fallen the task of bringing news of the merger across the Atlantic. This critical task had fallen to Garry for many reasons, including the fact that he was the sole bachelor on the HBC board and was, therefore, more free to travel than a married man of creature-comfort needs. Garry, clearly a skilled orator and business operative, also brought Simpson news of his friends on Great Tower Street, Colvile chief among them, and presented him with a letter of commission that promoted the late-twenty-something Scot from acting or substitute governor (*locum tenens*) to bona fide governor. If there had been any doubt about Simpson's future in the fur trade on his way into Athabasca Country the previous autumn, this vanished with the Committee's letter, which brought with it for Simpson a lifetime of both work and influence.

Garry did a remarkable job running this first joint Council and keeping NWC head man Simon McGillivray Sr. (the father of Simpson's rival, who had come out with Garry by canoe from Montreal) from hijacking the assignation of men to posts and posts to districts. McGillivray had done his best to keep the NWC's assets and agents busy with post-amalgamation trade. If the merger proved anything it was that with trade concentrated in the west it made economic sense to use posts on James Bay and Hudson Bay as entrepôts, rather than Montreal, which was just too far from the action. Why tie up money and goods for two seasons in transit back and forth when, through Hudson Bay, one could do the same transactions in one season, with less expenditure of time, energy, money and personnel? Even more remarkable, Garry had been able to finesse the aging former East Indiaman William Williams, on whom the last skirmishes of the fur wars had taken a toll both physically and

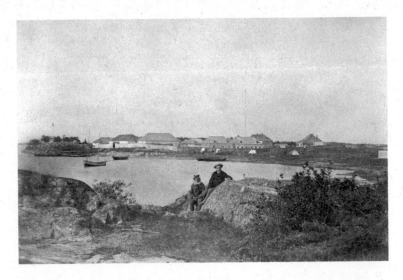

Annual meetings of the Northern Council were often convened at Norway House (seen here in an 1889 photograph), located on Playgreen Lake, just north of Lake Winnipeg, named for Norwegian workers who were brought to North America to build a winter road to transport settlers and supplies from York Factory to Assiniboia. It was here that Simpson usually made his northern headquarters when on his summer rounds.

psychically, into a job with the less consequential (because it was nearly trapped out) and newly created Southern Department, which included posts in the James Bay and St. Lawrence River watersheds. This move left Simpson with the position of northern governor, which meant he would oversee posts, personnel and operations north, south and west of a line between York Factory and the Selkirk settlement. Simpson participated in the Council, but largely as a spectator. Between hours at the table for meetings and meals, he had pored over clauses of the detailed legal agreement, the deed poll that spelled out categorically who would be where in the trade and how the merged company would work.[1] There had been bluster and discontent among the members of this first joint Council meeting, but considering that this was a meeting of men who years, months, days and even hours before had in some cases been ready to kill each other, the Council had been a triumph of Nicholas Garry's level-headed diplomacy.

Simpson was pleased that, on his suggestion, his arch NWC rival from Athabasca, Simon McGillivray Jr., and his most annoying colleague on the HBC side of the trade, John Clarke—both of whom, like Simpson, were lean and fighting fit after their winter in the northwest—were assigned leave "on the score of ill health," a year's time out of the trade for their sins. And Simpson had been especially impressed with Garry's face-to-face handling of young McGillivray's boisterous father, as he watched his son get sidelined for a year and his own plans to retain Montreal as a depot go up in smoke; but Simpson noted also with quiet glee that Garry engineered his upper hand over McGillivray Sr. in two particular minutes of Council:

> 59. That Simon McGillivray Esqre. having from courtesy and for
> the benefit of his advice been requested to be present at the Council
> of which the foregoing are the minutes, it is resolved that this instance
> of informality shall not be considered a precedent . . .
> 71. That a Letter addressed to Nicholas Garry Esqre. [containing
> a litany of McGillivray's discontents] has been read by the former
> Gentleman to the Council intimating Mr. McGillivray's dissent from
> certain resolutions passed and entered in their minutes, but (as they
> conceive it to be informal to receive any such communications) it is
> resolved that the Letter shall not be entered on record.[2]

But all that was behind him now. Simpson, with Miles, Taylor, Betsy Sinclair and a crew of hardy canoemen, renegotiated the thirty portages and was back in his express canoe for an uninterrupted float down the lower Hayes River to York Factory. The August breeze would have been warm on the travellers' weathered faces and, even though the days were getting shorter as they moved closer to the equinox, Simpson would have experienced a soothing wash of the familiar in the sounds of waterbirds or in the arc of the sun through the blue northern sky over the

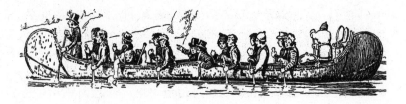

Artist C.W. Jeffreys's rendering of Sir George Simpson on the way to Fort William in a light express canoe. Although Simpson occasionally travelled in a canot du maître, *his personal canoe, the* Rob Roy, *and others he commonly used were smaller* canots du nord *paddled by seven or eight as opposed to fourteen* engagés, *as shown here. The Governor's beaver top hat, however, is exactly right.*

phosphorescent taiga greens. Time and time again as a boy he had seen that same solar sweep on similar hues of rock, water and heath halfway around the world, at Dingwall on the Cromarty Firth, latitude fifty-seven degrees north, the parallel he was crossing now. The fifteen-hour days and short summer nights filled with stars and the northern lights were just like those in the place he might have called home had they been kinder on his leaving. Here he was, on his way, while hand-picked *canadien* canoemen at his disposal rhythmically urged the boat forward. So much had transpired since breakup—a new position, a new address, new responsibilities, new friends, new enemies, new business opportunities. And waiting for him at river's end were the multifarious details to ensure passage of this year's outfit of trade supplies into the country and the previous winter's furs to market. But for now, he could ignore the challenges to come. Think terns and swallows wheeling overhead. Think for a moment of station. George Simpson, Northern Governor. The title had a pleasing ring.

Approaching York Factory, the Hayes River would have been alive with loaded boats propelled by stout Orcadians bent to the oars, hauling the year's supplies and trade goods up to Rock Depot and beyond. At Ten Shilling Creek, ten miles upstream from York Factory, they would have smelled the heady essence of freshly cut spruce, heard the ring of double-bitted axes or the rhythmic coughing of crosscut saws at places where firewood crews cut trees of decent size before the land around the factory gave way to a circle of barren scrub-tundra, whose stunted conifers had for over a century fuelled fur traders' fires. Finally, perhaps with cannon fire or the sound of a bell to herald the arrival of special visitors, Simpson would have landed at a wharf on the west shore of the Hayes River, not far from its mouth, and stumbled up the muddy clay bank to meet sundry personnel mustered to meet the new governor.

In his journal, Nicholas Garry (who likely arrived at York Factory with Governor Williams either with or just prior to Simpson) described the venerable installation as he found it that summer:

York Fort is situated on the West Side of the Hayes River on a Point of alluvial Land formed by this River and the Nelson or N[orth] River ... The Fort is built on Piles—but though drained on every side is still sinking. The Buildings are surrounded by Stockades and are of an Octagon Form, which appear to have been so erected to form Bastions but are now converted into dwelling Rooms and Warehouses. It is two Storeys high. The Roof which forms a Sort of Walk or look out is covered with Lead on which there is a Flag Staff, rigged as a Mast. In the Centre of the Building is the Hudson Bay Arms painted by Mr. Cooke. Within the Stockade are several Buildings, a small Garden and the Powder Magazine which is a wooden Erection covered with Lead ... The Fort may be about a hundred yards from the River. On landing there is a Warehouse to the right and one to the left. The former is called the Colony Warehouse. The Banks may be 60 or 70 Feet high and are of so loose and clayey a Nature that they are continually falling in. As a Fortification it is a Place of no Strength. There are twelve small Cannon within the Stockades and four six-pounders before the main Entrance, which were sent out for the Colony [at Red River] because of their Weight and the Shallow Navigation of the Rivers.[3]

What Garry's journal does not adequately convey is the crowd and bustle that Simpson would have encountered at York Factory at this busy time of year. There were the so-called home guard Indians with their sunny-faced children camped around the factory. These were the families that had gravitated from migrational life on the land to year-round residency and dependence on the HBC, drawn to those comforts of trade and convenience that they could acquire by bartering whitefish, partridge, venison and moose meat to feed the residents. And inside were clerks, coopers, blacksmith, boat builders, carpenters and cooks, each with jobs to do, mouths to feed and places to lay their heads.

Also coincident with Simpson's arrival was a continuing influx of European settlers, Scots displaced by the Highland clearances and other nationals drawn to promises of new beginnings in Assiniboia. Most of them seemed to have no idea of, or chose not to dwell on, the detail that from where they would disembark from their squalid transatlantic crossing there were still 385 miles and 30 portages upriver, and that distance again on the open expanses of Lake Winnipeg and on the Red River. But it was better than life at home, or so they'd been told.

That summer with the settlers came a flock of sheep that were to be lifted into boats and shipped up the portages. Until arrangements could be made for shipment to the colony, these unfortunate animals were corralled on an island in the river. But most of them mysteriously drowned, including all the rams, which, to add to the settlers' sorry circumstances, left no male seed to grow the herd. Nicholas Garry watched as Baymen loaded the year's crop of colonists and the remainder of their sheep, and described the unhappy scene:

> The Day was most unpropitious, cold North East Winds, foggy and incessant heavy Rain which must soon have drenched them to the very Skin. They had no Coverings to their Boats and altogether presented a Scene of Misery and a want of Comfort which pained the Heart. Their Situation is truly pitiable. After travelling so many thousand Miles from Switzerland to Dordrecht in Holland, cross the

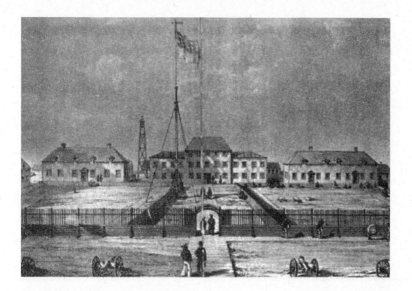

At York Factory, located at the mouth of the Hayes River, Simpson ordered the building of a separate entrance to his quarters so that he might spirit in and out his country consorts from the home guard Cree who camped around the fort.

Atlantic, encountering all the Misery and Danger of Icebergs, arriving at York Fort after a passage of three Months, expecting to find all the Preparations for their Departure ready but having to wait fourteen Days and losing this Time, so precious, when the Season is so short; and then starting to encounter all the Miseries of a Journey of nearly two months exposed to all the Inclemencies of the Weather, Rain, Fogs, Damp, Dews, Cold and intense Frost, with the Aged, the little Children and delicate Females, only a few of the Men appearing to be sufficiently strong to bear such Hardships, and all this on a Route subject to peculiar difficulties.[4]

In its chequered history, York Factory had been passed back and forth between the French and the English a number of times. Through it had passed sufficient peltry to make shareholders rich, but it was a

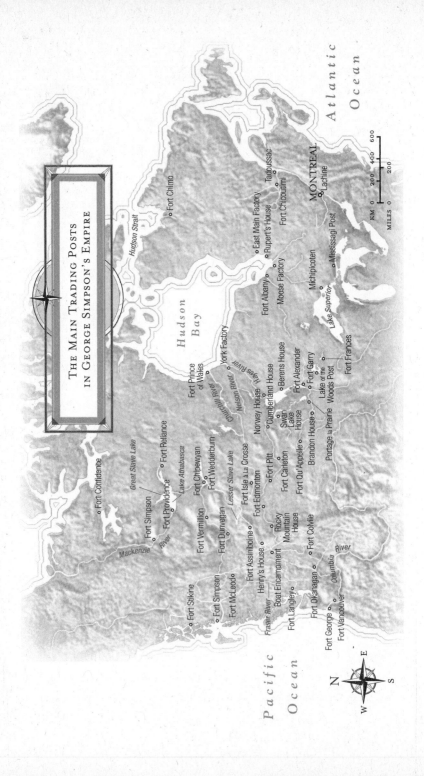

THE MAIN TRADING POSTS
IN GEORGE SIMPSON'S EMPIRE

Atlantic Ocean

Pacific Ocean

Hudson Bay

Hudson Strait

Lake Superior

MONTREAL
Lachine

Fort Chimo

East Main Factory
Rupert's House
Tadoussac
Fort Chicoutimi
Mistissagi Post

Fort Albany
Moose Factory
Michipicoten

York Factory
Fort Prince of Wales

Churchill River
Nelson River
Hayes River

Norway House
Cumberland House
Berens House
Fort Alexander
Fort Garry
Lake of the Woods Post
Fort Frances

Swan Lake House
Brandon House
Portage la Prairie

Fort Pitt
Fort Carleton
Fort Qu'Appelle

Fort Confidence
Great Slave Lake
Fort Reliance
Fort Providence
Lake Athabasca
Fort Chipewyan
Fort Wedderburn
Lesser Slave Lake
Fort Isle à La Crosse

Fort Simpson
Fort Vermillion
Fort Dunvegan
Fort Edmonton

Mackenzie River

Rocky Mountain House
Fort Assiniboine
Henry's House
Fort Colvile

Fort Stikine
Fort Simpson
Fort McLeod

Fraser River
Boat Encampment
Fort Langley
Fort Okanagan

Columbia River

Fort George
Fort Vancouver

Pacific Ocean

KM 0   200   400   600
MILES 0   200   400

N
W   E
S

contested structure in a difficult geographic location. It had been burned down at different times. Bits of it had been torn down, and other parts had collapsed. Some elements had been blown away by winds howling across the subarctic tidal flats. And all this destruction occurred as the buildings slowly sank on their wooden piles into the active layer of semi-continuous permafrost.

Evidence of these processes was always present at York Factory, giving it at the best of times a perennially tired lived-in feel. It was hot, moist and buggy for a few weeks in the summer, when the river would open and the ships would come. The rest of the year the place was drafty and dark, with scurvy and cabin fever never far from the door, the inside warmed only by sparse candles, fires of green wood—or coal if the residents were lucky—and the labours of its unlucky residents, the preponderance of whom were Orcadian. It may have been difficult to comprehend, but they were often better off here than they might have been at home.

Into this cloister of hardy officers and Baymen, misfits and miscreants, George Simpson strode in his beaver hat and his dirty, if well-tailored, Savile Row cape as if into the finest counting house on Great Tower Street. He was a man of style who carried his five-foot six-inch frame with surprising gravitas. He set to work interviewing employees and examining the journals and ledgers to assess the big picture of HBC and NWC operations across North America, gathering information from anyone and everyone in the vicinity of the fort, from the boatmen and the blacksmith's helpers, clerks and craftsmen, staffers and store keepers, right up to London governor Nicholas Garry, who awaited departure on a London-bound ship, and Simpson's now fellow governor and corporate equal William Williams, before the latter shipped off to Cumberland House for the winter to prepare for a subsequent move to Moose Factory.[5]

These deliberations would have drawn Simpson's attention to the full extent of his new domain and its 137 factories, forts and fur installations from York Factory south to the top of the Mississippi basin, west to the Pacific and north to Great Slave Lake and beyond. Amalgamation meant that many of these nodes in the Northern Department had multiple installations, such as the Nor'Westers' Fort Chipewyan on the north shore of Lake Athabasca and the HBC's Fort Wedderburn on an island just offshore. But before Simpson could begin the business of eliminating redundancies, he had first to get straight in his head what and who was where in his sprawling territory.

Not including minor posts like Rock Depot on the Hayes or Wedderburn's satellite stations on Lake Athabasca, upriver from York Factory was Norway House at the north end of Lake Winnipeg. West of that, in the Saskatchewan River system, was the HBC's first inland post, Cumberland House. Northwest from Cumberland, moving into the English (now Churchill) River and beyond was Fort Isle à La Crosse, where John Clarke had brooded during Simpson's winter at Fort Wedderburn; and north to Fort Chipewyan, beyond the Slave River, were Fort Resolution, Fort Reliance and Fort Providence on Great Slave Lake. West toward the Rockies from Lake Athabasca, up the Peace River, were Fort St. Mary, Fort Vermillion, Fort Dunvegan and Fort McLeod, and then, south through the snow-topped mountains, Fort George.

The other and more forgiving route through the Rockies, moving east and north from Fort Vancouver, led to Fort Okanagan and Fort Colvile, then Boat Encampment on the north-south switchback of the Columbia River, where traders on horseback would move over the height of land toward Rocky Mountain House and the watershed of the North Saskatchewan River. Downstream from Rocky Mountain House were Fort Edmonton, Fort Pitt and Fort Carleton, and far fewer posts on the south branch of the Saskatchewan than Simpson would have liked, linking up with Cumberland and back to the main river highway to the mouth of the Hayes River.

The original HBC charter also included the Assiniboine watershed and its posts, Fort Qu'Appelle and Fort Pelly in the upper reaches, as well as Brandon House and Portage la Prairie on the route down to Fort Garry and Fort Douglas, which were located at the junction of the Red and Assiniboine rivers in the heart of Assiniboia. North of that

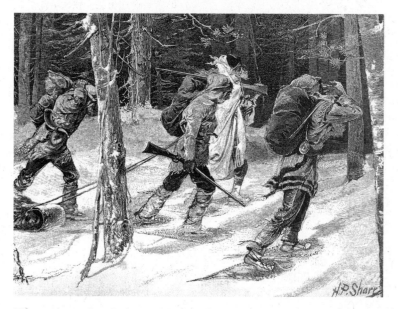

For nearly two hundred years HBC traders sat on the shores of Hudson Bay and waited for the furs to come to them, but with strong competition from the NWC as it moved west, the HBC was forced to move inland as well.

(although more often connected with the Southern Department of the HBC because it was on the main route west from Fort William, Fort Frances and Lake of the Woods Post) was Fort Alexander, sometimes called Fort Bas de la Rivière, at the outflow of the Winnipeg River on the eastern shore of Lake Winnipeg. Anyone heading north from the Selkirk settlement would always stop at Fort Alexander, and also at Berens House, at the mouth of the Berens River about halfway up Lake Winnipeg, before refreshing at Norway House and going on to York Factory.

In truth—and Simpson must have been well aware of this from the moment he entered the trade in Athabasca—the most potentially profitable parts of the Northern Department were actually outside the lands included in the original charter. The famously gruelling twelve-mile La Loche, or Methye, Portage in what is now the province of Saskatchewan marked the height of land between the Hudson Bay and

Arctic watersheds. Likewise, as soon as traders crossed out of the Peace River valley beyond Fort McLeod or out of the Saskatchewan River watershed beyond Rocky Mountain House, their activity was out of chartered territory. But by 1820 the beaver had been all but trapped out in large portions of Rupert's Land. Markets for other furs were developing, but to keep the core business in beaver hides robust, there was no other option than to move west and north into new terrain.

Equally aware of this situation were the London negotiators of the amalgamation deal, including former North West Company agent Edward Ellice, who was now an influential member of Parliament. Ellice supported the new company's business interests in the fur-rich lands outside the fur-depleted Rupert's Land watersheds, especially in the Pacific northwest and Columbia, where the Russians, Americans and Spanish were actively competing for footholds in the burgeoning Pacific-coast economy. The government, for its part, knew well the negative effects that fur traders' warring had on settlement. So Westminster actively encouraged the amalgamation deal and, in July 1821, to remove doubts about powers of the Canada Jurisdiction Act—a cause, or at least an exacerbating factor, in the fight in the first place—passed the Act for Regulating the Fur Trade and Establishing a Criminal and Civil Jurisdiction within Certain Parts of North America. Further, with Edward Ellice as chief cheerleader for the legislation in the House of Commons, it drafted a royal proclamation to give the new HBC exclusive right to the Indian trade in any part of British North America, except the two provinces of Canada and Rupert's Land. It would take until December 5, 1821, for the new king, George IV, to sign the proclamation into law but, for all intents and purposes, when Simpson became governor of the HBC's Northern Department in 1821, he assumed control over a vast territory that included the western half of Rupert's Land as well as Athabasca, Peace River, Mackenzie River, the Rockies and New Caledonia, Columbia and the Pacific-coast region (as modern-day British Columbia was known)—a domain larger than the Holy Roman Empire at its peak.[6]

With York Factory swollen with itinerant summer personnel, it is not clear where Simpson might have stayed when he moved temporarily into the fort, but we do know that he settled right in and, with only a rough table to sort his papers and another small writing desk and chair where Miles could take dictation, engaged in the correspondence of his new position with enthusiasm, enacting the wishes of the London Committee, interpreting the imperatives of the deed poll and making good the newly passed resolutions of the Northern Council.

Simpson's perfunctory do-this, get-that letters to officers of the trade are evidence of an encyclopedic mind for facts, figures and the minutiae of the trade and of a superb, possibly photographic, memory. Without question, they indicate that Simpson was a very quick study of detailed and complex business matters. Nicholas Garry was among those, for example, who complimented Simpson after he had been the only person present at the Northern Council at Norway House who was able to decipher clauses of the deed poll having to do with annual leave.

Simpson's more personal letters and occasionally "private" letters, of which there are a few in the public record, are much more revealing of the man behind the matter-of-fact business operative. He wrote often to his Nor'Wester friend from the *James Monroe*, now colleague in arms following the amalgamation of the two companies. John George McTavish, because of his senior position in the NWC, had been assigned the chief factorship of York Factory. While the two of them were there in the fall of 1821, their acquaintance developed into lifelong companionship and correspondence.

Illustrative of Simpson's early personal correspondence from York Factory is a long letter to his friend and mentor Andrew Colvile, dated September 8, 1821:

Dear Sir/
    ... Your much esteemed Letter of the 25th Feb[ruar]y gave me
the first indication of the recent happy arrangement and that of
the 28th March was handed to me from Fort William with various

other documents by Mr. Garry amongst which was my commission as one of the Governors; this mark of your good opinion and kind patronage has laid me under a thousand weighty obligations to you, I feel much flattered and honoured by it and shall ever entertain a grateful sense of the interest you have been pleased to take in me and I fondly trust you will find that I am not unworthy of the confidence thus reposed.—To you I feel that I am solely indebted for my advancement in Life and it will ever be my study to show that your good offices have not been misapplied.

From the Rock Depot where I went on my return from the interior for the purpose of arranging the Athabasca affairs I proceeded to Norway House in order to meet Mr. Garry and hold myself at his disposal, from this Gentleman I learnt all particulars relative to the coalition and arrangement with the N.W. [Company] which seems to give universal satisfaction to both parties and must under good management turn out a very profitable and important concern; the regulations are most salutory and the whole business seems founded on a solid basis which cannot fail of ensuring its prosperity . . . Mr. Garry's handsome and impartial conduct operated like Majick in removing all sort of jealousy he was open and easy of access with the nicest observance of strict honor, integrity and impartiality and so different in all these respects from his Travelling companion Mr. Simon McGillivray as to excite a general personal regard and respect for the one while the other was despised and this failing was prevalent among our fresh allies as our own party . . . Had McGillivray joined us alone armed with the commission which the committee so handsomely gave him he would have made a very improper use thereof and to gain his own selfish ends sacrificed the interests of the company but his intentions and plans had in an early stage of the business manifested themselves, and depending too much on his cunning and address, he overreached himself and put Mr. Garry completely on his guard, who foiled him at all points.[7]

Beyond its distinctive account of the first joint Council meeting and of the ways in which the old Nor'Wester distinguished himself, Simpson's letter to Colvile also reveals that he had taken advantage of his situation at York Factory to learn a great deal about the comings and goings in the Red River colony. The colony, of course, was a major bone of contention for almost anyone involved in the fur trade, including Simpson, who had learned the role that this move by the HBC had played in enraging the Nor'Westers. But Simpson, perhaps because of his connection to Lord Selkirk (who had just died), seemed to be aware that although this initiative did not advance the trade as such, it was an important indication that the HBC was taking seriously its responsibilities as laid out in its original royal charter—responsibilities that included settlement. In his short time at York Factory, he had also learned that the settlement had become a bit of a social cesspool, with a reprobate of a manager in charge. He described what he found to Colvile:

Red River at present I am sorry to say assumes more the appearance of a receptacle for free booters and infamous characters of all descriptions than a well regulated Colony, there is no law order or regularity, every man is his own Master and the strongest and most desperate is he who succeeds best.—Mr. West [John West, the clergyman at Red River] does all in his power to improve the morals of the people but with little success, on the contrary their habits are most vicious: they have not exactly committed Murder or Robbery but the next thing to it and frequently threatened both so that the well disposed feel themselves in continual danger. The population is now getting very considerable and such a mass of renegades and malcontents of disruptions are not to be constrained without the assistance of civil & military power; I therefore conceive it indispensibly necessary for its future welfare that a Code of Laws should be made, Magistrates appointed, constables sworn in and a small Military Establishment proved to give effect to the Civil Authorities,

and without something of this Kind in my humble opinion the
Settlement cannot flourish . . .

Mr. [Miles] MacDonnell I am concerned to say is extremely
despised and held in contempt by every person connected with the
place, he is accused of partiality, dishonesty, untruth, drunkenness, in
short a total dereliction of every moral and honorable feeling; without
certain grounds I would not bring such heavy charges against any
man altho' I have little doubt that there is a great deal of truth in what
is said of him . . . He carries on a very disgraceful Traffick in horses
&c, this is a trade which I am sure you would not countenance, of his
situation he must discontinue . . . He has contrived to get three near
Relations into the confidential situations about the establishment, they
are all men of bad character and dissipated habits and are supposed
to play into each other's hands; for instance Mr. Alley his Brother in
Law is Surveyor and Storekeeper, a Worthless Drunken blackguard,
McDonald his cousin, Storekeeper and Secty, of similar habits, and
Fletcher, another Brother in Law, Storekeeper &c, &c; these men
with the Governor are all "hale Fellows well met," Drink and carouse
together and I suspect bring things to very bad account.[8]

Continuing with news of the errant ways of the Red River colony and
its miscreant governor, Simpson moved on in the letter to what would
become his mantra, if not his second-favourite topic: "oeconomy," meaning efficiency and money-saving in all things with shareholder profit as
principal end. He pointed out to Andrew Colvile that the heavy guns and
the iron grist mill lying on the bluff at York Factory could not be moved
because there were no boats available that could carry cargo of such size
and weight. That was unfortunate. But what seemed to gall him the most
was that the settlement had purchased boats for £70 per craft that could
carry thirty-five 90-pound parcels, or "pieces," and could be navigated
by five men, while in his short time in North America he had learned
that the HBC's boats, which were built at Swan River post and in the
Red River settlement, cost only £30 to make and carried nearly twice as

much cargo with only six more men at the oars. This led Simpson to his main point: that in his opinion Miles Macdonell had to go, preferably to be replaced by a "man of superior judgment possessing a knowledge of the World and conciliatory manners in the prime of Life and full of energy and activity, and if a *married man* so much the better."[9]

The letter concludes with Simpson's own spin on the John Clarke story. He apparently convinced Clarke that on the basis of his despicable behaviour the previous winter he was going to be summarily dismissed from the trade. Unfortunately for Simpson, the deed poll had assigned Clarke a promotion from chief trader to chief factor and placed him in charge of Fort Garry; it was unlikely or perhaps impossible for Simpson, as new northern CEO, to fire Clarke, but the official appointment to Lower Red River would be delayed by a year, ostensibly for disciplinary reasons. However, as he explained the situation to Colvile in his letter of general appreciation, in which Clarke's punitive "sick leave" is trans-formed with the stroke of a quill pen into "visiting friends in Montreal," Clarke was greatly relieved to remain in the service of the HBC, to be promised a post after serving his time on "sick leave" during a winter in Montreal. In what is another example of his "smoothing" of recalcitrant underlings, Simpson clearly communicated his point to Clarke about who was boss and what was acceptable behaviour, but he also managed to issue what would have been for a senior hand in the trade like John Clarke a stern rebuke—yet one for which the offender was, in the end, grateful. Wrote Simpson to Colvile:

> Clarke did not come up to my expectations, on the contrary I found him not only extravagant but a more formidable opponent last season than the N.W. Co[mpan]y his conduct was in many respects most shameful as my Journal & report will fully explain and he expected to be dismissed from the service this season, indeed if the coalition had not taken place I intended to have taken the Isle à la Crosse [Clarke's post] and Athabasca Departments this Winter and made my arrange-ments accordingly.—He is highly satisfied with his appointment; ...

McGillivray attempted to bring him over to his party but he behaved well in communicating the circumstances to Mr. Garry who will give you all the particulars.—He has got leave of absence this winter to visit his friends in Montreal.[10]

Simpson's early correspondence as northern governor clearly shows his curiosity for all aspects of the trade and his remarkable drive to analyze the many strands and currents of supplies inward and furs outward that would allow him to engineer the corporation back to a position of profitability within the year. The goal of "oeconomy," which was that of the London Committee as well, would see dozens of smaller posts closed and the firm's workforce cut by 50 per cent.

This particular letter also shows Simpson's acute perception of his personal debt to Andrew Colvile and his almost servile gratitude toward his patron and mentor in London, who, in the fullness of time, would advance to chair of the London Committee on the back of the on-the-ground work Simpson conducted at his behest in North America. Although Simpson tended to be a harsh disciplinarian with his underlings in the trade, the lingering question for later historians was the extent to which the Rupert's Land martinet was more of a marionette for influential men in London, notably the well-born and well-placed Andrew Colvile.

—

CHAPTER VII

MANAGEMENT BY
WALKING AROUND

While another governor might have been content to settle into quarters at York Factory as mosquitoes and dampness gave way to dry cold and snow fleas in the fall of 1821, Simpson understood almost immediately that to manage the fur trade he should see for himself what was happening in his domain. He knew as well as anyone that what was contained in cursive stylings on pieces of paper sent to inform or impress could easily be different from what an observer might find on the ground. Lofty precepts of business notwithstanding, at its core the fur trade was a human undertaking: to understand the trade, one had to get the measure of its people. Reading their journals and ledgers was one road to understanding, but one had to meet the personnel of the trade on their ground, see them in action (or inaction), experience their habits and predilections. Ledger books and post journals, Simpson knew in his bones, could cover as many sins as they could reveal. And so much the better if he could drop by when people least expected a visit.

The nominal destination for what would be called his Inner Circle Tour was the Selkirk settlement at Red River, as he had identified this as one of the most serious impediments to the smooth operation of the fur trade. To get there, he would travel by snowshoe from York Factory upriver to Rock Depot, Oxford House and Norway House, across the top of Lake Winnipeg, and past Grand Rapids west to Cumberland House, where he would stay for a couple of weeks before moving south to Brandon House and Red River in time for spring. In June, he would set forth again, this time by canoe, paddling north via Fort Alexander and Norway House to be at York Factory in July, ready to convene the second meeting of the new Northern Council, his first as chair.

Simpson left York Factory in early December of 1821, about the time the royal proclamation that officially expanded his department to the Arctic and Pacific oceans came into effect. Wishing him adieu at the gate would have been his friend J.G. McTavish and McTavish's half-Scottish, half-Chipewyan country wife of many years, Nancy McKenzie, with several of their little daughters. Also there to say goodbye would have been Simpson's "washerwoman," Betsy Sinclair, who under her hide leggings, calico dress and blanket coat was roundly pregnant with Simpson's first child of the trade.

The journey was conducted with or in the manner of winter packeteers—the men who carried mail from post to post in the winter, travelling fast on snowshoes with their tent and supplies on a light wooden toboggan hauled by a long leather tump strap pulled across the chest or over one shoulder. Obviously comfortable in new hand-sewn leather moccasins and big Cree snowshoes with lampwick bindings, and more or less oblivious to cold and the staggering physical exertion of winter travel, Simpson and his Indian guide made Oxford House in near record time. At Norway House, however, the Governor's lightning progress was stopped so he could recover from a nasty burn on his neck caused by an eager post employee who applied *aqua fortis* (nitric acid) instead of hartshorn (an aqueous ammonia solution used like smelling salts) to remedy quinsy (a sore throat).

Sore throat or not, Simpson still managed to have a good look around the fort, which was now being run by the flamboyant Colin Robertson

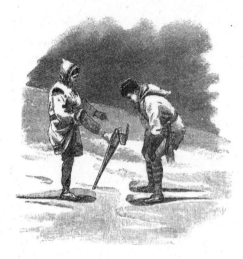

Even though snowshoeing was new to him, with instruction from his Aboriginal guides, Simpson took naturally to this mode of travel. As he had done in a canoe, he turned heads with his reputation for speed, distance and endurance.

who, after his arrest and subsequent return to England, had been delivered from personal bankruptcy by Andrew Colvile (who lent him the money needed to avoid debtor's prison) and by a deed-poll promotion to chief factor in the amalgamated company. Simpson never directly blamed the medicinal mix-up on Robertson, but this visit to Norway House did give him ample opportunity to see that the man who had been such an effective soldier of fortune in the fur trade war was a much less impressive post manager, information he tucked away for his own later use—and Robertson's future public humiliation.

After spending Hogmanay 1822 at Norway House, Simpson made his way around the frozen top of Lake Winnipeg to Cumberland House, where he and the Committee-castigated William Williams would again have spent time comparing notes. Among the correspondence Simpson wrote at Cumberland House was a letter back to his friend McTavish at York Factory regarding Betsy Sinclair, which, had he not referred to her in derogatory terms, might have contained a glimmer of earthly compassion. He told McTavish that he had made arrangements for Betsy to move to Rock Depot, where she would be with some of her relatives and where Chief Trader Thomas Bunn would look after her. He continued: "If my Article requires anything previous to her departure for the Rock pray let her be supplied (to my account) and if you will solace her with a little tea and sugar or any other necessary it will be obliging."[1] Two weeks later, on February 10, 1822, the York Factory journal recorded that "Mrs. Simpson was delivered of a daughter," whom she would name Maria—her first child of that name, Simpson's second.

Moving south from Cumberland House, with the strengthening sun in their faces, Simpson and his guide snowshoed through the snow-dusted evergreens of the Pasquia and Porcupine hills before stopping again, this time at Fort Hibernia, on the Swan River just west of Lake Winnipegosis. Here, in addition to thoroughly examining the workings of the post, Simpson noticed a handsome young man of Scottish-Cree extraction who impressed him mightily with his knowledge of history and of the country.

Others who met twenty-five-year-old Cuthbert Grant might have been cowed by his reputation as the notorious Métis leader of the renegades who had murdered Governor Robert Semple and twenty of Semple's Red River settlement men at Seven Oaks only five years before. But Simpson met Grant "as if a stranger to his character" and very quickly determined that, with his fine qualities as a leader and his intimate connections to the convoluted politics of Assiniboia, he might be a useful ally were the HBC to re-engage him. To the London Committee, and before inviting Grant to join him on his journey to Red River, Simpson wrote, "I am therefore of the opinion that it might be policy to overlook the past and if you did not object to it [he] might be smuggled quietly into the Service again."[2]

With Grant, Simpson made it to Red River and was even more unimpressed than he had thought he would be. In a private letter to McTavish, after only a few days in residence at the settlement, he wrote: "I am sick and tired of this place where all the blacklegs of Rupert's Land seem to be congregated." But he knew that he was into a good strategic alliance with Cuthbert Grant, and he told McTavish about arrangements he had made to help Grant, who had been acquitted of murder for his part in the deaths at Seven Oaks, find his way back into the trade.

Also in the letter to McTavish is ribald talk of Aboriginal women, this time of two unsuspecting "washerwomen" he was sending to York Factory for his future amusement: "Let them be kept inside the Stockades and distant from the young bucks otherways we shall have more ——ing than washing." And, as if thinking along these lines dragged him back to the realities of previous liaisons, he added, "If my Damsel is not gone pray send her to the Rock at once as I do not wish to be troubled with a Lady during the busy Season. I suspect my name will become as notorious as the late Govr. [William Williams] in regard to plurality of Wives."[3]

What might have prompted Simpson to comment at this time on his "plurality of wives," besides the oblique reference to Betsy Sinclair and the women he was sending to York Factory, was a liaison that was to produce a son—his first in the Old World or the New: James "Jordie" Keith Simpson, who was born in 1823 and who a number of scholars argue may have been conceived (by a wife or relative of Chief Factor James Keith) at Red River settlement sometime in 1822. Simpson's only time spent at Red River settlement during 1821 was on his Inner Circle Tour, which put him there from March to June in the spring of 1821, and he was not back at Red River until the September of the following year, when he went to spend the winter there, which would likely have been too late to sire a child born in 1823. Perhaps the most apt statement about Simpson in this regard is from novelist Fred Stenson, who in *The Trade* (2000) observed that, with Simpson's generous libido, "by God, if the Governor could find nothing else, he would stick his thing in a nest of bees. But given who he was, he stuck it where he pleased. For Halfbreed men the Governor had nothing but malice, wouldn't tolerate one above the office of clerk, but Halfbreed women? That was different. He was always on about their beauty."[4]

With a head full of facts learned and impressions gleaned on the Inner Circle Tour, and with a spring in his step and a gleam in his eye, Simpson was back in York Factory on July 2, 1822, to convene his first and most fabled meeting of the Northern Council. In a lively memoir written sixty years after the fact, HBC employee John Tod described the event:

At length the bell summoned us to dinner when forthwith in walked
the heterogeneous mass of human beings, but in perfect silence &
with the most solemn gravity . . . The Nor-Westers in one compact
body kept together & evidently had no inclination at first to mix
up with their old rivals in the trade. But that crafty fox Sir George
Simpson coming hastily to the rescue with his usual tact & dexter-
ity on such occasions succeeded, though partially, somewhat in
dispelling that reserve in which both parties had hitherto continued
to envelop themselves; it was to say the least of it a critical moment
requiring reconciliation & union of two irritable & powerful bodies
of men thus suddenly brought face to face after many long years of
strife, violence & fierce contention, & although now united in interest
were yet evidently adverse in feeling . . . It soon became evident that
[Simpson's] stratagems in bows and smiles alone would eventually
succeed in producing the desired effect on the exterior appearance of
his haughty guests. Their previously stiffened features began to relax
a little, they gradually but slowly mingled together, & a few of the
better disposed throwing themselves unreservedly in the midst of the
opposite party mutually shook each other by the hand. Then, & not
till then were they politely beckoned to their appointed places at the
mess-table . . . [There were] one or two awkward mistakes which it
had evidently been the Governor's intention from the first to prevent
by every possible means; for instance he whom they called blind
McDonnel [John MacDonald] all of a sudden found himself directly
in front of his mortal foe of Swan River the vivacious Chief Factor
[Alexander] Kennedy . . . [Kennedy] & he who now sat opposite to
him had hacked and slashed at each other with naked swords only a
few months before their present unintentional meeting. One of them
still bore the marks of a cut on his face, the other it was said on some
less conspicuous part of his body . . . I thought it fortunate that they
were without arms . . . It seemed not improbable they might yet renew
the combat, which probably was only prevented in time by a side

movement from the upper end of the table, where sat that plausible and most accomplished gentleman Simon McGilliavery [*sic*] who used to talk of the "glorious uncertainty of the law" & the "nullity of the H.B.C. Charter"; . . . Immediately on the right of McGilliavary sat that flexible character McIntosh [William MacIntosh]; his ever shifting countenance & restless black eye might seem that nature had designed him the harbinger of plots, treasons & stratagems. I allude to the same who, some years before, in Peace River tried to poison poor little Yale, but could not succeed, so invulnerable had the integuments of the latter's stomach become by long acquaintance with the rough fare of the inhospitable stepmother New Caledonia, that the diabolical attempt failed. Directly in front of McIntosh sat his gallant enemy of the preceding winter, the pompous but good natured John Clarke . . . During the rivalship of the two companies Clarke & McIntosh, now confronting each other at the same table, were for many years close neighbours & in fact, always considered as forming part of the advance guard of the two opposing bodies which had kept the country in a state of civil war so long, consequently they had unavoidably come often in collision together & it was only some time during the winter immediately preceding the period now referred to & at the close of a long day's march together on snow-shoes that they agreed to end a dispute which had arisen between them on the way by a round of pistol shots, which they actually & deliberately discharged at each other over the bright blaze of a winter night's camp fire, separated merely by the burning element; Clarke, it was said, cheering on his antagonist all the while to continue the combat until either one or both should fall. But these were the rugging & the riving times when might was right & a man's life was valued at naught.[5]

Sadly, close examination of Tod's colourful account reveals troubling inaccuracies. To begin with, Tod was a junior clerk in 1822 and very likely not at the formal dinner table with the senior officers. Next, while Bayman Alexander Kennnedy and Nor'Wester John "One-Eye" MacDonald did spar at Swan River at the height of the fur trade war, if their glaring match at the dinner table in 1822 did happen, it could not have been broken up by Simon McGillivray because no McGillivray—Junior or Senior—was present at the meeting. Further, while John Clarke and Nor'Wester William MacIntosh certainly did have their moments in the Athabasca campaign, according to the minutes of the 1821 and 1822 Northern Council meetings Clarke was present but MacIntosh was not. And readers of this account should also keep in mind that six of the eleven chief factors present at the Northern Department Council in 1822 had been at the meeting the previous year, the first after amalgamation, and would either have worked out their frustrations then or had time for their angst regarding the enemy to dissipate. But those quibbles notwithstanding, the spirit of Simpson's "smoothing" of the gathering is entirely consistent with his nature, and this account by John Tod, written though it was in the 1880s, documents as much the emergence of George Simpson the myth as the behaviour of George Simpson the man.

Even in the opening paragraph of the minutes of this first meeting, Simpson's firm hand on the tiller is evident. With Nicholas Garry at the helm the previous year, the minutes had begun perfunctorily with what, where, when and who (Norway House, Rupert's Land, August 11–13, 1821, Nicholas Garry, etc.). But with Simpson in charge, specificity and purpose were added to the opening paragraph, as if to ensure brevity and confirm direction in the deliberations: "Minutes of a Council held at York Factory, Northern Department of Rupert's Land this 8th day of July, 1822 for the purpose of establishing such rules and regulations as may be considered expedient for conducting the business of the said Department and in order to investigate the result of the Trade of last year and determine the Outfits and general arrangements of the Trade of the Current year conformable to the provision of a deed poll under seal of The Governor and Company of Adventurers of England trading into Hudson's Bay, bearing the date the 26th day of March 1821, at which the following members were present, vizt. . . ."

One-third of the 115 resolutions made that day had to do with personnel matters—who was going on leave as dictated by the deed poll, and who would be appointed to what district. Having completed his "time out" for bad behaviour in Montreal, for example, Chief Factor John Clarke was back in the game and appointed to Lower Red River District. Colin Robertson, having spent his first season back in the trade at Norway House with a less-than-stellar managerial performance that Simpson had witnessed first hand, was appointed in absentia (because he had not deigned to get himself to York Factory for the Council) to the North Branch of the Saskatchewan District. But several resolutions later, having already dispatched a hunting party to examine the trade potential of the South Branch of the Saskatchewan because he thought that might be a better place for the company to be, Simpson engineered a move that forced an ominous make-or-break scenario for Robertson—resolution 55: "That George Simpson Esquire Governor, be impowered to cause the Establishments of the North Branch of the Saskatchewan District to be abandoned next Spring, in the event of his receiving information . . . which may render it expedient to do so."[6] Robertson would need to move again.

Other resolutions shaped the day-to-day economies of the trade. To make sure John Clarke's hoarding exercise at Isle à La Crosse was not repeated, resolution 42 stipulated that the Athabasca District be supplied with 30 bags of pemmican at Isle à La Crosse, furnished by the English River District. To ensure the separation of the needs of the Red River settlement and the needs of the trade—always a contentious issue—Simpson sent three boats and eighteen men to Lower Red River with 180 pieces of goods, 35 of which were to be used for trade, the rest to be used to stock a retail shop for the settlers. Clarke was instructed in another resolution to keep the accounts of the colony shop and the trading store separate at all costs, and to sell goods to the settlers at not lower than a 58 per cent markup over the York Factory prices.

Also passed by a two-thirds majority of members present were myriad resolutions to increase efficiency, reduce waste and increase profits. With

John Clarke's faux pas of unloading his canoe the previous year in order to accommodate his country wife in mind, it was resolved that no chief trader, chief factor or clerk would be permitted to travel in a light boat or canoe; they must proceed instead with full cargo, at least ten pieces of baggage, which is "not to be transferred to other craft, exchanged for other lading, or left along the route." Annual salaries for inland servants and boatmen were adjusted downward, and their allowances of spirits discontinued. Officers were to get three years' use out of one tent or, unless a tent was "lost by accident in the dangers of the navigation," they would have to purchase a new one from stores as penance for not looking after the first one. In a measure that was as much for austerity as it was to break the cycle of alcohol dependency that had crippled the trade during the height of the war in Athabasca, officers in charge of all posts in the district were directed "to give Indians no more than one half the quantity of Spirits they have been accustomed to receive in the way of presents, and that no furs be traded for that article."[7]

Most instructive of the change to the way business was going to be done in the Northern Department with George Simpson in charge were two items among the last resolutions to be voted into the record. Resolution 110 stipulated, on pain of a £10 penalty (keeping in mind that this was about the annual salary of a Canadian voyageur), that officers in charge of districts would "within 48 hours of their arrival at the Depot deliver into the hands of the General Accountant the District Books, Servants accounts, Journal, Report, List of Engaged and unengaged men, and general account Current."[8] The last resolution contained in the minutes of the 1822 meeting of the Northern Council, number 115, when it was passed with at least a two-thirds majority of members present voting in its favour, quietly but effectively concentrated unilateral control in the new administrator's hands: "That Governor Simpson be fully impowered to decide upon whatever steps he may consider necessary to be adopted for the Interest of the general Concern, both at this place and Inland, from the breaking up of this Council until the meeting of the Council next year."[9]

Almost from the moment that resolution was signed, grumbling began about just how much input the officers had in creating the minutes of their meetings. One of the progressive perks of the deed poll, along with a profit-sharing scheme designed to keep officers of the trade interested in the outcomes of their labours, was participation in governance through the Southern and Northern Department Councils. Some would observe in later years, however, that the minutes seemed to be written before the Councils actually met, causing at least one disgruntled chief factor to call the Council exercise "impotent make-believe."[10]

Simpson was aware that his officers' engagement in the decision-making process was important to them, but he trusted his own judgment most and endeavoured to concentrate in himself as much power as possible as quickly as possible while still maintaining at least the illusion of participation on the part of the chief traders and chief factors. But the real decision-making within the company happened officially through the aegis of the London Committee.

And just as Simpson was realizing that, as the only senior administrator of the corporation on the ground in North America, he could manipulate his underlings in the field, he also realized he could sway the London Committee too, with carefully crafted dispatches from Rupert's Land. Within hours of the adjournment of his first meeting of the Council of Factors, he was dictating detailed letters to the home office, responding to their concerns expressed in dispatches that arrived with the boats of the season and providing his account of affairs in the Northern Department.

Simpson's observations at Wedderburn the previous winter and his first-hand learnings from his time at York Factory and from his Inner Circle Tour had shown him just how slipshod the record keeping at most HBC installations was. There were far more women and children attached to men of the trade than anyone had ever imagined, and there had been unwritten rules about quiet care for these unofficial partners in the trade. With Simpson's concurrence, the London Committee made arrangements to start charging individual employees for the food and clothing consumed by their dependents. And while the chief factors at Council had passed a resolution about stepped-up expectations for record keeping, it is safe to say most of them had no idea with what level of detail the new governor was considering the matter. In a lengthy letter to the Committee dated September 1, 1822, Simpson detailed nineteen types of documents that he thought should be "the objects of primary attention and of the most consequence" for arranging the general accounts of the Northern Department:

1st A Ledger, for the European Servant to be balanced every year after the District accounts are made out up to 1st of June with Interest upon all Balances exceeding £10. A correct Balance Sheet from which ought to be sent home shewing the Book Debt, Bills & Wages, whatever extra may come to the Cr. of a/ct. [Credit of accounts] such as Hunts &c. the preceding Winter's residence, remarks on Deaths &c. &c. & the Balance Dr. or Cr. in Sterling Money.

2nd A [ledger] for Canadian Servant to be Balanced in the same manner and Balance sheet sent home made up on the same principle, in Livres, Quebec Currency; but if thought advisable it would make but little difference to keep their accounts in Sterling Money.

3rd A [ledger] for Free Hunters throughout the Country shewing their Book Debts, hunts and Balances up to 1st June—a Balance Sheet from which ought to go home also.

4th An Inventory Book shewing the Stock on hand 1st June in every District throughout the Country, a copy of which ought annually to go home.

5th A Transfer Book shewing the particulars of all property &c. transferred from one District to another. Accounts one Outfit versus another, Copy of which ought to go home.

6th An Acct. Currt. of Districts Book; Copy of which ought to go home.

7th The Invoice of Outfits Book: Copy of which ought to go home.

8th The Abstract of Packages for Outfit Book and Abstracts of returns of Districts, shewing the number of men employed, Craft &c. ingoing with their number of Packs &c. outcoming.

9th Tariff Book of Importations from England annually.

10th General Account Book of Northern Deptmt. on the present plan.

11th Invoice Book of Importations from England.

12th [Invoice Book] of Shipments to England.

13th Bill of Lading Book of Craft leaving York for different Districts.

14th A Petty Ledger for Officers' Shop.

15th Regular and District Books for each District of Men's Advances in Gen[era]l Shop at York Factory.[11]

16th Bill Book.

17th Scheme Book for Outfits, shewing from the Districts' Indents the Goods necessary to form a general Outfit, and from which the home Order is made out.

18th Order Book shewing the annual Indents sent home.

19th Minutes of Council Book, Copies of which to be sent home annually.[12]

That there was not a more regular bookkeeping system in place within the North American operations of the HBC speaks to the company's history of hiring adventurers like Colin Robertson and sea captains like William Williams to execute and oversee its trading. As the first bona fide businessman to enter the North American trade, Simpson saw immediately that he had to systematize it. But for all the accounting elegance and dispassionate regularity he could bring, there was still between the lines of Simpson's moves to modernize accounting practices and principles an old boys' system of checks and balances—even in the new system, there was room to reward favour with favour.

A case in point is contained in the text of the same letter as the litany of new accounting documents. Simpson is explaining to the Committee that any record-keeping system is only as strong as the men who do the accounting and that, on this score, there is less talent than necessary to keep things running in the Northern Department: "Our counting house requires a head man who can not only fag himself but enforce it on those employed under him."[13] Having been unimpressed with a clerk called Spencer, who was working in the York Factory accounting office, he told the London Committee about the fine qualities of Robert Miles, who was with him in Athabasca and whom he had, with his new authority, promoted to principal clerk in the counting house. He wrote: "Mr. Miles I have not the least doubt after one Winter's Experience here, will be better able to take charge of this branch of the business than any young Gentleman in the Country."[14]

Simpson then went on to recommend a one-year leave for Miles to do an accounting internship in the London office, provided he return the following year and agree to enter into a five-year contract at £150 per annum. Coincidentally, it wouldn't be long before Miles would "choose" to take up with Betsy Sinclair and her baby, entering with feast and dance a marriage *à la façon du pays* that would see seven or eight more children born, as half-siblings to his illustrious governor's first child of the country, in a relationship that would last the rest of their lives.

Eager to continue his management strategy, Simpson left York Factory that summer in a specially constructed light carvel-built York boat called *Eclipse*, which McTavish had built for the Governor in the depot boat shop. In this Outer Circle Tour, Simpson again moved with inhuman speed, working west from York Factory to Norway House and Cumberland House, and on to Isle à La Crosse. Waiting for freeze-up, so that he might continue on snowshoes for a second winter, he drafted another private letter to McTavish, in which he stroked his friend for his prowess in boat design before asking him for a couple of more favours of the family kind:

My Dear Sir

I had the pleasure of addressing you so fully of Yesterday's Date [in an official letter] that I have scarcely left myself anything to say but must endeavour to pick up some Parish news for your amusement. It is my intention next Season to vote you a Patent for Boat building; the *Eclipse* performed Wonders, under Sail she is a prodigy and with 8 Good men she will beat any light canoe in the Country from York to Cumberland; it was a Neck & Neck race between her & the Saskatchewan canoe to Norway House in 10 days with strong head Winds and from thence to Cumberland we gained three Days; the Orkneymen however have no ambition to Travel in the *Govrs. Barge* again . . .

My Family concerns I leave entirely to your kind management, if you can dispose of the Lady it will be satisfactory as she is an unnecessary & expensive appendage, I see no fun in keeping a Woman without enjoying her charms which my present rambling Life does not enable me to do; but if she is unmarketable I have no wish that she should be a general accommodation shop to all the young bucks at the Factory and in addition to her own chastity a padlock may be useful . . .

I have jumbled a great deal of nonsense into this apology for a Letter the whole of which is in confidence for your perusal & thereafter to be committed to the Flames. Dinner Bell is ringing I shall therefore conclude with sentiments of much regard believe me always

> My Dear Sir
> Your truly & sincerely,
> Geo. Simpson

On this Outer Circle Tour of posts in the Northern District, in addition to achieving the inspection objectives, Simpson also likely travelled with and met along the way Cree and Chipewyan Indians who were going about their end of the trade, trapping fur. Surprisingly, in all the minutes, reports and correspondence that crossed the Governor's work tables as he made his way around the district, there was little about the actual procurement of fur, the labour at the foundation of the entire enterprise. Yet the reason for moving the HBC west and north into Athabasca was the continuing European demand for beaver hides, in particular the

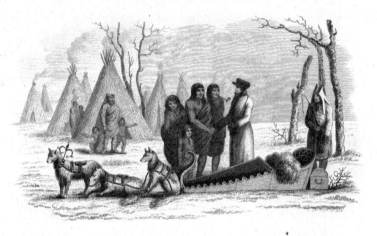

*For some of his winter journeys, when conditions would permit, Simpson trav-
elled in the manner of the country with dogs, often bundled up as a passenger
inside a well-ornamented Cree or Métis carriole. Though colourful and well
padded with buffalo hides, these still made for very cold and bumpy travelling.
This example of a carriole is in an image that depicts Rev. John West, the
HBC's first chaplain in "Indian Country," visiting an encampment west of
Red River in 1821.*

ultra-fine and lightly barbed underfur of the rodent, which was manufactured into the stylish hats so coveted by the British aristocracy and
growing middle class.

Choosing to break their own trail (a tiring activity) as little as possible
to help maintain their speed, Simpson and his travelling companions
would very likely have travelled on paths packed down by Aboriginal
trappers. Simpson, then, would have learned about the trapping side
of the business, as well as about the Indians themselves. This particular year, in places where beaver populations were not yet stressed by
overtrapping, beaver numbers were down because of low water levels,
forcing trappers to move to sets for smaller animals, like marten and
muskrat, that also traded well—though not as well as the beaver.

Once winter had firmly set in, Simpson continued—likely wrapped
up in blankets tucked inside a carriole, or canvas-sided toboggan, pulled

by dogs with a Chipewyan handler who, by turns, would be out front breaking trail or, on old snow or packed trail, kicking the sled along from behind. They continued on from Isle à La Crosse over the Methye Portage, west on the Clearwater River and north on the Athabasca River to Lake Athabasca, where they travelled past Fort Wedderburn on Coal Island, abandoned since amalgamation, and straight to Fort Chipewyan, where Simpson's Nor'Wester rivals had holed up just two years earlier. If the Governor felt even a whiff of nostalgia in returning to the place where he had spent his first winter in the trade, where he had sired his first known child in North America, where he had been a player in the denouement of the fur trade war, it is not evident in the historical record.

Simpson teamed up with Chief Trader Peter Warren Dease (whom he had met at the 1821 Council of Factors and who would be seconded in 1825–27 to Sir John Franklin's second overland expedition and thus become something of a northern legend in his own time), and the two of them, with a guide and two other Chipewyan men, bundled up in blanket capotes, hats, scarves, embroidered mitts, duffle socks and long-legged moosehide moccasins, turned the dog train north and in a scant nine days dropped in out of the blue at Fort Resolution, on the south shore of Great Slave Lake. Chief Trader Robert McVicar noted the arrival of guests in the post journal:

1822

13 December . . . At 8 P.M. we were agreeably surprised by the arrival of Governor Simpson and Mr. Dease who made their appearance in the Hall while we were playing a Game at Whist, with their Blankets and Buffalo Robes about them and so much did they resemble Indians by their Dress and manners that all the Gentlemen called out "there are more Indians," but before we had time to present them with the customary salute of a Dram and a Pipe of Tobacco the Governor discovered himself by taking the Blanket off his head (which was before covered) which excited an equal degree of surprise and astonishment. They have three men along with them, and this is their ninth

Day from Athabasca Lake which is considered at this season of the year extraordinary travelling.[15]

Never one to do anything by half, Simpson threw a dance for the people of the fort the following night and toured the surrounding area for five days more before scuttling back to Fort Chipewyan. On February 1, 1823, he started up the Peace River to Fort Dunvegan and over to Lesser Slave Lake and Fort Edmonton, where, before and after a quick side trip up the North Saskatchewan River to Rocky Mountain House, he took the measure of Colin Robertson, and definitely didn't like what he saw with respect to how the post was being run. He was at Fort Edmonton through the month of April until breakup, at which point he struck out with the loaded boats for Fort Carleton, Cumberland House, Muddy Lake and Norway House, and eventually made it back to York Factory by July 2. He had completed another grand circle of some 3,800 miles and deepened his understanding of the trade—and his contempt for Colin Robertson, among others.

One of the best characterizations of Simpson's modus operandi when on these tours is found in a letter to Lord Selkirk's widow from inside the trade: "[Simpson] has such tact in seeing people's characters that there is not a man in the country that he can not lay down on paper at once, and tell what they are good for. In visiting a post he first has his talk with the chief in command, then with each of the under strappers down to the guides and interpreters, and never omits to go and have a gossip with the old women, so that before the canoe is gummed up and in the water again, he is up to everything great and small that has happened at the post for a twelvemonth past, or since his last visit."[16]

That summer there was ferment in the room as the chief factors gathered for the annual Council at York Factory. It had not been easy getting used to the mixed HBC and NWC personnel in their districts. Implementing all the economy measures dictated by Simpson and the London Committee had also not been without its problems. And the dramatic cutback in liquor rations for trading gifts and keeping the men happy through the long winter had left some very cranky fur traders, to the point that a goodly number of the Canadian boatmen—the voyageurs, many of whom had learned to paddle on high wine and rations of rum—threatened mutiny if this restriction was not eased in their favour. The amalgamation honeymoon was over, and they were all a bit nervous about the Red River settlement. The very idea of settlement was for many a liability. With Colin Robertson leading the charge, they pointed out that in every one of their contracts with the new HBC, there was a clause—a promise—that no expenses of the settlement would be charged to the fur trade. But they knew that the salaries of Miles Macdonell, governor of Assiniboia, and of clergyman John West (who had been sent to Red River to minister but also to see what he could do about schooling the growing ranks of mixed-blood children who were congregating there) were being paid by the company.

Initially at least, as he had learned about Robertson's antics from Robert Miles, who had been with the ex-Nor'Wester in Athabasca, Simpson quite liked the man. However, after the neck-burning incident, the administrative squalor at Norway House and Fort Edmonton, Robertson's bankruptcy and bailout in England, and the intimation that Simpson had somehow stolen credit for success in Athabasca when it was Robertson who should have had it, the Governor made a strategic decision when faced with a room full of angry chief factors.

With Robertson openly challenging his leadership, the little governor pulled himself up to his full five-foot-six height, his sun-freckled face blanching under his thinning red hair and collar-length mutton chops, and dressed Robertson down in front of the assembled company. Simpson almost gloated as he related this memorable incident to his mentor Andrew Colvile:

> By the Deed Poll or rather the Original Deed between the Contracting parties it is provided that no expense relating to Colonization will affect the Fur Trade. The salaries to the Governor and Clergyman therefore gave them [the chief factors] a hand to break out violently;

it kept them in ferment the whole season, and altho' I used every means to bring them into good humour it was for a length of time impossible; they looked upon me with suspicion, had private meetings in Councils day after day, and were about to have written the Committee in a strain which must have given offence. Robertson was one of the leading malcontents, but his blustering folly knocked the whole on the head, and in order to make himself pass for a man of weight came out with all their secrets which gave me an opportunity of bringing them to their senses; in short I found it necessary to show my power and authority and in full Council gave them a lecture which had the desired effect, made them look on each other with suspicion and restored their confidence in myself. Instead of writing themselves they left the whole to me and attended to their other business. No man ever took greater pains or labour to please and give satisfaction than I have done, but some of our Chief Factors are so much accustomed to grumble that a Saint could scarcely keep them in humour. This last season however I found it necessary to act with firmness, convinced them that I could talk loud also, and made an example of Robertson to begin with. He was more noisy about the Colony than any other, talked of rights and privileges, getting Council's opinion on the Deed Poll, in short wished to be a Leader, but I have made such an exposure this season of his maladministration in the Saskatchawaine and told him so many home truths in presence of the whole Council that he was quite crestfallen and will I think give no more trouble. McDonald [John "One-Eye" MacDonald, who duelled with Alexander Kennedy at Swan River] was likewise inclined to be violent about the expenses incurrent on account of the Colony, and was to have given me a set down or prepared speech thereon at the close of the sittings, but the lecture to Robertson had the desired effect, none seemed inclined to enter the Lists with me again, and on the whole we all separated on excellent terms and I believe they now have a greater respect for me than ever.[17]

Thus spake an emerging Emperor.

CHAPTER VIII

COLUMBIA

A nyone who has spent time on the southwestern shores of Hudson Bay knows that summer, such as it is, effectively ends about mid-August. By that time in the year, warm dry westerlies give way to wet nor'easterlies, howling in off the water and stealing heat and hope from every warm crevice. This is a time to be stockpiling food and wood and maybe readying for the fall goose hunt; it is not an ideal time for a cross-country canoe trip.

But in August 1824 that is exactly what George Simpson was embarking on. At thirty-two years of age, he had been in the country for just over four years and had told the London Committee of his hunger to return to England in order to, among other things, seek a wife. The Committee for its part, despite its incredulity about what Simpson had achieved, was far more interested in its energetic governor's continuing his grand circles through company territory. Marriage would have to wait—especially if they believed the gossip that had filtered back to the London office about the young governor's uncanny ability to sate at least his carnal needs with resources in the field.

Prior to amalgamation, the North West Company had had to be far more proactive than the HBC in the west. In fact, NWC agent Edward

Ellice had brought to the negotiating table a constellation of forts in the Columbia District that represented business opportunities that simply could not be overlooked. With Andrew Colvile buttressing the Committee's request that Simpson make an inspection tour of Columbia, the governor set aside his desire to return to the UK and set his sights instead on the west coast.

Simpson's intelligence from the Indian guides, voyageurs, boatmen and officers who had been to the Rockies or farther west was that the probability of completing such a journey by canoe dropped precipitously starting about the tenth of August. After that, the tedium of winter travel on foot, with sparse food (Simpson would have been well acquainted by now with the ubiquitous trail condiment called "Hudson's Bay sauce"—meaning hunger), or with bickering dogs on unpredictable ice would rule the day. Snow or ice in the mountains could bar the way, or the hostilities of the Blackfoot or other Plains tribes, who themselves would be moving into winter hunting grounds, would force detours that could slow a travelling party even more.

With his annual deliberations with the Council of Factors done and transcribed into the record books, and with calculation and transshipment of returns for the year underway and in J.G. McTavish's capable hands by early August, the only item left on the northern governor's to-do list was to review the London Committee's instructions for the year. These were supposed to arrive any day by ship from England. Waiting for the sound of the bell from the top of the rickety watch tower that looked out to sea from York Factory, Simpson saw the tenth of August come and go. Then the eleventh and the twelfth. Each day checking the readiness of his travelling partner, James McMillan, his servant, Tom Taylor, and his hand-picked express canoe crews, Simpson paced and fussed, knowing that the likelihood of his getting stuck for another winter in Athabasca or Peace River country increased with each passing minute.

His worry was not so much the cold and privation that such a winter would unquestionably bring—it was that a business opportunity would be missed. Columbia would go unsupervised, unexamined, un-Simpsonized, for another winter. And from what he had heard, that would just extend the life of indolence and excess lived by company officers who had, since the War of 1812 and the takeover of Astoria, done more or less what they pleased in the absence of administrative scrutiny or interference from the east.

By the fifteenth, Simpson could wait no longer and, in spite of a nasty onshore wind, he ordered his party to embark. And so began the most incredible canoe journey in Canadian history.

As mindful of the geography of Rupert's Land as he was about the business topography of the fur trade, Simpson was only too aware that York Factory was located on a low isthmus of land separating the Hayes River from the Nelson River, though it was the Nelson, not the Hayes, that actually drained Lake Winnipeg. It chafed at his sense of efficiency and economy that the Hayes, which had become the main route to the interior, was longer than the Nelson and had more portages. And yet he had been told repeatedly by men with long experience in actually doing the backbreaking work of trade freighting that the Nelson was far too swift and dangerous for safe travel with loaded York boats or bark canoes. Nevertheless, Simpson was intent on experiencing the differences for himself—and on demonstrating that he was again correct in his own assessment of what was best for HBC profits. With that goal in mind, Simpson and his party settled into two four-fathom *canots du nord* and headed downriver from York Factory, instead of up—out to sea, as it were, to round Point au Marsh before starting up the Nelson and heading west to Columbia.

The wind, waves and tide that August day were of such contrarian force that the embattled crews had not even doubled back on the point before both canoes had to head for shore lest they all perish. To stop the craft from breaking up in the surf, both crews, including Simpson and McMillan, were forced to abandon ship in ice-cold neck-deep water and usher their craft onto the beach by hand. But so hell-bent was Simpson to get this journey underway that rather than wait out the storm he ordered the party to continue over the marshy tundra point on foot, which must have gone over like scurvy with the lads.

The Governor's doggedness in this pursuit is evident in his description of what happened next: "We therefore shouldered our Craft and Baggage for Fifteen long Miles which was a tedious Service on account of the badness of the road and strength of the Wind rendering it necessary to employ Six Men in the transport of the Canoe alone, two being the usual number in short and Four in long Portages; by great exertion however and some danger, having re-embarked before the Storm abated by Wading through the Surf in like manner as on landing, we had the satisfaction of finding ourselves at liberty to prosecute the Voyage in defiance of the Weather, having got within the shelter of the banks of Nelson River."[1]

It is not clear whether the "we" who shouldered the craft included the governor—likely not, especially given that at five foot six he was probably shorter than his Canadian (part French, part Mohawk) canoemen and thereby unable to do anything other than trot along beside or under the canoe when it was "shouldered" by taller men. Simpson's journal does reveal, though, that on this journey he had divested himself of more executive habiliments in favour of a checked cloth chemise and green blanket coat, and that these garments, in concert with traditional moccasins and the long beard he was sporting at the time, made him look enough like a man of the country to be mistaken for one at a number of stops along the way. And the pace of travel with Simpson bordered on the insane:

> Weather permitting, our slumbers would be broken about one in the morning by the cry of "Lève, lève, lève!" In five minutes, woe to the inmates that were slow in dressing; the tents were tumbling about our ears; and within half an hour, the camp would be raised, the canoes laden, and the paddles keeping time to some merry old song. About eight o'clock, a convenient place would be selected for breakfast, about three quarters of an hour being allotted for the multifarious

operations of unpacking and repacking the equipage, laying and removing the cloth, boiling and frying, eating and drinking; and, while the preliminaries were arranging, the hardier among us would wash and shave, each person carrying soap and towel in his pocket, and finding a mirror in the same sandy or rocky basin that held the water. About two in the afternoon we usually put ashore for dinner; and, as this meal needed no fire, or at least got none, it was not allowed to occupy more than twenty minutes or half an hour ... Such was the routine of our journey, the day, generally speaking, being divided into six hours of rest and eighteen hours of labour. This almost incredible toil the voyageurs bore without a murmur, and generally with such a hilarity of spirit as few other men could sustain for a single forenoon.[2]

In August, water levels are usually at their lowest, and yet one of the features of the Nelson River—in contrast to the Hayes, which drains only land between Lake Winnipeg and Hudson Bay—is that it carries the combined volume of the Saskatchewan, Assiniboine, Red and Winnipeg rivers. Even in August the Nelson had a formidable current. Though the river's seven-hundred-foot drop in four hundred miles would not have been a steep gradient for upriver travel, in narrow stretches it would have slowed the normal six- to eight-mile-per-hour speed of Simpson's canoes to one or two miles per hour. Between meals and camps, the Governor would have had interminable hours—perched amidships on the soft cargo of canvas tarp–covered tents and blankets and shifting carefully to avoid upsetting the dynamic balance of the paddlers—to ruminate on things great and small to the sixty-stroke-per-minute rhythm of bent backs and vermillion blades.

At Split Lake Post, from where, he hoped, subsequent Athabasca brigades would carry on west up the Burntwood River, thereby completing one side of a geographic triangle to Isle à La Crosse instead of two had they gone the old route up the Hayes to Norway and Cumberland houses en route to Frog Portage, Simpson had a look at the books. He noticed a long-faced clerk who wasn't pulling his weight—

and summarily fired him and sent him packing for York Factory and the first boat back to England. But eager to proceed with dispatch toward the west, lest the season run out under their bark canoe hulls, the Governor oversaw the repair of one canoe that had been damaged coming up the Nelson, then declared that they would move on.

The only problem was that, this being an unconventional, unused and unpopular route, they had no one in their party who could guide them over the height of land to the Churchill River and west to Frog Portage. This oversight required a side trip to Nelson House where, to Simpson's utter dismay, they found no likely suspects.[3] Reluctantly, the party struck out again, with Simpson almost resigned to having to continue on the conventional Norway House–Grand Rapids–Cumberland House route.

They had come to the end of a portage in the upper reaches of the Nelson River, northeast of Lake Winnipeg, when Simpson spied an Indian canoe disappearing behind an island far down the lake. Without waiting to load his canoe, he instructed his canoemen to catch the canoe at all costs and, if there happened to be in it a person who could guide the way west, to apprehend the man and employ him as a guide. This turn of events caused Simpson to exhort in his journal that this find "afforded me greater satisfaction than the sight of an Indian ever did before."[4] By the end of the month they were at Frog Portage on the Churchill River, and back on the beaten track.

Besides staying ahead of the season, Simpson's haste on this journey—as in all his journeys—was driven as much by his Napoleonic ego as by anything else. He was a man who wanted to be in command and to move faster, farther and with more authority than anyone who had come before, impressing people as he went, putting his own performance on display and doling out reward and punishment as he saw fit. His old nemesis from Athabasca, John Clarke, had the misfortune of being caught at Frog Portage in an express canoe with his country wife again, instead of travelling with his Lesser Slave Lake brigade, as stipulated in a resolution that had been passed at Council. On learning that Clarke's

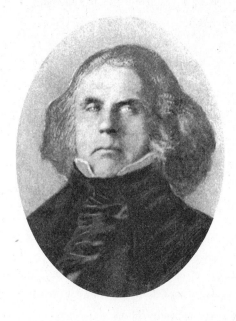

Physically, factor Dr. John McLoughlin dwarfed the diminutive Simpson, who described him as "such a figure as I should not like to meet in a dark Night in one of the by- lanes in the neighbourhood of London."

brigade had suffered losses from another canoe being overturned after Clarke had gone ahead, Simpson made a note then and there to bring the matter again before Council and to summarily "move the loss and expense occasioned thereby [to Clarke's] private account."[5]

But there was nothing on this journey that made the tenderfoot Simpson happier than catching up with old Nor'Wester, now senior HBC factor, Dr. John McLoughlin, also on his way to Columbia. McLoughlin had left York Factory on the conventional Hayes River route on July 26, twenty days before Simpson. In his journal, Simpson painted a vivid picture of the wily McLoughlin, which becomes all the more intriguing with the knowledge that in later life these two would come to blows—the "pawky little bantam" versus the "grizzled giant." For now, though, it was an amicable meeting, with Simpson very pleased that he had caught the old Nor'Wester. Simpson wrote:

Came up with the Dr before his people had left their Encampment altho we had by that early hour come from his Breakfasting place of the preceding Day; himself and people were heartily tired of the Voyage and his Surprise and vexation at being overtaken . . . is not to be described; he was such a figure as I should not like to meet in a dark Night in one of the by-lanes in the neighbourhood of London, dressed [in] Clothes that had once been fashionable, but now covered with a thousand patches of different Colours, his beard would do honor to the chin of a Grizzly Bear, his face and hands evidently Shewing that he had not lost much time on his Toilette, loaded with Arms and his own Herculean dimensions for a *tout ensemble* that would convey a good idea of the highwaymen of former Days.[6]

A significant part of the delight in this encounter was that Simpson and his crew had done in a frenetic forty-two days what had taken McLoughlin a leisurely sixty-one.

The two men travelled on together after they met, working their way up the Athabasca River to Fort Assiniboine. There were maps of the area at the time, but, in the long tradition of the First Nations, the sum total of navigational information that was with the chief factor and the Governor on this journey was carried in the heads of their guide and the other expeditionaries who'd been this way before. Simpson, of course, had been in Athabasca during his first winter in the trade, and he had travelled again this way during his Outer Circle Tour, en route to Fort Edmonton, but the reaches of the boreal forest through which they travelled, its uniform green broken only by frost sprinklings and occasional gold patches of larch, would have had a sameness that might have confused less aware travellers. Among his considerable talents, Simpson possessed uncanny observational skills, which allowed him to place himself in the larger geographical picture with enviable accuracy.

At Fort Assiniboine, for example, near a crook where the Athabasca River swings from west- to north-flowing, he ruminated in his journal about getting a winter road cut across country to Fort Edmonton and the North Saskatchewan River, a distance of some seventy-five miles or so. In the event that this route could be proved workable, all of the freight for the area from the Lesser Slave Lake District to the north and Columbia to the west could be moved up the mighty North Saskatchewan River in York boats, instead of being dragged through the swamps and mud bogs of the Beaver River and over the time- and energy-consuming Methye Portage.

That Simpson saw a shorter and less arduous route involving a switch of freight from boat to horseback and back to boat was not in itself all that remarkable. Of note, however, were his willingness to challenge conventional thinking and his ability to hold in his head the relative positions and distances between key points in the supply line without detailed maps of any kind. Indeed, on the way back east from Columbia the following spring, Simpson himself would try out this alternate route. Although his intuition about the Nelson River–Split Lake–Burntwood River route would prove totally impractical for the movement of freight (one of Simpson's few colossally bad ideas), one of the legacies of this epic cross-country canoe voyage would be the building of a thoroughfare from Fort Edmonton to Jasper House and the discontinuation of the muddy Beaver River–Methye Portage route as a major supply line.

After fifty days of upriver paddling through all manner of nasty fall weather (seventy for McLoughlin's men), it must have come as something of a relief when the expedition reached Jasper House and the eastern end of the Athabasca Pass. Here Simpson ordered seven of his men out of the boats and onto the backs of skinny horses that would take them up into the mountains and eventually down to the Wood River, a tributary of the mighty Columbia River, on a route pioneered by the great Nor'Wester David Thompson in 1811. Their instructions were to travel the 120 precarious miles to Boat Encampment on the Columbia with dispatch, and to build a new canoe to supplement the two already there to take the party downstream to Columbia. The rest of the *engagés* followed on horseback, with James McMillan in charge. But Simpson and McLoughlin kept two canoemen behind to paddle them in a small canoe another 50 miles up the Athabasca River,[7] on water too shallow for the loaded *canots du nord*, to Henry's House, where they too eventually

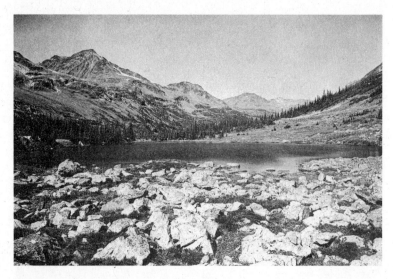

Labelled for the first time on John Arrowsmith's 1832 map of British North America, the Committee's Punch Bowl, flowing east and west, was named by Simpson in honour of the London Committee on his way through the Athabasca Pass in 1825. On the height of land on the border of what is now Alberta and British Columbia, Simpson treated his men to a bottle of wine as they had "neither time nor convenience to make a bowl of punch, although a glass of it would have been acceptable."

stashed their craft for the return journey and continued up a rocky trail with a cavalcade of 21 more horses, headed west.

With the imposing deltoid chock of Mount Brown[8] seemingly right in their way and the sheared crags and shadowed scree slopes of lesser peaks making short days even shorter, snow was the order of the day as these three parties trickled up through the Athabasca Pass. Oblivious to physical discomfort, passing through country he called "beautifully wild and romantic,"[9] Simpson seems in his journal as taken with the wildlife they saw (and roasted over evening fires) along the way, especially the Dall sheep and mountain goats, as with the difficulty of the terrain. Once fully into the pass, however, where the October sun could be seen only as slivers of light for scant parts of the day, he was prompted to laud David Thompson, his Nor'Wester forebear, by asking how any human being could have stumbled on a pass through such a formidable barrier.[10] And, when with McLoughlin he climbed to the two little marshy lakes that combine to form the height of land between the Pacific and Arctic watersheds at six thousand feet above sea level, he was as moved toward public sentimentality as ever in his life, choosing to name this small but consequential body of water in honour of the London governors:

> At the very top of the pass or height of Land is a small circular Lake or Basin of Water which empties itself in opposite directions and may be said to be the source of the Columbia & Athabasca Rivers as it bestows its favours on both these prodigious Streams, the former falling into the Pacific at Lat. 46 ½ north and the latter after passing through Athabasca and Great Slave Lakes falling into the Frozen Ocean at about 69 North Lat. That this basin should send its Waters to each side of the Continent and give birth to two of the principal Rivers in North America is no less strange than true both the Dr. & myself having examined the currents flowing from it east & West and the circumstance appearing remarkable I thought it should be honored by a distinguishing title and it was forthwith named the "Committee's Punch Bowl."

Descending the other side of the pass in the shadow of McGillivray's Rock, a conical massif named by Thompson for founding winterer of the NWC William McGillivray, Simpson and McLoughlin's horse cavalcade took six days to fumble its way through Athabasca Pass and down through four thousand vertical feet to Boat Encampment, crossing and re-crossing the Whirlpool River, on the way up, and the cascading Wood River dozens of times as they switched back and forth to avoid sliding or falling to certain injury or death. For their part in the crossing, three horses were slaughtered at Boat Encampment to feed the crew, which was running perilously close to a steady diet of "Hudson's Bay sauce."

Simpson later noted in his journal that he had written to John Rowand, the chief factor at Fort Edmonton who had succeeded the indolent Colin Robertson, with some comments and observations about fine-tuning the logistics of horse husbandry for the proposed new Assiniboine crossing and, as well, here at Athabasca Pass. There was seemingly no detail, large or small, that escaped Simpson's purview.

It is not clear whether the advance crew under James McMillan's leadership actually made a canoe at Boat Encampment. Given the very short head start they had been given, and especially with freezing conditions at this altitude and at this time of the year, it is unlikely that a canoe was built by the time Simpson and McLoughlin caught up to the others there. When they arrived, they found McMillan with three canoes, two made of sewn-together boards and one cedar dugout, that had likely come up from the coast as part of Aboriginal trade on the Columbia. The two clinker-built craft Simpson noted to be from a different design tradition from the bark canoes he had used on the other side of the divide; they more properly might be considered "Bateaux wrought by Paddles instead of Oars."[11] Simpson learned from McMillan that, in terms of transportation, they were comparable to conventional *canots du nord*, but smaller. Nonetheless, to Simpson's dismay, they still employed eight paddlers. "I do not know whether this innovation is meant as an indulgence to the Masters or the Men," he wrote, "but suspect it is agreeable to both altho' injurious to the Comp[an]y as thereby one third more people are employed in transport than necessary. I shall however take care that this evil is remedied before my departure and endeavour to improve on the original plan, Seven Men being in my opinion quite sufficient to Navigate a Boat containing Fifty pieces Cargo and the Crews of two Boats equal to the transport of One across the Portages."[12]

In these large craft, on a river that pours more water into the Pacific Ocean than any other in North or South America, Simpson and his party headed south and downstream on October 21, 1824. Had they been there in spring or summer, they might have seen against a blue sky the Monashee Mountains flanking the river on the west and the

Selkirks on the eastern rim of the valley. As it was, all Simpson's expedition experienced at river level over these mid-autumn days was rain, rain and more rain, the grey sinews of the deep Columbia and its sleeping eddies shrouded most days in swirling wet mist. The clammy feel of the air might have reminded Simpson of the Cromarty Firth, as might have the sight of dead and dying salmon that had come up the river to spawn, had he not had bigger things to occupy his active mind.

———

Tales of the Pacific northwest may have been among Simpson's first memories of exploration and conquest, as stories of his Black Isle kinsman Alexander Mackenzie were told around the dinner table in Dingwall. That family narrative would have been stitched into Alexander Simpson's school lessons about James Cook dropping anchor in Nootka Sound on March 30, 1778, and finding untold riches in furs to be traded there. He would have learned as well about the East India Company's trade in China and the Far East, and of James Cook's protégé, George Vancouver, and his re-entry into the Juan de Fuca Strait, to try to convince the Spanish that lands around what is now Vancouver Island and the Olympic Peninsula were rightly British.

All of that formative knowledge would have been background to Simpson's new attentions to the west when it became part of his purview in the expanded Northern Department. As he floated down the Columbia River, his mind may well have been racing through the historical chronology that had led him to an unparalleled business opportunity west of the Rockies. Following the American Revolution, relations between the British government and the fledgling American government had not been the best, but the government had worked out compromises and accommodations. US chief justice John Jay's treaty of 1794 had settled some issues and put in place mechanisms for delineating the border between the new United States and British North America. Decisions made in this process had forced the North West Company to move its inland headquarters from Grand Portage, which was now on American soil, north to the mouth of the Kaministiquia River, and it seemed as if forty-nine degrees north latitude was going to be the line of separation, at least east of the Rocky Mountains. West of the mountains it was a different story.

Mackenzie had shown in 1793 that it was possible to get to the Pacific overland, although it didn't look as if this route would be ideal for trade. President Thomas Jefferson had given explorers Meriwether Lewis and William Clark a mandate to work their way west to the Pacific via the Missouri River to see what kind of economic opportunities that route might bring to the fledgling American confederation. In 1808, Nor'Wester Simon Fraser had, by the skin of his teeth, walked to the Pacific beside the river (too wild to paddle) that now bears his name. It was North American–born Nor'Wester Fraser who had named the region, which essentially comprises the interior of what is now the province of British Columbia, "New Caledonia," because, think some historians, it matched his mother's descriptions of the Scottish Highlands.[13] And map-maker David Thompson, the lad who had learned his trade through the HBC but plied it to most advantage when he switched allegiances to the NWC, had pushed his way to the mouth of the Columbia in 1811, only to find that John Jacob Astor had made it there first and established his commercial enterprise, Astoria, on the south shore of the great river's estuary.

In the same year, the Governor's friend, now chief factor at York Factory, J.G. McTavish, had been dispatched to go west of the Rockies to resupply Thompson. It was he who took news to the Astorians of renewed fighting between the Americans and the British, and warned that ships were on their way to capture Astor's valuable western outpost. That information, along with the wily negotiating skills of a true Nor'Wester, allowed McTavish to purchase Astoria for $58,000 (the NWC would eventually have to return it as unfair spoils of war) and rename it Fort George. It was in the west that McTavish met and married in the manner of the country Nancy McKenzie, who was now the respected mixed-blood "Madam" of York Factory, and who at the moment Simpson made his way down the Columbia might well have been negotiating Betsy Sinclair's future with Robert Miles on behalf of her husband and his procreative boss and confidant, George Simpson.

By 1818, border issues east of the Rockies between the Americans and the British had more or less coalesced around the forty-ninth parallel, but west of the mountains, where things were much less certain (largely because of the huge distances involved), provisional joint claim had been established for all of the territory between forty-two degrees north, below which the Spanish held sway, and fifty-four degrees, forty minutes north, above which the Russians had been operating for longer than anyone could remember. On September 16, 1821, while Simpson was holed up to winter at Fort Wedderburn, the Russian czar, knowing that his days of uninterrupted trade and commerce in the American northwest were numbered, had issued an *ukase* (proclamation). It claimed exclusive control of the northwest coast as far south as fifty-one degrees north, including a hundred-mile exclusion zone off all islands and the mainland of what is now the Alaska panhandle that was to pertain to all foreign vessels, regardless of their flag.

The territory west of the Rockies was vast—at 58 million hectares, the Columbia River watershed alone was the size of France, and this was not the whole of the contested parcel. North of Fraser's river was the region of New Caledonia, famous for its black-furred beaver, the area to which Simpson had tried unsuccessfully to send his old classmate Duncan Finlayson to reconnoitre for possible HBC development during the winter of 1820–21. To the south was the Columbia District, an area that generally included the lands north and south of the mighty river. And reaching southeast out of Columbia was Snake River Country, into which American free traders were travelling in increasing numbers from the Missouri River system, through the deepest gorge in North America (7,900 feet), and into which the Nor'Westers were flooding from the west. The southern edge of New Caledonia and the whole of Columbia and Snake River Country was often referred to as Oregon Country, for lack of a more specific term.

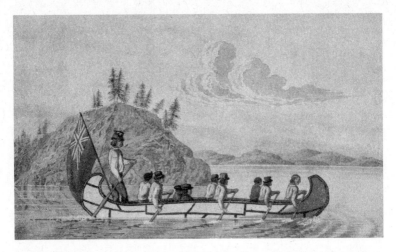

George Simpson and his band of willing Caughnawaga voyageurs can claim to this day the record for the fastest and longest canoe voyage in one season, travelling from York Factory to the mouth of the Columbia River in eighty-four days, August 15 to November 8, 1824.

Back on the Columbia, with a five- to six-knot current adding to the speed of his eight-paddle-power Columbia-style bateau, George Simpson was slipping in the autumn of 1824 into Oregon Country at about twelve miles per hour—twelve miles every hour for eighteen hours a day, with time out for portaging, gulping scant meals and bedding down for short four-hour sleeps. This was fast, but not half as fast as he would have liked.

To make the most of time spent en route, he thought, some business might be done, and he suggested that Dr. McLoughlin might enjoy some company from one of the other vessels, instead of travelling alone in his own canoe—Chief Trader James McMillan, perhaps? In vintage Simpsonian style, he had previously explained the situation in Oregon Country (as he understood it) to McMillan, pointing out that after careful examination of the Snake River Expedition fur results over the last few seasons, he had learned that, for whatever reasons (American free traders, declining stocks, hostile Indians), returns were diminishing in this contested area, and that however the conflict over who owned the territory might ultimately be resolved, the Honourable Company would be well advised to think about moving its operation north, perhaps setting up a post at the mouth of the Fraser River as a forward-thinking alternative to Fort George. Secretly, he hoped McMillan would take the bait and get interested in this bit of corporate forechecking.

Unfortunately, McMillan, who was obviously in a totally different frame of mind—perhaps trying to stay warm or dry or both or, if the sun happening to be shining for a brief period, drinking in the spectacular mountain scenery—"did not see my drift or would not take the hint."[14] Simpson was looking for him to volunteer his services to lead an expedition that winter to see about a possible site for such a post. Around the fire that evening, it was only when Simpson suggested that the HBC's lack of knowledge of the district was "a disgrace to the whole concern," and that he, the northern governor, was thinking of checking out the Fraser River post idea himself, that McMillan twigged to what his boss was asking and "immediately offered his services on this dangerous and unpleasant mission."[15] But making a connection between McMillan and McLoughlin was crucial. Internal politics were every bit as important as external politics in the trade, and no one, it seemed, had a more acute appreciation of that than George Simpson.

Aside from regular contact with First Nations groups camping along the Columbia, the first direct communication with the Pacific end of this protracted canoe journey came when Simpson's party met Chief Trader Peter Skene Ogden and a group of thirty men who were on their way inland from Fort George with the year's outfit for Spokane House, on the Kootenay River. These supplies had been unloaded from the HBC vessel *Vigilant*, which had arrived at the mouth of the Columbia a week before. Taking advantage of horses for transportation and of the legendary Oregon trader Ogden to guide them, Simpson left the canoes for a sixty-mile side trip east up the Columbia tributary to inspect Spokane House.

Through Ogden, at Spokane House, Simpson learned more than he perhaps really wanted to hear about the Snake River Expedition and the somewhat unorthodox ways in which the trade was orchestrated in Oregon Country. Contrary to the practice in the districts east of the Rockies, where Aboriginal people did the trapping and Europeans did the trading, in many cases in the west the situation was reversed: Europeans did the trapping and traded with the well-developed Indian cultures of the west coast for food, produce and other considerations that they were otherwise without. The object of the exercise remained the acquisition of furs that would make their way to the European markets, but on the west side of the mountains, in Oregon Country, competition between English and American traders, as well as intermingling and internecine fighting among Aboriginal peoples, gave the resource economy a very different look and feel.

The previous year's aggregate returns for Spokane House had been about 9,000 beaver, which was fairly impressive compared to harvests from similarly sized districts in the east, but Simpson could not help thinking that the involvement of free trappers and traders in the conduct of the trade was not really in keeping with the way things were done in the Honourable Company. The returns to date for the district that Ogden was able to show them looked even better than the year before. Yet Simpson looked carefully at what he saw of the lifestyle of these western gentlemen and wondered if, in sum, the whole effort was worthwhile from the HBC's point of view. Making the computation that he had made at every post along the way, Simpson reckoned that at most it would take two boats to carry inland the 80 to 100 pieces of trade items needed to "purchase" the number of skins that were showing on the books at Spokane House. And yet records showed that for the previous three years it had taken five and sometimes six boats to do the job. On inspection of the waistlines and habits of Ogden and his men, Simpson surmised that these extra 240- to 390-pound packs of freight comprised "Eatables, Drinkables and other Domestic Comforts" for the personal consumption of company personnel whose eastern and London-based bosses had no idea, until Simpson started managing, what was going on in the hinterland of Oregon Country.

And if he needed more proof that this department had gone unsupervised too long, everyone he talked to on the Lower Columbia had things to say about difficulties the traders had encountered with each other and with local Indian bands. At the junction of the Snake River and the Columbia, he heard the sad tale of an NWC clerk, one Mr. Reed, and eight or ten other men, killed in revenge for the hanging of one of their own, who had been caught stealing several articles from an officer's table. That officer, Simpson learned, was Chief Factor John Clarke, then a clerk, who seemed to have had as poor judgment as a junior officer as he did when Simpson cut his trail in Athabasca seven winters later. Simpson's journey had begun with the inappropriate behaviour of John Clarke, and still the man's foibles were haunting him. In his journal Simpson scoffed, "The only remark I shall offer on this affair is that it is to be lamented that the innocent should have suffered instead of the guilty."

After three months in transit, Simpson and his party paddled into the final gorge of the Columbia, with the white-dusted Cascade Mountain sentinels of Wy'east (Mount Hood) to the south and Loowit (Mount St. Helen's) off to the north. On the eighty-fourth day out from York Factory, at about 5 p.m. on November 8, they reached Fort George. Simpson's relentless pace had knocked twenty days off the record time.

Musing in his journal, he reckoned that with eight good men in an express canoe on the Saskatchewan route (which would mean crossing from Fort Edmonton to Fort Assiniboine on the Athabasca instead of dragging up through the "circuitous and tedious" Beaver River–La Loche Portage route), he could do the same journey in just two months. To save time, instead of stopping during the day to change into fancy dress prior to the final sprint to the end, Simpson and his voyageurs put on their best clothes in the morning of that last day. Further to the Governor's suspicions about company personnel living a gilded life out of sight and mind of the London Committee, Chief Factor Alexander Kennedy and a fellow officer were languishing in a sailing skiff in the evening sun when their chief administrative officer paddled into view of Fort George. Simpson was singularly unimpressed. But now that this amazing transcontinental canoe journey was done, he had all winter to clean house.

CHAPTER IX

VICEREGAL CEO

Besides the changes wrought in George Simpson's knowledge and confidence, and notwithstanding the enhancement of his image in the eyes of his underlings as a result of his having travelled the breadth of North America in one season, faster than anyone else, another, more subtle shift began on this journey. The Governor was now able to see and appreciate his role in the Hudson's Bay Company as proxy for the British government in North America (and especially in New Caledonia and Columbia). His role as the HBC's northern governor was tantamount to being the unofficial government agent representing British interests on what was fundamentally an international stage.

As niggling as he was with the minutiae of economy and the trade when he was at Fort George during the winter of 1824–25, he was equally expansive in his far-reaching illusions of grandeur for the HBC and of himself as master of that domain. If there was ever a moment when Simpson accepted or assumed a mantle of leadership larger than that of a conventional business operative, it was during that first winter in Columbia.

Surprisingly, the London Committee had no real expectations of profit from Columbia. It had inherited the NWC's head start in the region and had seen promising results in numbers and quality of furs, but managing an operation a mountain range away from the main depot on Hudson Bay had costs that seemed to eat up most of the profits. Sending supplies around Cape Horn, at the tip of South America, and maintaining a resupply base in the Sandwich Islands (Hawaii) also ate up time and money. Hostile Indians in the area and competition with the Russians to the north, the Spanish to the south and the Americans throughout the region had further conspired to keep the expectations of the London governors low.

Simpson, however, felt differently. His travel west with James McMillan and John McLoughlin, both of whom had experience in the west and both of whom had knowledge about and judgments of trade that Simpson, at the time, respected, only increased his resolve to surprise Andrew Colvile and the rest of the London Committee with his ability to make profit where none was anticipated.

Arriving at Fort George, he found "little to commend and much to reform" in the ways in which trade was being conducted, but these problems were not any different from those he had encountered at every other post he'd examined during his four years in the trade. Though the solutions had local nuances, they would be much the same as those he had engineered elsewhere in Rupert's Land and in the northwest.

A quick scan of the Columbia Department and its four units—Fort George, Fort Nez Percés (later known as Old Fort Walla Walla), Thompson's River House and Spokane House—as well as the Snake River Expedition, combined with what he witnessed of waste and excess on his trip down the river from Boat Encampment, was all he needed to know in order to cut the company payroll from 151 men (2 chief factors, 3 chief traders, 10 clerks and 136 men) to 83 (2 chief factors, 3 chief traders, 6 clerks and 72 men). And these efficiencies, combined with enforced lifestyle reductions for the officers and other economies down through the ranks to the trading floors, would, he reckoned, allow the company to realize an immediate profit of about £5,000, with annual improvements to follow. By now, decisive managerial action was almost

routine for Simpson. He may even have enjoyed making unilateral decisions, unclouded by emotion, that cut inefficiencies in the system but
that surely landed like anvils on the lives of people who were transferred
or summarily relieved of their duties. He seemed not to care if people
liked him or feared him, provided they bent to his will.

From the moment he entered this contested territory, however, and
cagily inquired of James McMillan if he would consider an expedition to explore the possibilities of setting up a post at the mouth of the
Fraser River, it was evident that Simpson was thinking strategically and
beyond the narrow confines of profit. Letters and journals indicate
that he was well aware of the ongoing disputes of the government of
the fledgling American confederation with the British government in
Whitehall and its representatives in Canada. He was also fully aware
of President Thomas Jefferson's commission to his military officer
Meriwether Lewis (inspired by Alexander Mackenzie's successful overland crossing of North America), which had as much to do with claiming territory as with finding opportunities for settlement and economic
development. Ever the pragmatist, Simpson predicted that the logical
place for a provisional border to be drawn was the Columbia River, and
that he, as chief officer of a British company operating under royal charter, was the de facto government agent in Columbia, there to do the on-
the-ground manoeuvring on Whitehall's behalf. To Chief Factor John
McLoughlin's great chagrin, one of the first major strategic decisions
Simpson made that winter was to move the company's western headquarters to the north side of the river.

It hadn't escaped Simpson that the fabulous snow-covered volcanic
mountains in the Cascade Range were surrounded by almost desert-like
ground. And if, like the Indians of the region, the HBC was going to
decrease its expensive reliance on European food by growing its own,
it would be well advised to locate its fort in a place where better soil
might support more robust agriculture. The place he chose, apparently
with the help of local intelligence, including from a Chinook chief called
Concomely, was Belle Vue Point, upstream of the Columbia River Gorge,

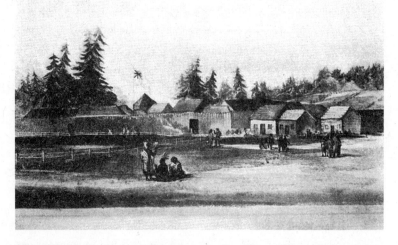

The HBC's first outpost in Columbia was Fort George (formerly Astoria) on the south bank of the Columbia River. Simpson, seeing that it was only a matter of time until the Americans would claim that land, decided to move the company's installation inland and onto the north side of the river, calling the new location (shown here) Fort Vancouver.

a location that had not only excellent crop and grazing possibilities but other advantages as well, including the fact that it was on the north side of the river, on land that the Americans, at least in the short run, might concede rightfully belonged to King George IV. He would call the new establishment Fort Vancouver.

Nor had it escaped Simpson that the natural market for the bounty of the northwest coast of North America—be it fur, fish, lumber or agricultural produce—was not Europe but East Asia, China in particular. John Jacob Astor may have been ousted from Columbia by the North West Company, but his inclination toward Asian trade had been 100 per cent correct: ships laden with resources from Columbia could be traded for a tidy profit in Canton (Guangzhou), with ships returning with tea, spices and other comestibles that would readily sell to the colonies in the east. Simpson may have learned a version of this story from Astor himself, or from Colonel Perkins, on his way through New York City in 1820. The only difference between the American free traders and the Russians, who had done well with sea otter pelts on the Canton market, was that just as the HBC had a monopoly on the North American trade, the East India Company had a unilateral grip on the China trade. If the HBC was going to take advantage of economic opportunities in the Pacific, it would have to not only outmanoeuvre the Americans and the Russians but also find a way to work profitably with the East India Company's monopoly.

George Simpson, with his brief history in the trade buttressed by a decade or more in the London sugar trade, knew that this was as much a political as a business proposition. In any case, he had it all worked out in his head, down to the smallest detail, as he described in a letter to the London Committee:

> In order to see the whole machine put in motion I should wish to
> pass one or two Winters on this side, indeed if the Honble Committee
> thought that my Services on the other side could be dispensed with
> for a whole year, say 1826/27, I have the vanity to think that much ben-
> efit would be derived by my presence and I shall here take the liberty
> of pointing out how I conceive my time could be turned to best advan-
> tage. The Vessel intended for the China trade would leave England
> in November or December 1825 so as to reach Fort George in June or
> July 1826, deliver the Outfit, take in the Furs for China and be in readi-
> ness to take her departure from and after the 20th October. I should
> propose starting from York Factory after the arrival of the Bay Ship
> from the 20th of August to the 1st of September and be at Fort George
> by the 1st of November, accompanying the Ship to Canton, dispose
> of the Cargo either by delivery to the E.I. Co^y [East India Company]
> Agent, bringing it immediately to Sale or putting it into the hands of
> respectable mercantile House to be disposed of afterwards as the state
> of the market or other circumstances might render expedient; take
> in a cargo of China Goods, proceed to Lima, Acapulco or some port
> on that Coast most likely to present an advantageous market which

the Honble Committee would be able to ascertain from some of the
London Mercantile Houses in that line and of which I should have
information by the Bay Ships; dispose of the Cargo and remit the
proceeds or leave it (the Cargo) in the hands of a respectable House of
business to be disposed of afterwards as the state of the market would
authorize; take in the goods required for the outfit of the following
year and reach the Columbia in June or July 1827 by which time the
interior Brigades would have delivered their returns and gone inland
with their outfits. Embark the Furs, people & property and proceed
to the mouth of Frazers River; remain there until the 1st November
by which time our Establishment would be completed and the York
Factory Express arrived; dispatch the large Vessel for China and then
proceed in the small Vessel along the Coast on a Trading Expedition,
touch at the Russian Settlement in Norfolk Sound and see if any business could be done there, return to Frazers River in March, proceed
from thence to the mountains meet the different Brigades from the
interior going with their returns and for their outfits to the Depot, and
be at Norway House by the opening of Navigation about the middle
of June 1828 thereby being absent from the Councilling business at
York only one Season.[1]

Implicit in Simpson's thinking about the China trade and how to make
it all work was the understanding that active occupancy of the Columbia
District would not only honour the company's charter responsibilities
but also show the HBC making good use of lands on the west side of the
Rockies ceded to them by the recent royal proclamation that extended
HBC operations to the Pacific. With the increasing scrutiny in Britain
of any and all government-linked monopolies, Simpson knew that the
London Committee was interested in doing—or, more important, being
seen to be doing—the right thing with respect to meeting its statutory
obligations. But also implicit in Simpson's thinking was the clear understanding that the company's actions in Oregon Country were the de
facto activity of the British government, with significant implications

for holding its place in border disputes with the upstart Americans and, to a lesser extent, with the Russians above fifty-four-forty and with the Spanish below forty-six degrees north latitude. Historian Frederick Merk says, of this assertion of power, "By reason of Simpson's elimination of major losses the Company had found it possible to remain in the valley of the lower Columbia, that by the vigour and energy of the new administration it had succeeded in reversing American domination of the coast, that it had compelled American competitors one by one to withdraw from the field, and that in the interior, no less than on the coast, it had completely carried the day. What George Simpson had achieved by his reforms was to reduce Oregon to economic vassalage to a British corporation. He had converted the Columbia Department into a new principality of the Hudson's Bay Company, ruled over from Fort Vancouver as by the viceroy of a king."[2]

George Simpson intuitively grasped the mantle of corporate leadership and saw himself as a leader of men—preferably men of European stock—but, with a racist attitude toward non-whites, he did not believe in advancing the HBC's charter responsibility toward North American Indian tribes.[3] In early correspondence with his mentor, Andrew Colvile, Simpson talked bluntly of his frustrations with indolence and alcohol abuse among the First Nations and Métis populations (he had the exact same complaints of many of the HBC employees he met) but said that effort in educating these people about other lifestyles was a waste of time, because "an enlightened Indian is good for nothing." He was at least, though, aware that this sentiment—a lingering bias from the days of slavery, and one that still prevailed among the British ruling classes—was contentious ("I give you my ideas thus freely for your private information in case the subject should come up before the Committee, if they were known by the very pious I might be looked upon as a true North Wester")[4] but he was unrepentant. This view may have softened slightly during the first winter he spent in Columbia.

Simpson may have paid closer attention to the Chinook Indians while at Fort George because these communities along the Columbia

River were highly organized and of more economic significance to the HBC than were other Indian communities he had known. They encompassed trapping of fur species, fishing, agriculture, building technology and social conventions, including a hierarchical system of slavery. The Chinooks intrigued Simpson and, unlike the more dark-skinned Cree and Chipewyan Indians he had encountered east of the Rockies, they had another endearing characteristic: "Their looks on the whole are pleasing being more fair and their features more resembling those of the Whites than any other tribe I have seen."[5]

Simpson devoted a good many pages in his journal that winter to recording ethnographic details of the Chinook people, beginning with a description of how the masters distinguish themselves from the slaves: "They have however a strange practise of flattening the upper part of the Head which at an early age disfigures them very much but as they advance in Life it is not offensive to the Eye, at least not so to me at first sight, and as none but the wretched slaves have round heads I begin to fall into the Chinook way of thinking that they do not look as well (particularly the Ladies) with round as with Flat Heads . . . This operation does not seem to give pain as the children rarely cry and it certainly does not affect the brain or understanding as they are without exception the most intelligent Indians and the most acute and finished bargain Makers I have fallen in with." But lest his readers get the idea he was actually connecting strongly with the Chinook as equal human beings, Simpson (always conscious that his journal had an audience) added, "A couple of these Heads will be sent to the Hon[ble] Committee next Season as a curiosity."[6]

Simpson seems to have developed something of a friendship with a number of the Chinook who lived in the vicinity of Fort George that winter. Among them was Chief Concomely—"His One Eyed Majesty"—who helped him choose the location for Fort Vancouver and whose daughter, Chowie, may have been offered to the randy Scotsman to keep him warm in the evening hours. In his usually elliptical style when it came to writing of such matters, Simpson said this: "The Young

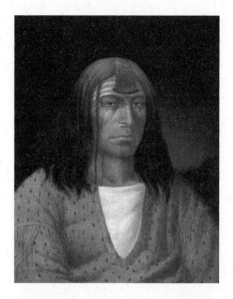

Artist Paul Kane visited George Simpson in autumn 1845 and got approval to travel in spring 1846 with HBC brigades to Fort Vancouver, meeting many of the same people the Governor had encountered and creating one of the most important ethnographic records of his day. Kane made a sketch of this Aboriginal man near Fort Colvile on his way back east in July 1847. Whether or not he was a member of the Nez Percé tribe, Kane added a pierced nasal septum, which was not part of the original sketch, in the final painting.

Women previous to Marriage are allowed to indulge the full scope of their inclinations, and chastity is not looked upon as a virtue except in regard to the Ladies of the very first rank when the parents are desirous that they should be allied to White great men, in which cases they are closely watched indeed and are never allowed to cross the Door except after Dark and then attended by Slaves. It however strangely happens that these precautions are of little avail as the Young Ladies are in this respect very much disposed to disregard the injunctions of their parents and have sufficient address to elude the vigilance of their guards."[7]

Simpson found that although Concomely was the titular head of the tribe, in this matriarchal society most of the main decisions were made by the women. As had been the case since the very beginning of the trade—a point that the French understood much better than the English—strategic alliances with First Nations through relationships with their women were a way to ensure smooth commerce between the two societies. But in Columbia, Simpson soon learned that just as there were politics between groups, so also there were internal politics. In this case, the wife of the third-ranking man in Concomely's group believed that her daughter, "a buxom Damsel of 18 or 20 who has never yet seen Day light," should be with Simpson instead of the chief's daughter. Wrote Simpson, "I have therefore a difficult card to play, being equally desirous to keep clear of the Daughter and continue on good terms with the Mother, and by management I hope to succeed in both altho her Ladyship is most pressing & persevering, tempting me with fresh offers and inducements every succeeding Day." The Governor's desire to keep on good terms with the highly placed women of the tribe was connected with his insatiable need to know what was going on at the post. Referring to the second-ranking woman in the tribe, he wrote, "She is the best News Monger in the Parish and through her I know more of the Scandal, Secrets & politics both of the out & inside of the Fort than from any other Source."[8]

The point to be made here is that as Simpson warmed to the Chinooks he also reconsidered his previously harsh views about Indians generally. The HBC charter mandate called for effective stewardship of the Aboriginal populations of Rupert's Land and now on the west side of the Rockies. When he first arrived in Columbia, he might well have subscribed to the mantra of the hard-bitten American free traders coming up the Missouri River from St. Louis for whom "the only good Indian" was "a dead Indian." Instead he appeared to adopt the corporate paternalism of the HBC, which—in Columbia, at least—sat in stark contrast to American individualism. No one was more surprised than George Simpson himself when he ended up taking two of Concomely's adolescent grandsons with him to the east to be educated.

George Simpson may indeed have been starting to understand and appreciate more fully his custodial role as governor of the Columbia District, and he may indeed have harboured whispers of viceregal yearnings alongside his natural savvy as a chief executive officer. But when it came to the day-to-day, he would rather be doing something active and physical than lingering too long over the ledgers. With his trusted confidant James McMillan (who had completed his survey of the mouth of the Fraser River) again in tow, Simpson moved east on March 16, 1825. On the shore at Fort George as they left were Chinook chief Concomely and his daughter "the fair Princess Chowie," both in tears.

Always up for a little ceremony, they dropped John McLoughlin amid the ongoing construction at Fort Vancouver. (McLoughlin, in his distinguished career as chief factor there, which began on this day, would become the "Father of Oregon.") The following morning Simpson called everyone together and christened the new headquarters with a service that finished with a bottle of his finest HBC rum being smashed on the flag staff as he pronounced, "On behalf of the Honble Hudsons Bay Co^{y} I hereby name this Establishment *Fort Vancouver* God Save King George the 4th," followed by three hearty cheers. Then, with no time to dally, on up the Columbia he went.[9]

On April 22, 1825, Simpson was back at Boat Encampment, the western end of the hundred-mile Athabasca Pass portage. After five hard weeks working their way up the Columbia River, Simpson and his men were counting on finding extra provisions and horses to carry them at this staging point. There were neither. Simpson had left word on the way west that there were to be horses and fresh victuals left on or before the twenty-fifth. Knowing he was three days early, he expected that they might have to make at least part of the way up the Wood River on foot, but, in a letter from François-Antoine Laroque from Jasper House, dated April 2, at the east end of this gut-busting portage (of which he said that he "never saw a document in which there is such a dearth of news or interesting matter")[10] he learned that there would be no provisions and that horses would only be starting their way west near the end of the month. They would have to walk and, to boot, cover the territory without food. Simpson sent ahead two of his best voyageurs, Cadotte and Grand Louis, with only light loads, in the hope that they would get to the other end and ready the canoes that had been left the previous fall. Baggage for the others, which amounted to "their own property and provisions to about 60 lbs. p[er] Man,"[11] was shouldered, and off they went, crossing and re-crossing the Wood River, through waist- and at times chest-deep glacial water.

In almost no time at all, some of the group (likely including Concomely's nine- and ten-year-old grandsons) fell behind, and the rest got spread out on the snow-covered trail. On the second day, some of the Iroquois (who had come west from Canada) who were helping with the transport convinced some of Simpson's men to open a keg of rum they were carrying. Simpson sat and waited for these stragglers, who by the time they staggered in were so drunk that they could not proceed any farther. To add to the insult, Simpson learned that one of the tipplers, in a moment of drunken rage, had tossed his load into the river, sending it cascading back toward the Columbia and further decreasing the available provisions for the rest of the journey. Simpson was so incensed that "on the impulse of the moment" he "was induced to descend to the disagreeable duty of chastising him on the spot with the first stick that came to hand."[12] His fit of temper not yet sated, Simpson smashed a hatchet into another rum keg and poured its contents into the river, apparently conveying unequivocally to the group their leader's resolve to carry on regardless.

It was a four-thousand-foot climb to the peak of Athabasca Pass. As if the problems with food shortages, drunken men, exhausted Chinook children and ice-cold running water weren't enough, the snow deepened as they reached the summit of the pass, leaving them slogging—without snowshoes—in steps that sank eighteen inches to two feet into wet snow over rough rock shingle that chewed up the bottom of their moccasins and left them lame and exhausted. The spring avalanches that boomed all around them only added to the general feeling of foreboding.

But, maniacally focused on leading by example, Simpson called

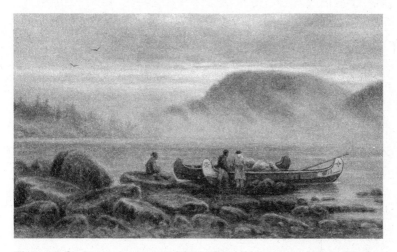

Simpson's business acumen notwithstanding, this was a man who loved to travel and who, often before sunrise, would thunder naked into the water for a quick swim as the men were loading the canoes.

for each man to be issued a glass of rum (though two kegs had been destroyed and they had no food to speak of, they still apparently had wine and spirits in good supply), and together at the Committee's Punch Bowl they raised three cheers and toasted the "Health of their Honours" and carried on—every one of them now capable of moving only with the help of rough aspen walking sticks. Simpson dispatched two more good men, Lesperence and François, to forge ahead to speed the horses, should they encounter them, and to assist with the re-gumming of the canoes at the other end.

On the fifth day of this nasty slog through the mountains, they were once again waist deep in fast-flowing water, as the trail switched back and forth across the Whirlpool River. It was during the twenty-seventh ford of the day, at about ten o'clock in the morning of April 26, that one of the men at the front of the sorry line of stragglers let loose with the best half-hearted whoop he could muster, to let the Governor know that the horses were in sight. With that happy sight came news from the east, including an update on Simpson's old classmate Duncan Finlayson, who had been mortally wounded by the accidental discharge of a gun at Fort Dunvegan and, worse still, news of a fire that had destroyed Norway House and all its contents. Undaunted, Simpson and his faithful servant Tom Taylor, with what men and boys he could muster verbally or otherwise to the continuing task, loaded up the canoes and struck off down the Athabasca River.

With a better response from Laroque at Athabasca Pass, as a result of gubernatorial instructions left on the way west, Simpson was very pleased to learn at Fort Assiniboine that the improved cross-country trail to Fort Edmonton had been substantially cut and that Chief Factor MacIntosh had already left for Edmonton and for the North Saskatchewan route with his returns. Simpson left the newly gummed canoes and once again took to horseback for the eighty-mile trek to Edmonton. In a journal entry written near the completion of this overland crossing, he crowed about his own brilliance in coming up with this revolutionary idea:

> I am now from experience enabled to say that New Caledonia and Lesser Slave Lake can be supplied by this route instead of Athabasca and the Beaver river which will be a very great Saving in Men's Wages, Provisions &c &c; indeed the change of routes I have determined on will on these two Districts alone yield a saving to the Company of at least 12 to £1500 p[er] Annum if the company determine on continuing transport business of New Caledonia with York Factory and further I am satisfied that this discovery of Mine (as I alone can claim the merit thereof, it never having been even dreamt of by any other) will enable us to do the Peace River business at a reduction of one third on the usual expenses of that place as the Peace River outfits & returns can be taken by Horses in 5 Days between Dunvegan & Lesser Slave Lake, by Boats in 4 or 5 Days between Lesser Slave Lake and Fort Assiniboine, by Horses between the latter place and Edmonton in 3 or 4 Days and by Boats between that and York Factory and the difference of Expense between Boat and Canoe transport is at a fair estimate 33 1/3^d p Cent.[13]

Still pushing the season at Fort Edmonton, on May Day he learned from guides there that the brigades were not scheduled to head east for another fortnight, due to ice and low water in the running parts of the river and to ice that remained on the lakes. But Simpson struck out anyway, intent on walking over ice and dragging through or carrying his canoe beside shallows, the party now hunting as it went to keep loads light and mouths more or less fed along the way.

The tough physical circumstances of this journey did not seem to interfere with Simpson's thinking about the management and organization of the company. At Edmonton he received a variety of other mail—more about the Norway House fire, but also about crop failure the previous year at Red River. Although when he had first heard news of the fire he had intended to go as quickly as possible straight across country on the North Saskatchewan to Norway House, the events at Red River make him change his mind. He decided instead to turn southeast at Fort Carleton and travel five hundred miles (he pegged it as eight hundred in his journal) overland to Red River instead of following the voyageur highway.

The story of this crossing is as harrowing as the group's ascent of Athabasca Pass, with hostile Indian groups and navigational problems layered on top of harsh weather, exhaustion, periodic starvation and now, with the advance of spring, "muschetoes [mosquitoes] . . . most tormenting." Measure of Simpson's resolve to carry on is evidenced in accounts of this journey that describe his servant, Tom Taylor, and George Bird getting lost on a side trip to hunt birds to feed the party and that note Simpson's decision to leave them behind to an uncertain fate after just one half-day of looking. On another occasion they came to an impossibly deep ford in the Qu'Appelle River, after getting lost. Some of Simpson's party, of course, could not swim, and there was no wood available on the prairie to build a raft. They had nearly decided to kill a few horses to make skin canoes of their hides, when, without further discussion, Simpson stripped and, with a few of his things, swam the river. Three others who could swim followed suit. The non-swimmers, inspired or shamed by Simpson's example, held onto the tails of the remaining horses for dear life with one hand as they whipped the skinny horses across deep waters with the other. There was no way they were going to be left behind by this madman of a leader.

Not long after that—with Taylor and Bird still unaccounted for, the Chinook boys in unknown condition and the rest of the party cold, hungry and totally worn out—Simpson decided that he and James McMillan should forge ahead alone to see if they might reach White Horse Plain and the home of Simpson's friend Cuthbert Grant. That plan too went from bad to worse. The two emaciated officers wallowed into a nine-mile-long swamp complex that put them again into waist-deep water, but instead of snow, this time they faced mud. When they did arrive, Grant, as luck would have it, was not home, but they were able to hire a nearby Indian to go to Fort Garry to alert the officers there of the Governor's approach and to send back fresh horses and clothes.

So eager was Simpson to finish the journey that when the horses arrived, without checking the saddle bags (which contained food), he left McMillan and galloped to Fort Garry, announcing his arrival by pounding on the door of the stockade at midnight on Saturday, May 28, 1825, having performed in eighty-two days "one of the most dangerous and harassing Journeys ever undertaken in the Country through which thank God I have got with no injury or inconvenience worthy of Notice"[14] (as long as you don't count the dead horses or the exhausted and missing men scattered all along the route).

After tending to the business of the settlement for a week or so, Simpson boarded another express canoe and made his way to the site of the rebuilding at Norway House, where, thanks to Providence and a dollop of good luck, he was reunited with Tom Taylor, though he thought not to mention it in his journal of the day. It was only in a subsequent volume, detailing travels of 1842–43, that he thought to tell the real story of "injury and inconvenience" that very nearly resulted in the death of his most trusted servant. Here, for the record, is that account:

After abandoning all hope of falling upon the track of our party, they set themselves seriously to work in order to find their way to some encampment of the savages, or to one of the Company's posts. After a day or two, their ammunition was expended, and their flints became useless, while their feet were lacerated by the thorns, timber, stones, and prickly grass. They had no other clothing than their trousers and shirts, having parted from us in the heat of the day; so that they were now exposed to the chills of the night, without even the comfort of a fire—a privation which placed them, as it were, at the mercy of the wolves. From day to day, they lived on whatever the chances of the wilderness afforded them, such as roots and bark, and eggs in every stage of progress.

At length, after fourteen days of intense suffering, despair began to take possession of their minds, and they were strongly tempted to lie down and die. Next morning, however, the instinctive love of life prevailed, and they slowly and painfully crept forward, when suddenly the sight of our track revived their energies and their hopes. Almost intoxicated with joy, they followed the clue of safety; till at length, after growing more and more indistinct for a time, it entirely disappeared from their eyes. At this awful moment of disappointment and despondency, Tom Taylor, as if led by a merciful Providence to the spot, slowly recognized the scenes of his infant rambles, though he had never seen them since his childhood.

Life was now in the one scale almost as certainly as death was in the other; and under the influence of this definite motive of exertion, the two famished and lacerated wanderers reached before night the Company's establishment on Swan River. Being well acquainted with Mr. [Miles] MacDonnell, the gentleman in charge, they crawled rather than walked to his private room, standing before him with their torn and emaciated limbs, while their haggard cheeks and glaring eyes gave them the appearance of maniacs. After a minute inspection of his visitors, Mr. MacDonnell, with the aid of sundry expletives, ascertained by degrees that one of his friends was "The Governor's Tom"; and having thus penetrated to the bottom of the mystery, he nursed them back into condition, with the kindness of a father and the skill of a doctor, and then carried them to Norway House.[15]

———

In some ways it was a very different George Simpson who boarded the HBC ship at York Factory that fall and, finally, made his way back across the Atlantic and home to Scotland for the first time in over five years. Correspondence shows that he stopped in Stromness en route, and spent time with his aunt Mary in Dingwall (her husband, Simpson's former teacher Alexander, had died some years before), where he encouraged his cousins Thomas, who was at Aberdeen University, Alexander and Aemilius to consider careers in North America with the HBC. And, having very likely seen son Jordie at Red River or Fort Alexander and daughter Maria with Betsy at York Factory, he would likely have checked in with his Scottish progeny as well. Maria Louisa would have been eleven and Isabella nine, and, if they were not with Aunt Mary in Dingwall, they may well have been with Simpson's uncle Duncan and his wife in the comfortable country house and gardens at Bellevue overlooking the Beauly Firth, a short carriage ride across the uplands of Black Isle from the Cromarty Firth.

But Simpson was never fully a parent, never a doting father or uncle. He was a business operative who, through his own efforts and with his own bootstraps and a bit of luck, had tasted power and influence of near royal dimension. When he did get to London and sit down with Andrew Colvile and the rest of the Committee, they reinforced the thirty-six-year-old governor's success with news that they had recalled William Williams altogether and that the "bastard son of Dingwall" was now in charge of both the Southern and the Northern departments. Although this new charge would not be made official until the following year, and it would not be until 1839 that the two departments would be officially merged into one, this turn of events put George Simpson in charge of a massive business operation with more than a hundred forts (smaller than the number he had inherited immediately following amalgamation of the two companies) spanning a domain that included fully one-twelfth of the earth's land surface.

———

PART II

THE LITTLE EMPEROR

CHAPTER X

A Man on the Ground

The London George Simpson entered in December 1825 would have been every bit as close as the bustling city he had hurriedly left nearly six years before. Five years of pure snows and fragrant conifers in Rupert's Land would have made the experience of a winter rain as stark a contrast as that described by Charles Dickens in *Little Dorrit*: "In the country, the rain would have developed a thousand fresh scents, and every drop would have had its bright association with some beautiful form of growth or life. In the city, it developed only foul stale smells, and was a sickly, lukewarm, dirt-stained, wretched addition to the gutters."[1] Though he was anything but a sentimental man, there must have been for Simpson at least some nostalgia for his decade spent in London town as he made his way from the Thames-side docks past the Tower of London and up St. Dunstan's, St. Mary's or Fish Street Hill toward his old haunts on Great Tower Street.

Before any kind of formal audience with the London Committee, however, Simpson would have found lodging, if not with his friend and mentor Andrew Colvile, who lived five minutes' walk east of Hudson's Bay House on Fenchurch Street, then with his uncle Geddes at New Grove House in Bromley. And for the returning governor there would

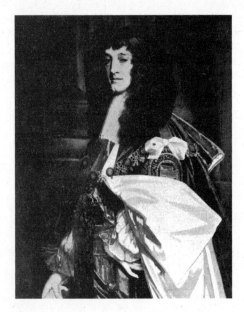

*Prince Rupert of the Rhine,
first governor of the Company
of Adventurers of England
Trading into Hudson's Bay,
whose portrait hung in the
boardroom at 3/4 Fenchurch
Street.*

also have been an early stop at his London tailor or a fine haberdasher who, in outfitting him with shirts, collars, cuffs, vests, trousers and jackets in the latest style, might have commented in generous terms about what five years in the fur trade had done to improve the compact governor's physique. The clothier might have also noticed a slightly more officious bearing to the man who had come back from Rupert's Land, thinking back to the young clerk he had come to know during his years at the sugar brokerage. Had Simpson stayed with his uncle Geddes, these new clothes might have been appreciated by his young cousin Frances, as her father and his nephew shared stories of the fur trade and the sugar trade over post-prandial cigars and brandy by the fire. Thirteen-year-old Frances was fragile and shy but beautiful in her own way and, at this point in her privileged life, blissfully unaware that in five years she would be married to this balding red-headed little dandy who'd just blown in off the North Atlantic.

The London Committee gathered at noon on Wednesdays to review the week's business of the Hudson's Bay Company at Hudson's Bay

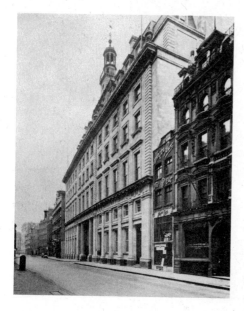

When the HBC outgrew its headquarters at Scrivener's Hall in 1696 it moved to the home of a former lord mayor, Sir John Fleet. The building, seen here after a new facade was installed in 1930, has since been demolished to make way for newer structures in the heart of what is still the bustling business district of central London.

House, at numbers 3 and 4 Fenchurch Street, where their predecessors had met for more than a century to direct from afar the operations in Rupert's Land. When the company had been formed by royal charter in 1670, its first governor, Prince Rupert of the Rhine, had convened meetings of directors in his home. But by 1682, the Company of Adventurers of England Trading into Hudson's Bay had grown sufficiently to warrant the lease of Scrivener's Hall and a small warehouse off Cheapside to conduct its London affairs. By 1696, the company had outgrown these first official premises as well, and an agreement was made to take over the stately downtown home of former lord mayor of London Sir John Fleet at 3/4 Fenchurch Street.[2]

Inside, Hudson's Bay House would have smelled like lemon oil, dust, old leather and men, with a whiff of unseasoned fur thrown in for good measure. Descriptions of the interior mention high white plaster ceilings, tall doors and dark mahogany woodwork, brass lamps and green velvet swags up the broad main staircase. One late-nineteenth-century description calls the upstairs Court Room "dark and dirty" (which

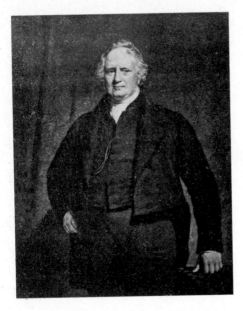

John Henry Pelly, who was governor of the HBC during Simpson's tenure, from 1822 to 1852, was held in high regard by George Simpson. Simpson's only son with his wife Frances was named after Pelly.

makes sense given the north-facing windows that opened onto a narrow street lined with similarly imposing multi-storey buildings), its straight-backed wooden chairs darkened to near black from decades of tobacco-stained air inside that was worse some days than the coal-smoked air outside. Gazing down from a place of prominence on an interior wall was a portrait of the HBC's first governor, Prince Rupert, resplendent in lace ruffles and finery, looking with his shoulder-length black curls as woolly as the standard poodle called Boye that he reputedly took with him into battle on some occasions as a commander of the royalist cavalry during the English Civil War. But lest anyone think this London hub of all fur trade operations in North America was bereft of vestiges of the land that was its raison d'être, an 1867 book about the curiosities of London notes that in this main meeting room of Hudson's Bay House hung a "vast pair" of moose antlers weighing 56 pounds and a near-life-sized painting of a 1,229-pound elk in all its ungual glory.

During Simpson's absence, the chair of the London Committee, Joseph Berens Jr.—son of Joseph Berens Sr. and grandson of Herman

Berens, both of whom had also been on the Committee—had departed, and former East India Company sea captain John Henry Pelly had become governor,[3] the latest of generations of Pellys to serve the HBC. As Simpson sat down at the big board table in the Court Room to receive congratulations for his five remarkable years of work in Rupert's Land, along with Berens and Pelly there were seven other Committee members—all of whom were shareholders, and most of whom had deep roots in the company through either family or marriage. Simpson, for his part, given his taste for gossip and insatiable need to know the nature of his friends, allies and possible enemies, had probably made it his business to know at least as much about each of them as they did about him.

Benjamin Harrison, a cousin and brother-in-law to John Henry Pelly, had been brought onto the Committee in 1809 as an outspoken social reformer and member of the Clapham Sect; the Quaker libertarian views might have curried favour for the British government's perpetuation of the HBC charter through his natural and convincing push toward good works with North American Aboriginal peoples. Nicholas Garry, the bachelor of the Committee, whom Simpson had met during the post-amalgamation Councils at Norway House and York Factory in the summer of 1821, was there as well. By now, Simpson would have learned that Garry was, like himself, a bastard, raised by his father's brother, Thomas Langley. The latter, a long-standing member of the London Committee, had convinced Garry to invest in the HBC and subsequently to join its governance group. Also at the table were Thomas Pitt, descendant of Benjamin Pitt, the eighth governor; John Halkett, business associate and brother-in-law to the newly departed Thomas Douglas, 5th earl of Selkirk; and William Smith, parliamentarian and long-standing secretary of the London Committee.

But Simpson's strongest connection to the London Committee was through his friend, mentor and manipulator Andrew Colvile. Colvile had come onto the Committee in the spring of 1810, at a time during the early days of the war with the NWC when HBC stock was seriously depressed, and had almost single-handedly worked out a "retrench-ment system" to see the HBC back to profitability. The final and most important element in that system was the installation on the ground in Rupert's Land of a person who could translate the plans of a distant directorate into results in a complex and far-flung wilderness business operation. Colvile had found George Simpson and brought him to the Committee.

The Committee had given Simpson his charge and sent him packing to Rupert's Land. And by all indications Simpson had delivered. To appreciate the measure of the Committee's effusive welcome back to its polished wooden table at Hudson's Bay House in the winter of 1825–26, one needs to get some measure of how the HBC functioned before Colvile's retrenchment system was proposed.

———

Prior to Colvile's arrival, there had been really only one simple credit/ debit method of accounting or budgeting. Budgets, such as they were, were a balance of "outfits" and "indents." Indents consisted of a wish list of items for trade and consumption by HBC personnel in Rupert's Land that was sent with the season's fur returns on (preferably) the last ship of the year heading for England from York Factory or any of the posts on James Bay. Outfits consisted of a shipment of actual goods to be traded or consumed in the course of the year that, providing ice and weather made it possible, arrived on the first ship of the year from England. Even with the vagaries of fur sales on English and European markets, the indent/outfit system had worked reasonably well, especially during the first century of HBC operations, when the company had only coastal posts and when margins of difference between the cost of the outfit and the monies received for the sale of furs, even if delayed by surpluses or sluggish markets, were sufficient to absorb any inefficiencies in the sys-tem and still allow acceptable dividends to be paid to shareholders.

When the HBC opened inland posts in order to compete with the NWC, its financial operations became much more complex. The company now had to keep track of a much bigger network of men and goods over larger and larger distances. There were increasing delays in shipping and financial transactions. Trade with Aboriginal trappers carried its own complications. A move to divide the inland operation into districts, each associated with one or other of the bayside posts, helped, but as expansion continued, the affairs of the HBC remained an accounting nightmare. The London Committee, which apparently had no interest in actually setting foot in Rupert's Land, flailed away with "seriously incomplete information"[4] about the business mechanics of the actual trade.

The extent of the problems created by competition from the NWC was reflected in the HBC's bottom line almost from the moment the Montreal traders started getting seriously organized in the 1770s. A successful naval attack on York Factory by a French commander, the comte de La Pérouse, in 1781 further complicated matters to the point that in 1783, for the first time in sixty-five years, the Committee paid no dividends at all. The HBC returned to modest dividend payments during the remaining years of the eighteenth century, but often these were paid not by returns of a given year but from balances built up in the monopoly years. Evidence of financial trouble was even more obvious by 1806, when a 4 per cent dividend was paid—in spite of the fact that the company owed £25,000 to three Committee members and a further £17,000 to the Bank of England on a company capitalized at only about twice that amount of debt. Further financial relief was sought from the Bank of England in 1808, and in 1809, acknowledging the seriousness of its situation, the Committee again suspended dividend payments altogether, which remained more or less the financial story of the HBC until Simpson's arrival in 1820.[5]

Before Simpson's arrival and the amalgamation of the two companies, however, Colvile's retrenchment system added clarity to the indent/outfit budgeting system, which helped quench the hemorrhage of value that resulted from waste and inefficiency inside the North American operations of the HBC. Most significant among Colvile's recommendations was the establishment of a workable standard of trade, which was a more complicated problem than it might at first appear.

The actual "trade" on which the Hudson's Bay Company had been built was an exchange of manufactured goods for dried animal skins. For the first 140 years of the company's existence, HBC trade was as simple as that. The standard of trade was, in the early days, the hide of a beaver: so many prime beaver pelts were exchanged for a blanket or a gun. In 1733 at Fort Albany on James Bay, for example, one prime beaver from one family's winter inventory of, say, three hundred such pelts would buy one pound of tobacco, or two pounds of sugar, or five pounds of shot, or twelve dozen buttons or a gallon of brandy. A blanket cost one beaver, the same as two yards of cotton broadcloth, while a gun cost ten times that.

As the beaver was trapped out in areas within easy reach of Hudson Bay at York Factory, and as the market shifted to mink, marten, otter, wolf and muskrat, equivalencies in these other furs were expressed in terms of "made beaver." For example, by the 1806 standard of trade, a prime buck deer pelt was equivalent to one made beaver (MB), while it took two well-stretched winter weasels or otters, six muskrats or twenty squirrels to reach the equivalent of one MB. Rarer and more valuable furs tipped the equivalencies the other way: a wolverine, for example, was worth two MB and a good-sized black bear was worth up to five MB. And, as one might expect with increased numbers of forts and trading establishments, the HBC recognized and delivered simple coinage in the MB standard as well, which was convenient for the trappers but caused accountancy havoc. The issuing post, which received the furs and issued the credit, had to somehow reconcile financially with the accounts of the post at which the credit was spent.

But the real problem with the MB standard of trade was not so much the unit itself (although this was changed to actual currency values about the time Simpson arrived in fur country) as the way in which its value was determined—in England, by the London Committee. The distant establishment of a standard of trade had worked reasonably well when both furs and manufactured goods and comestibles were traded in posts along the shores of James and Hudson bays, but as soon as the HBC moved inland, complexities and inequalities were added to the business equation, not least the cost of shipping. A fur in the warehouse at Fort Chipewyan, for example, had to be transported south by canoe, over the La Loche (Methye) Portage, down to Cumberland House and east to York Factory and London before it could be sold at auction, whereas a fur traded directly at York Factory would have only a small portion of that handling and shipping expense attached to it. The same applied to trade goods, especially bulky or heavy items like blankets and guns, that the HBC had to lug upriver and inland. Economists Gary Spraakman and Alison Wilkie have described how Colvile's retrenchment system made important improvements to the HBC's trade standard by abolishing the old standard and replacing it with a more adaptable and realistic convention:

> Instead [of the old system,] the traders responsible for posts were allowed to trade with the aborigines with the standard judged most advisable and suitable to local circumstances. They were provided with the invoiced costs to port (i.e. York) for all articles consigned. From the landed costs they were to add an "advance" markup for all expenses, risk, and a reasonable profit to the Company. The Committee provided a list of recent fur prices to serve "to regulate you in some measure in trading with the aborigines at the same time . . . you must add the officers' and men's wages and all other expenses." In effect, the standard of trade from 1810 that pertained into the 1820s and for decades thereafter was just as demanding as the rigid committee-imposed standard of trade that had existed for 140 years, but it became flexible or adjustable for costs which differed in line with distances from ports.[6]

This flexible standard of trade was, in theory and (to a smaller extent) in practice, a workable way for the HBC to keep track of business activity in Rupert's Land, but Colvile went beyond this, with other new management accounting techniques. First among these was an instruction to start keeping systematic track of inventories at the individual post level—not only of outfits as they arrived and were traded out, but also of fur stocks as they came in and were baled for storage and transit. Balance books at each of the trading rooms across Rupert's Land thus helped to keep track of what went in and out of the warehouses, and goods damaged in transit or given as part of a deal-sweetening gift to encourage a trader were also recorded. In addition to providing a day-to-day measure of operating efficiencies at each post, this inventory, in concert with other record books, also helped post managers make more informed assessments of needs when it came time to write up their indents for the following season. For if there was one thing the London Committee had noticed, and the situation was exaggerated even more by the time Andrew Colvile came on board in 1810, it was that with the profusion of inland posts and the increasing competition with the Nor'Westers, post managers' wish lists had very quickly exceeded the company's maximum capacity to ship goods across the Atlantic. More sophisticated budgeting, flexible standards of trade, inventory records and operating records were all ways to reel in the freewheeling trade and return the HBC to steady profitability.

The only problem with Colvile's retrenchment system, for all its theoretical strengths and proposed improvements to the way business could be conducted in the field, was that control of the whole effort was situated an ocean away. London Committee secretary William Smith came up with some standard forms and specially designed record books, but the long and the short of it was that there was a scarcity of on-the-ground accounting knowledge in Rupert's Land. In even shorter supply, it seemed, was motivation. Why should traders care about matters that would generate profits for shareholders but have very little if any effect on their daily lives? A profit-sharing system for chief factors and chief traders, inspired by the Nor'Westers' ways of doing business, was one part of Colvile's revitalization plan, but this too failed.

What the HBC needed under Colvile's retrenchment system was a man on the ground in Rupert's Land. And this is why Andrew Colvile, having considered the best and brightest young businessmen in London, recruited George Simpson, and why Simpson, with his business acumen and his head for figures and detail, coupled with his insatiable drive to see for himself the day-to-day operations of the trade, had such a lasting impact on the fortunes of the HBC after 1821.

The sugar trade had taught Simpson about balance sheets, standards and the importance of keeping meticulous records of a business operation. It had also impressed upon him the value of time management, which became the main pillar in his fixation on "oeconomy," as characterized by his dashing like a madman around North America by snowshoe and canoe. And just as he had read and interpreted the minutiae of the deed poll for Nicholas Garry and the assembled chief factors in the first meetings of the new HBC after amalgamation with the NWC, so he attacked with similar zeal not only the challenge of imposing Colvile's retrenchment system, but also the business of teaching the officers of the trade the value of these numbers. And, unlike any previous HBC operative on the west side of the Atlantic Ocean, Simpson made it his business to know by all means available to him—from gossip to unabashed interrogation—who was who and what was happening in the trade. Simpson knew the processes of business management well enough to know that his own authority to enforce the London Committee's rules or to make up new ones to fit what he learned on his travels had to be institutionalized in the written proceedings of the company. Even more important, his authority had to be seen to be enforced—hence his very theatrical and carefully orchestrated dressing down of Colin Robertson at one of his first Northern Councils.

Simpson chose a velvet-gloved approach for some, a lead pipe for others. It seemed not to matter to him how he achieved his ends. Knowing it would please the London Committee—and his mentor, Andrew Colvile—Simpson raised the standards of record keeping in the trade with Machiavellian vigour. For example, in the minutes of his fifth and last Council before his triumphant return to London to receive the congratulations of the Committee, he drafted an innocuous-looking resolution designed to "prevent all misapprehension irregularity or inattention on the subject of Accounts":

> 95. That all Commissioned Officers be directed and considered
> bound to keep regular and satisfactory Accounts as hereinafter
> pointed out in special Resolves, of the business under their respective
> managements to be annually transmitted to the person superintend-
> ing such District and through him to the Accountant at the Depot in
> order that the same be examined and entered, and where defective be
> produced for the inspection and determination of Council.[7]

When it came to getting things done, though, Simpson was never a one-punch manager. Resolution 95 was a tap on the jaw compared to the roundhouse punch that he slipped into the end of the minutes. By then the Governor, through his Inner and Outer Circle tours and his run to Columbia and back, knew that there was a problem with the field implementation of the London Committee's retrenchment plans. For too long the Committee had shipped across the ocean edicts that either missed the point or were too easy to ignore with impunity by the men of the trade. The Committee's credibility was spent, and Simpson knew that to regain control he had to regain the attention, if not the trust, of his officers. So he blew into their places of residence with bluster and flair to set them an example to follow, but he also set into the minutes mechanisms to punish any and all who would stray from the company way. To wit, the final text and resolutions in the 1825 minutes—which were part of the post-amalgamation policy of inclusion written by and for the men themselves. The devious Simpson had engineered a way for the men to essentially scold themselves and set up a regimen of con-sequences for continued bad behaviour. The last two resolutions were prefaced as follows:

> Much irregularity inconvenience & loss having been experienced
> from a general inattention to neglect of & deviation from the minutes

of Council on the part of Commissioned Gentlemen, instances whereof are too numerous & generally admitted to require examples [it is resolved]

145. That wherever a recurrence is detected unsupported by such forcible reasons or unavoidable causes as may be conclusive in the estimation of Council as to the propriety thereof, such deviations will be most exemplarily noticed & suitable Mulcts [fines] or other estimated damages imposed on this individual trespasser as the council may determine.

And in order that no plea of ignorance be adduced by those unavoidably prevented from taking copies thereof on this ground.

146. That a Compend or Epitomé comprehending the substance thereof be transmitted from hence accompanying the other requisite public documents for each District p[er] winter express.

This missive was duly signed by all in attendance, including Colin Robertson and the illustrious John Clarke.

Simpson's strength as a manager went well beyond the simple application of accounting principles from head office or working to inspire, cajole, scare and—with luck—win the respect if not the admiration of his unit heads. He seemed to understand implicitly that with the move inland came increasing amounts of business uncertainty from a host of sources, an uncertainty that was consuming the momentum of the trade. New policies might have some effect on systemic waste in the system, but they could never improve the attitudes of the Aboriginal trading partners toward the company as a result of the fur trade war. They could never increase the capacity of chief traders and chief factors to understand the large-scale mechanics of the trade. They could never overcome opportunism on the part of "suppliers" spoiled by extravagant gifts from the last days of competition, or on the part of Baymen, from the woodcutter to the chief factor, who would, because of human nature, place self-interest over company interest almost every time. George Simpson understood in his bones that all these less tangible sources of business loss—factors considered "transaction costs"—were killing profits for the HBC. Until George Simpson arrived, the London Committee saw the financial effects of friction on the operation but had no way of knowing exactly the causes or sources of that resistance. Simpson changed that.

Simpson's other gift as a business leader was equally mercurial and difficult to define: the man had charisma. After five years in the trade, there was no one he had not affected. He had summarily closed forts. He had reduced the workforce by nearly half, often through less than gentle means. He had pounded on tables and hammered on people with his fists—whatever it took to get the job done. He had set a pace that had run lesser men into the ground. He had set policies that he himself had contravened. He had niggled over minute details and driven some colleagues to despair with his preoccupations with "oeconomy" (for example, he had insisted on smaller and smaller boat crews and larger and larger loads, making the canoes and York boats more sluggish and dangerous in rapids and on portages).

And yet George Simpson had charmed the men of the trade. As he left for London in the fall of 1825, he had in his pocket a letter signed by the entire Council, who had just reproved themselves for bad behaviour, which read as follows:

York Factory 9th July 1825

Dear Sir

Happy of having an opportunity of assembling together for the purpose of publickly expressing our sentiments, on a subject on which there exists such perfect unanimity: and equally unmoved by flattery as uninfluenced by example—We the undersigned, composing the majority of the Chief Factors and Chief Traders of the Northern Department, on closing the more important business and public discussions of the season at which you so ably presided, do most cordially congratulate you on your safe return to this place,

and tender you our most grateful acknowledgements for the devoted
attention and unremitting exertions you have so uniformly evinced
throughout your whole management, more particularly for the great
retrenchment and amelioration introduced by your trip inland in
1822; the spirited and disinterested manner in which you undertook
that of last year to Columbia, in which District your Personal influence, masterly arrangements and decisive measures, have already
been productive of the happiest effects and have opened a field on
which to act with confidence and when to look forward with expectation. Still are you conferring additional obligations and about to
expose yourself to the most painful sacrifices, by the handsome
tender of your services, personally to superintend and direct the
execution of measures, so ably planned embracing such a variety
of objects and involving such important results and although your
temporary absence may excite a feeling of regret, yet we are fully convinced much benefit will be derived from your extensive Knowledge
and personal representations to the Honorable Committee, whose
late gratuity and augmentation of your Salary[8] preceded, as well as
accompanied by their most unqualified approbation of your conduct reflect equal credit on you as they are honorable to them—and
wishing you a pleasant and auspicious voyage and happy return to
head and direct our Councils. And in the fond expectations that
the Honorable Committee will permit this blunt and unvarnished
expression of our sentiments, to be recorded in the Minute Book of
their Honorable Board annexed to the minutes of the season, and
implicitly relying on such indulgence and meantime favored with
your permission we would feel much gratified to record the same in
the public Minute Book of this place.

We remain with much respect and unfeigned regard

> Dear Sir
> Your most Obedient
> and very faithful Servants (signed)

In due course, when this letter was written into the minutes of the fall 1825 deliberations of the London Committee along with notes on meetings that Simpson himself attended, this apparently unanimous vote of support from Simpson's immediate underlings would have made the London governors just that much more sure that their intuitions about his performance and their expressions of reward for increased profitability—in the form of a one-time 25 per cent bonus and a permanent 20 per cent raise on a salary that was a hundred times the pay of the HBC's least remunerated employees in Rupert's Land—had been 100 per cent correct. And with the continuing class distinctions between men of the trade and men of the London Committee, and the continuing disconnect between what was really going on in Rupert's Land and the picture painted for London in the correspondence of the trade, there was really no way the Committee could have read this letter as anything other than complimentary—albeit overwritten to the point of fawning, perhaps—especially without benefit of actually talking to the likes of Colin Robertson and John Clarke. But they knew how the game was played, as did Simpson when he wrote back to the Council members, for the benefit of the record books, on the same day he received his letter:

Gentlemen

The very handsome and complimentary expression of your approbation of my public conduct, conveyed in a Letter I had the honor to receive from you of this date, inspires a feeling of pleasure and satisfaction in my mind which I am at a loss for language to express.

My humble exertions to promote the general interests which you are pleased to estimate so highly, could have done little towards attaining the object in view, had I not been favored with your liberal and Friendly support and uniformly steady co-operation, for which my most grateful acknowledgements are due, and to *our joint* endeavours under the enlightened direction of the Honorable Committee can alone be ascribed the present flattering appearance of our affairs.

The toils of business are to me a pleasure, situated as I have the good fortune to be, in the confidence of Employers whose high respectability, honor and talent are so eminently conspicuous, and in the estimation of coadjutors who from possessing every good quality I shall ever be proud to call Friends, and I trust you will believe me sincere, when I assure you that I am at the summit of my ambition in the place I hold in their confidence and your esteem, which I shall endeavour to retain by the utmost exertions of which my body and mind are capable to promote the general interests.

It is but fair to admit that I am too vain of the honor you have done me, to affect an unwillingness that the same should be recorded in our Minute Book, but must at the same time take the liberty of entreating that this humble tribute of the heavy obligations I am under towards you, be annexed thereto; and with sentiments of the highest regard

> I have the honor to be
> Gentlemen
> Your faithful & obliged Servt.
> (signed) GEO. SIMPSON

CHAPTER XI

"THE CHIEF
WHOSE DOG SINGS"

With the endorsement of the commissioned officers of the trade, and with a raise in pay and a near doubling of his responsibilities from the Committee, it was a different George Simpson who sent for a carriage on February 26, 1826, to take him from Fenchurch Street west through the still green English winter countryside back to Liverpool and the noisy wharf where the packet ship *Manchester* was being loaded. Instead of wondering how the fur trade might have been different from the sugar trade and trying to imagine life in the wilderness of Rupert's Land, as he had on departure almost six years to the day before, he now had a working knowledge of North America from coast to coast—places, names, faces, the rush of white water, the pungency of dried pelts, the crunch of snowshoes on crusted snow, the squeak of hand-split cedar ribs on dusky white bark, the drafty chills of winter nights and the warmth and wordless satisfaction of covert liaisons with women he'd spirited in and out of his tents and quarters hither and yon.

Added to his visceral memories of the trade were the political realities of the HBC's place in North American politics. While in London, the Committee had been impressed with his detailed replies to questions posed by Henry Addington, permanent undersecretary for foreign affairs, on behalf of his minister of the Crown, regarding the state of affairs in Oregon Country. This trip to London had deeply underscored Simpson's pivotal position, in the absence of any other agents of the British government, in developing strategies to maintain Britain's hold on contested territories west of Lake Superior, in Columbia. There was really no one else with George Simpson's detailed intelligence of North America. Lord Bathurst, British secretary of state for war and the colonies, like the London Committee was in his own way grappling with the situation from a distance. Simpson's pivotal role as information gatherer and on-the-ground creator/enactor of British foreign policy no doubt put a jaunty cock to his beaver topper as he boarded the westbound packet.

Evidence that he was taking the American negotiations seriously was the presence of his cousin by marriage Aemilius Simpson on the Liverpool wharf that day. The other Simpson boys from Dingwall were intrigued with George's stories. Thomas, a bright young man who was at Aberdeen University and showing much promise, declined his cousin's invitation initially but would eventually catch up with Simpson in North America, as would his younger brother, Alexander. Aemilius, however, jumped at the chance for a new adventure.

George and Aemilius had been classmates at Dingwall Academy. Just before his father married George's aunt Mary, Aemilius had joined the Royal Navy and served throughout the Napoleonic Wars. But like so many bright young officers, just as his career was taking off, the conflict subsided and the lure of standing shoulder to shoulder with Nelson at the bridge was replaced with half pay and moping around home in Dingwall awaiting recall to active service. Simpson offered Aemilius a post as a hydrographer and surveyor for the HBC, with the express task of ground-proofing the line of the forty-ninth parallel at Pembina, east of the Rockies, to prevent HBC traders from running afoul of the Americans (and vice versa). After that Aemilius would go to Oregon

Country, and maybe put his seamanship skills to work on the Pacific Coast. And so it was that the two Simpsons settled into the salon of the *Manchester* for another fast (five-week) but chilly winter crossing of the North Atlantic.

Later correspondence with his friend from his previous westward packet crossing, J.G. McTavish, would reveal that even with his hefty salary, Simpson himself admitted to being penny wise and pound foolish when it came to personal expenditures. On what the Governor might have spent these sums of money one might guess—speculative investments, support for his daughters in the UK and for his growing "family" in Rupert's Land—but by all accounts, especially at this juncture in his life when he became the lord and master of all HBC affairs in North America, a goodly sum would have been spent on his wardrobe: tailored suits and hand-stitched percale cotton shirts with starched detachable collars and cuffs affixed with tortoiseshell studs and engraved golden cufflinks; silk cravats and brocade vests; beaver hats with monogrammed leather travelling hat cases; custom-made shoes with silver buckles; classic capes, at least one of which was made of rich red Royal Stuart[1] tartan lined with blue Bath coating.

With these accoutrements and his personal complements of fine wines, French brandy (available again on the British market following the end of the Napoleonic Wars), Cheshire cheese, boiled eggs and pickled meats from the London markets all neatly packed up in brass-cornered mahogany travelling cases, Simpson and his cousin landed in New York, steamered north on the Hudson and bumped their way through mud and spring snow to La Prairie and Lachine, where in due course, with a coterie of the finest Caughnawaga Mohawks and the most able *engagés*, they would transfer their loads to express canoes and continue west through Lake of Two Mountains and on up the Ottawa River to Rupert's Land.

Although he was, as always, in a hurry, Simpson was energized by Montreal, and spent twelve days there on company business before actually moving on (he may even have made a few inquiries as to where a man of his new station might take up residence)—enough to confirm a notion in the back of his mind that Lachine, rather than the social back-waters of York Factory, Moose Factory or Red River, might be a place for the HBC's chief man in North America to spend his winters directing the proceedings of the trade in relative comfort.

By June they were at Fort Douglas, in the Red River settlement. Aemilius continued on to execute his first survey but, because of his affiliation with the Governor, he did not enter the service of the HBC as anything like a neutral player in company politics.

Beneath the polite smiles as John McLoughlin had taken the helm at Fort Vancouver a year previous was a fundamental disagreement with Simpson about how subsequent trade could and should be done on the west coast. While they both agreed that moving company headquarters to the north side of the river was advantageous and that using the Snake River Expedition to essentially trap out the country south and east of the Columbia was wise (because American free traders would be less likely to inhabit a territory with no fur), McLoughlin held the view that other trade should be done from established posts, such as Fort Langley, which James McMillan was just getting started on the lower Fraser River after his 1824–25 survey. With his first-hand knowledge of the lay of the land and its relationship to the sea, of the many regional Aboriginal tribes and their enmity for Europeans and for each other, and of the Russians, who, despite their *ukase*, were half a world away from their resupply points, Simpson thought that the Pacific trade should be con-ducted from the decks of ships plying the coast. Appointing Aemilius to go west as "surveyor and hydrographer" was necessary for its own sake, but, even better, it meant that Simpson would have an ally in Columbia with Royal Navy experience who could oversee the construction of, and perhaps eventually captain, a dedicated trade vessel on the west coast.

Travelling with the 1826 Columbia brigade, Aemilius completed his survey that summer. The surveying activity was suspended that winter while he supervised the building of two vessels at Fort Vancouver. The following spring, he took command of a ship called *Cadboro* that had brought supplies from England, and sailed north with materials and protection for the crews building Fort Langley on the Fraser. Several years later, Aemilius Simpson, not surprisingly, was appointed superintendent of the Marine Department of the HBC on the Pacific.

Simpson himself, after Aemilius's departure for the west, headed back north from Fort Douglas down the Red River and along the shore of Lake Winnipeg to Fort Alexander, at the mouth of the Winnipeg River, where in all likelihood he reconnected with his long-time servant Tom Taylor, who, once again, could take personal responsibility for the Governor's day-to-day comfort. Only this time, having been for nearly four months in transit and bereft of intimate female companionship since London, Simpson took a shine to Taylor's sister Margaret (or Peggy, as she was known), who wintered there with her brother and her sister, Mary, who was married *à la façon du pays* to Chief Factor John Stuart. A rise in power and increased responsibility had done nothing to diminish the Governor's passion: almost as soon as they were together, Margaret became pregnant with Simpson's third known child in North America, his second with an Aboriginal woman.

Now comfortable with the parameters and routines of the trade, Simpson mused that summer, as he chaired the Northern Council meeting at York Factory, about images of himself as governor of all things in North America, perhaps even conjuring up heroic imaginings of himself as Napoleon in a birchbark canoe.[2] But he knew that in the fullness of time he would be required to settle for one woman, who would become First Lady of the Trade.

On the domestic front, he had the example of J.G. McTavish at York Factory, whose long-time Chipewyan partner, Matooskie, had been with him since they married in the manner of the country in 1813 in Columbia. Matooskie was of mixed blood, the product of a conjugal union between an HBC trader, Roderick McKenzie, and an unidentified Aboriginal woman in Athabasca. But unlike most country wives, whom fate relegated to second-tier social status, she had risen through the ranks with McTavish and, after the union of the two fur companies, had taken a place on the top rung of the social ladder at York Factory as "Madam," wife and partner of the bourgeois (the senior officer). They had several daughters together and, by the mores of Rupert's Land, were a leading couple of the trade.

In contrast, Simpson's Great Tower Street friends and colleagues and the members of the honourable London Committee of the HBC had married daughters of distinction who, in their silks and fineries, managed some of the finest houses in London. Men of the sugar trade, whom he knew best, might have dalliances on the side, especially with black women in the West Indies, but these were encounters to satisfy sexual appetites rather than to advance their social standing.

Simpson had such appetites, of that there was no doubt, but he also carried in his bones—from the moment of his inauspicious birth—a hunger to measure up, to be somebody. George Simpson craved power and authority and, by the mid-1820s, that was coming to him. He also craved to be accepted by the landed gentry, by the London toffs and courtiers. He was smart. He was aggressive. He was physically and mentally tough. But with each passing day in the trade, especially now that on his trip back to London he had been reminded of how the others lived, he realized that there were other things he needed to get in order to rise socially.

Competitive in the extreme, George Simpson was also a pragmatist. Having tasted for the first time ultimate business power and authority, he now realized that to beat the gentry at their own game, he would at some point soon have to marry well. Colvile had cautioned him in a letter, "A wife I fear would be an embarrassment to you until the business gets into more complete order & until the necessity of those distant journeys is over & if it be delayed one or two years you will be able to accumulate something before the expense of a family comes to you."[3] Meanwhile, there were his "bits of brown," as Simpson described his female companions.

That winter, as he went about his business in Lachine, his efforts to construct a proper governor's image continued. The fact that at this

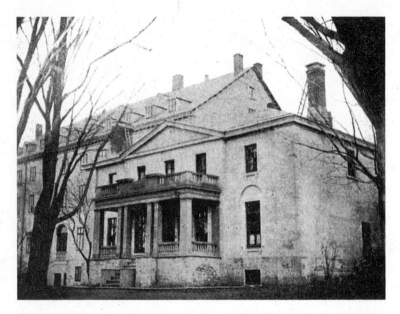

All HBC affairs were conducted in what was at the time the most palatial house in Lachine, located across the street from the Lachine Canal and the HBC warehouse (which is now a national historic site), from which canoe brigades headed west to fur country.

juncture in his HBC career, soon after assuming the top job in North America, he would choose Lachine over, say, the Red River settlement, is revealing. The amalgamation of the NWC and the HBC had consolidated the fur trade's shift to the west, making an eastern base far less attractive or efficient. But the exciting nation-building energy in northern North America was emanating from the many political and business interests, including the HBC, in Montreal.

The social scene among the lonely traders in the frigid confines of York Factory (a separate entrance for spiriting women in and out of his quarters notwithstanding) was now not all that appealing. And life at the Selkirk settlement was grim, a bit too Calvinist to match Simpson's tastes. Montreal, by contrast, was home to many French Canadians, Catholics all, who had joie de vivre. Montreal was also home to the remnants of the NWC and their agents, who were known for their free spirits, their colour and their love of frivolity and the finer things in life.

Eventually Simpson would purchase a handsome house across the canal from the old NWC depot at Lachine—a place he would call Hudson's Bay House, just like the august hall on Fenchurch Street—but in November 1826, he finished his travels in Montreal, where he leased quarters to continue his affairs. One of the first letters he wrote from there was to his friend McTavish at York Factory, inquiring of his latest love, Margaret Taylor: "Pray keep an Eye on the commodity and if she bring forth anything in the proper time & of the right color let them be taken care of but if anything be amiss let the whole be bundled about their business."[4]

No doubt Simpson had heard from his many Nor'Wester friends in the trade about legendary nights of debauchery in Montreal at the Beaver Club. Formed originally by winterers of the NWC who gathered there to consume their prodigious weights in fine food and alcoholic beverages,[5] the club had struggled after amalgamation, but in the winter of 1827, as a way of announcing his arrival onto the social scene in Montreal, Simpson made an effort to revive the institution. He engineered a meeting of ten of the aging original club members at the home of William Blackwood, where recruits James Keith, Hugh Faries and George Simpson were duly inducted.

While that was going on in Montreal, Simpson wrote to John Rae Sr., the HBC's agent in Stromness, to see if he couldn't round up a piper "from whom not a little service may be expected"[6] to join his Rupert's Land entourage. Rae, the father of Arctic explorer Dr. John Rae, made a suggestion to the London Committee, but even his written description of the nominee fell far short of the requirements the Committee knew the man would need to keep up with their North American governor. Secretary William Smith wrote back to Rae with a curt assessment and a suggestion: "I am now to acknowledge the receipt of your letter of the 5th inst. and in reply to inform you that the Committee do not consider the Piper you allude to will suit Govr. Simpson as he seems deficient in

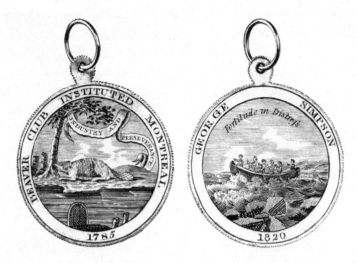

Eager to work his way into Montreal fur society, Simpson attempted to resurrect the Beaver Club in 1827, having cast for himself a club medal indicating that his first winter in the country was 1820.

two very necessary qualifications—youth and strength . . . Under these circumstances you will have the goodness to communicate with your friends in Caithness and you may as well at the same time write to the Governor's Father at Ullapool—giving him an extract from the original letter from the Governor to you and mentioning should he be successful the time at which it would be requisite for the Man to be at Stromness."[7]

With smacks going up and down the coast from London to Orkney, with regular packets now crossing the Atlantic and with Simpson himself in Lachine and within range of regular communications from New York during the winter, correspondence on the matter of the piper took on a frenzied pace, relative to the usual letter-in-the-fall, reply-in-the-spring pace of communication throughout much of Rupert's Land. Interestingly, however, there is no record of direct correspondence between Simpson and his father in Ullapool.

Nevertheless, by April George Simpson Sr. had found a likely candidate in Colin Fraser (possibly a relative through Clan Fraser), who was prepared to work for £30 per annum and who had the requisite youth and spring of step to handle travel with his "worthy Son." At first Simpson thought he might catch up with the new piper at Moose Factory, knowing he was heading here in the coming season to do a full assessment of operations of the Southern Department. But by May that had changed. Secretary Smith wrote again to John Rae Sr.: "I have lately from our friend Governor Simpson in which he mentions it will be requisite for the Piper he expects to be engaged for him to go to York instead of Moose Factory. I have therefore to request you will put him on board the Prince of Wales when she arrives in Stromness."[8]

A letter written in May from Hudson's Bay House in London to Simpson Sr. tweaked the plan even further:

> I beg to acquaint you that I have recently received a letter from your worthy Son in which he mentions that he wishes the Piper that might be engaged for the Company to be sent to York Factory to winter there and obtain a little insight of the Service prior to the Governor's arrival in Spring 1828. The Ships will sail from Gravesend the 2d. prox. and if they have a tolerably fair Passage may be expected to reach the Orkneys by the 10th. I must therefore request you will direct Colin Frazer to start from your neighbourhood in sufficient time to be at Stromness by the latter date, he need not take a large stock of clothing with him (what he does should be stout and warm calculated to protect him from the cold) as he can be supplied on moderate terms with proper necessaries from the Company's Stores, it will be necessary to transmit an account of his advances with him to York Factory, you will therefore advise Mr. Rae the amount you may pay, and should he require a small supply at Stromness, Mr. R. has been instructed to let him have it.[9]

While Simpson tended to these labours in Lachine, "the commodity" gave birth at York Factory in February 1827 to a bouncing baby boy, whom she named George Stewart Simpson. Simpson met the child for the first time that summer, during the Northern Council at the Depot, just before he hurried back south to make his way via Osnaburgh House, Martin Falls and Fort Albany to Moose Factory, where, having completed somewhat parallel inner and outer circles in this domain, he prepared a detailed report on the Southern Department (which, as we would expect, he found rife with waste, sullen and unmotivated Indians, and indolent, extravagant, irresponsible HBC employees). On his way back upriver in September, to return to Lachine, he jotted off another quick private note to McTavish, in which his paternal responsibilities were given their usual shrug: "Pray keep a sharp look out upon Madam, if she behaves well let her be treated accordingly but on the contrary [be] sent about her business and the child taken from her. Should any accident happen to me and that the youngster lives until 4 or 5 years old he will in all probability be claimed by some of my friends in England or Scotland."[10]

———

The danger inherent in the winter and summer travels Simpson was undertaking was far from trivial. Each summer, voyageurs died of ailments, such as strangulated hernias, brought about by the prodigious loads and back-breaking eighteen- and twenty-hour days they spent in harness, to say nothing of the occasional internecine knife fight. And each winter, people in the country starved or froze to death for want of adequate food or shelter. Although Simpson was always travelling with Aboriginal men and women who in most instances had all the right knowledge, kit, sustenance and travelling methods and camping techniques, the pace for a man who, after all, had sat for more than a decade at a desk in London was starting to take its toll.

The men of the Committee—especially Andrew Colvile, who knew Simpson long and well—had noticed signs of physical wear and tear that concerned them. They knew the benefits of his peripatetic management style, but they were also keenly aware of the firm's vulnerabilities should Simpson suddenly become incapacitated. After receiving his report on this whirlwind assessment of the Southern Department, they admonished him: "Your friends in the Committee are not quite satisfied with your proceedings, as they consider that you run more risks and exert yourself more than is absolutely necessary for the service, allow me therefore to recommend you take more care of your health and not expose yourself unnecessarily; on this subject you may shortly expect a jobation from your sincere friend the Deputy Governor."[11]

Although he suffered from time to time from noticeable headaches and bouts of dizziness, and although his usual response to London edicts was to comply, Simpson appears to have taken absolutely no heed of this rebuff. Life in Montreal was good, so much so that on or about a wild Hogmanay that year, he sired yet another child with yet another woman, this time a white woman named Ann Foster.[12] In November 1828, when the irrepressible traveller was on his way to Columbia for a second time, having started in Lachine and attended the Council of the Southern Department at Michipicoten on Lake Superior and the Council of the Northern Department at York Factory, the following record was written in the register of St. Gabriel Street Presbyterian Church in Montreal: "A. SIMPSON BAPTISM George Simpson Esq. of this [parish], The Hudson's Bay Company, lately resident at La Chine, and Ann Foster, both unmarried persons, had a child born on the third day of October last, [baptized] this thirteenth day of November one thousand eight hundred twenty-eight, named ANN. Father absent, (signed) Ann her + mark Foster, witness Mary Campbell, Jane her + mark Robison."[13]

Given that she had not the wherewithal to sign her own name on the baptismal record, we can assume that Ann Foster was illiterate. She may well have been a domestic, a white "washerwoman" who, perhaps like her Aboriginal equivalents, had not the station or power to resist the advances of her employer, or who maybe thought that bedding the master might be her ticket up in the world. In any case, by the time the child was born, Aemilius Simpson was back in Montreal, meeting up with his brother Thomas, who had come out to take up Cousin George on his offer of employment with the HBC. Aemilius could not resist teasing his cousin (as no one else in the trade, save McTavish, could have done): "It appears that under your own roof you have divided your occupation. Accidents will happen in the best regulated family, but I do not think it improves the arrangement of your domestic economy to have a mistress attached to your establishment—rather have her elsewhere."[14]

Simpson's own rather spartan account of his second epic cross-continent trip[15] is augmented by that of a second journal keeper, HBC officer Archibald McDonald. This account adds substantially to our understanding of the peripatetic governor. McDonald had come to Rupert's Land as the leader of one of the Scottish parties of Selkirk colonists, and had an observer's eye. On amalgamation of the companies he joined the HBC and was sent to the Columbia District as a senior clerk. He had come east for the Northern Department Council meeting of 1828, at which he had been promoted to chief trader, and was headed back to take command of Fort Langley on the Fraser River when he had the good fortune to join Simpson and his entourage, who were also heading west.

Interestingly, we learn from McDonald's account that the party did not use the Athabasca Pass, as Simpson had in 1824–25; instead they travelled through the mountains on the Peace River, 225 miles farther north. It was not until nearly five decades later, when the Canadian government was debating which pass to use for a transcontinental railway, that McDonald's journal, supporting the choice of the Peace River route, was published. *Peace River: A Canoe Voyage from Hudson's Bay to Pacific* is not the most obvious source of information about Simpson, because the book was edited by Malcolm McLeod, son of a Bayman who had been a boy at Norway House in 1828 when the party passed through, with Simpson's and McDonald's names buried in the subtitles.

The journal is delightful both for McDonald's observations and for editor McLeod's insights in his voluminous notes (in fact, if a person wants to read only one slim volume on the nature of George Simpson and the fur trade, this would be it). It paints a picture of the flamboyant

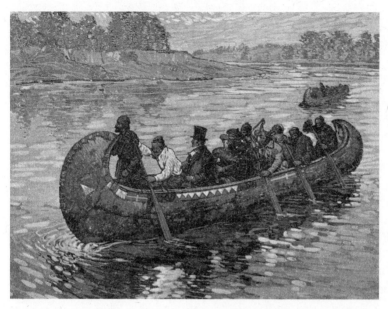

A consummate showman: the Emperor of the North with his personal piper, Colin Fraser, approaching an unsuspecting HBC installation.

gubernatorial character that Simpson had been actively creating. The leather-lunged piper Colin Fraser had spent his winter at York Factory and was now part of the entourage, and on this journey the skirl of Fraser's pipes was augmented by a military bugle blown at any opportune moment by McDonald himself or by the other officer on the trip, Dr. Julian Richard Hamlyn, who was also on his way west. Here is McDonald's account of this noisy, colourful party arriving at Norway House. (Neither McDonald nor Simpson, who did not like to be proven wrong in anything, says anything about the fact that the Governor had finally come to the same conclusion as everyone else regarding the Nelson River–Split Lake route: that it is difficult to navigate and, even if shorter in distance, much harder on men, equipment and often time.) They have come up the Hayes River in the second week of July 1828 and have stopped to change into their finery before moving in their two express canoes into sight of Norway House:

As we waft along under easy sail, the men with a clean change and
mounting new feathers, the Highland bagpipes in the Governor's
canoe was echoed by the bugle in mine; then these were laid aside,
on nearer approach to port, to give free scope of the vocal organs of
about eighteen Canadians (French) to chant one of those voyageur
airs peculiar to them, and always so perfectly rendered. Our entry into
[Norway House] about seven p.m., was certainly more imposing than
anything hitherto seen in this part of Indian country. Immediately on
landing, His Excellency was preceded by the piper from the water to
the Fort, while we were received with all welcome by Messrs. Chief
Trader McLeod [editor McLeod's father] and [Peter Warren] Dease
[who had just come from Fort Good Hope on the Mackenzie River,
having served on Franklin's second overland expedition in 1824–25],
Mr. Robert Clouston, and a whole host of ladies. We here got some
little things arranged for the voyage. The Governor was occupied in
writing the whole of the evening.[16]

McDonald's account provides other glimmers of insight into
Simpson's character and his particular way of looking at the world.
They kept the same eighteen-hour-a-day pace, only here we learn that it
fell to McDonald and Hamlyn to "watch time" so that they might rise at
the Governor's appointed moment.

In his journal, Simpson says nothing about the physical hardship of
Peace River Pass, which McDonald paints as a slog through difficult terrain: "By four [a.m.], the canoes were underway. Reached the top of the
last high bank and breakfasted at eleven. About a mile of the worst road in
Christendom. After midday, resumed the journey, and with unspeakable
misery to the poor men got to a small swamp, a little more than another
mile. Ourselves, however, with the necessary baggage, pushed on to a
little clear stream ahead, not quite half a mile, and encamped late."[17]

McDonald also gives a fuller idea of their interactions with Indian
peoples along the route and of Simpson's response. Recognizing a man
of importance, both by reputation and by his fancy dress, the head man

would smoke with Simpson, have a dram or receive gifts as from the head of one nation to another. On one occasion, high up in the Peace River Pass, they encountered a group of Indians, probably Sekani, who asked that the Governor adjudicate a dispute between one man and the man he had assaulted under suspicion of "tampering" with his wife. McDonald describes Simpson in all his finery listening carefully with aid of the spotty interpretation provided by one of his guides. When the arguments were made, Simpson, with as much gravitas as he could muster, declared the trial *scoticé*—not proven—strongly recommended to the accused that he not do this again and suggested, under the benign doctrine of the Scottish law, that both pay into a joint pot a modest *solatium*, a compensation for hurt feelings. The judge may well have suggested that this might be used to purchase all concerned a dram to help wash away the hurt. What's even more humorous about the account is that McDonald includes a snippet of poetry by Robert Burns, with the intimation that Simpson himself may have recited this as a solemn chant to mark the conclusion of the trial:

When neebours anger at a plea,
And are as wud [angry] as wud can be,
It's ae the lawyer's cheapest fee,
To taste the barley bree.[18]

"The beauty of the Judgement," wrote Archibald McDonald, "in its pre-eminence from the top of the Rocky Mountains, whence delivered, was, that it pleased not either party, and, not a little, frightened both out of their impropriety and evil doing in their respective ways, and on all, had a most wholesome moral effect. Most rightful Judge! Most learned Judge!! (Shylock, Merchant of Venice)."[19]

Soon after his account of this mock trial, McDonald details the loads that each man carried on the portage from the headwaters of the Peace River to the headwaters of the Fraser on the other side: La Course carried a keg of madeira wine; Delorme had a bag of pickled tongues;

Anawagon carried a wooden cassette containing McDonald's and Hamlyn's personal effects; Martin carried the Governor's paper trunk; Larante carried another cassette of clothes; St. Denis had a bag of biscuit; Houle shouldered blankets and canvas ground sheets for the two junior officers; Lasard tumped a keg of port wine; Charpentier carried one roll with two canvas tents; Hoog carried a large basket of food; Desguilars and Peter had each one heavy piece of pemmican; Nicholas carried the Governor's cassette; Tomma, the singer of the group, hefted Simpson's bed; the guide, Jean Baptiste Bernard, carried dried meat, shoes and two skins; Colin Fraser carried a cooking kettle, tea kettle, saucepan, gumpot and, of course, his pipes; and Tom Taylor, Simpson's personal servant, carried guns, greatcoats and any other bits and pieces that were left.

The only mystery item on this list was a person detailed as M——, who carried the Governor's little travelling case with his medicines, razor and other items of personal hygiene. Who "M" might be and why McDonald was hesitant to mention the name is a curiosity. In the opening of his journal, McDonald was very clear that when they began with two express canoes, they had eighteen "men" and three officers. And, indeed, if one enumerates the Peace River Pass portage list, there were eighteen people carrying loads to begin the hundred-mile carry toward Stuart Lake. The officers, of course, travelled on horseback. With such detailed attention to names and loads, it is odd that the person carrying the lightest load, the Governor's "case," does not benefit mention by surname like all the others. Nowhere in Simpson's own journal or in McDonald's is it mentioned that with them on this journey was Tom Taylor's sister Margaret, with whom Simpson had had a child on return from London in 1826–27. Indeed, Simpson had earlier castigated officers for doing exactly what he was doing on this trip: filling a space in a canoe that might have been filled with cargo or another able-bodied man with his country woman. The M—— who carried the travelling case had to be Margaret, also known as Peggy Taylor, who kept the chief warm in his private tent throughout the trip.

Even on horseback, Simpson described this five-day overland trek as "a very fatigueing part of our Journey,"[20] which, in translation and taking into account the Governor's usual stoicism and reticence regarding matters of the flesh, meant that he was feeling very poorly indeed. But appearances had to be kept up as they neared Fort St. James on Stuart Lake. This was, after all, the district headquarters of New Caledonia, and it was proving in only a few years of operation to be one of the most significant profit-producing posts of the whole HBC operation. Simpson ordered a halt so that they might "dress," and Archibald McDonald describes the parade these tired travellers were able to muster:

> The day, as yet, being fine, the flag was put up; the piper in full
> Highland costume; and every arrangement was made to arrive at
> Fort St. James in the most imposing manner we could, for the sake
> of the Indians. Accordingly, when within about a thousand yards of
> the establishment, descending a gentle hill, a gun was fired, the bugle
> sounded, and soon after, the piper[21] commenced the celebrated march
> of the clans—"Si coma leum cogadh na shea," (Peace: or War, if you
> will it otherwise) . . . The guide, with the British ensign, led the van,
> followed by the band; then the Governor, on horseback, supported
> behind by Doctor Hamlyn and myself on our chargers, two deep;
> twenty men, with their burdens next formed the line . . . During
> a brisk discharge of small arms and wall pieces from the Fort, Mr.
> [James] Douglas . . . met us a short distance in advance, and in this
> order we made our *entrée* into the Capital of Western Caledonia.[22]

Simpson's character seeps into the public record through Archibald McDonald's journal. We learn that he had with him as they travelled through the mountains a dog. Whether this dog was one brought all the way from Lachine, or even from York Factory, is unknown. But we do know that Simpson had a dog called Boxer during his first winter at Fort Wedderburn, the protagonist in his famous boundary-line dispute with Simon McGillivray in the winter of 1820–21. It may be that although

Fort Wedderburn on Coal Island had been abandoned in favour of the more substantial quarters at Fort Chipewyan on the mainland since amalgamation, Boxer had survived and may in fact have been pleased to greet his old master on his way through a few years later. It is easy to imagine that Simpson had some history with this dog because he also had with him a wind-up music box that he managed to play in a way that gave the impression that the dog was making the sound. McDonald writes about an encounter with a group of Carrier Indians at a campsite near McLeod Lake, in what is now northern British Columbia: "The bagpipes pleased them to admiration, as well as the bugle, but it was the musical box that excited their astonishment most, especially when it was made to appear to be the Governor's Dog that performed the whole secret."[23] As a result, Simpson was known among the Crees, Chipewyan, Sekani and Carriers of the west after this particular journey as "the chief whose dog sings."

CHAPTER XII

———

ITCHING TO MARRY

W hen Simpson arrived at Fort Vancouver on October 25, 1828, he wrote of "having between that Date, and the first of May performed the longest Voyage ever attempted in North America in one Season, about 7000 Miles."[1] He is entitled to self-congratulation, as this was indeed, at least in the written record, the longest North American canoe voyage ever completed in one season—a record that stands to this day. His estimation of distance, however, was exaggerated. The trip—though still a feat of speed and endurance—was closer to five thousand than seven thousand miles.

Having already set something of a land speed record of eighty-four days from York Factory to Columbia on his first journey in 1824, Simpson had predicted that he could do the same journey in a scant two months. Archibald McDonald's detailed account of this second trip to Columbia shows that it took them ninety days to travel 3,261 miles from York Factory to Fort Langley, including sixteen days spent reviewing the books at posts along the way and another nine days at the forks of the Fraser and Thompson rivers, waiting for a split party to reach the same junction.[2] So the total travelling time in canoes was sixty-five days, nineteen days faster than he'd done the trip the first time, at an average speed (including portages and vast distances of upstream paddling) of fully fifty miles per day. And of course that prodigious feat of travel and endurance does not include the two-thousand-plus-mile earlier leg of Simpson's journey, from Lachine to York Factory, which had begun in May, as soon as the ice was out.

All told, from Lachine to the west coast, Simpson had been in hard physical transit for five months, and in McDonald's journal are recorded the first hard observations of the health problems that would plague the Governor for the rest of his days. Early on in the journal, editor Malcolm McLeod describes the man he remembered seeing as a boy, leaving Norway House: "George Simpson was, though not tall, say about five feet seven at most, of rather imposing mien, stout, well knit frame, and of great expanse and fulness of chest, and with an eye brightly blue, and ever ablaze in peace or war, with an address which ever combined the *suaviter in modo, et fortiter in imperio* ["gentle in manner, resolute in execution"]. He was, indeed, on such an occasion, an address to strike awe on his hearers."[3] That bearing was very much diminished, as the party struggled on horseback between the Fraser and Thompson rivers. For three days in late September, Simpson was barely able to travel but apparently bulled his way through. Complaints he would admit to having in later years had to do with eyesight that was starting to fail and symptoms associated with apoplexy; yet although the beginnings of these slowed him down on this second journey to Columbia, his indomitable will was able to rise above any physical imperfections, at least for now.

Whatever the state of the Governor's health on the way back from Columbia in the spring of 1829, it was the usually stalwart Peggy Taylor who slowed the group down—or at least that was the complaint of the man whose child she was carrying. Under normal circumstances, a Chipewyan woman could and probably would carry, pound for pound, more weight than any man, as well as being expected to cook and sew to keep the expedition moving, but on this journey, in addition to having the libidinous governor's attentions by night and his outbursts of temper brought on by the party's slow pace by day, she was also carrying her second child with Simpson. In fact, she had re-crossed through the April snows of the treacherous Athabasca Pass when well into her second trimester. Ninety miles on foot or on horseback slogging over her beloved governor's muddy winter road between Fort Assiniboine and the North Saskatchewan likely did nothing to improve her feeling of well-being. By the time they made Edmonton House, Simpson was fed up and decided to leave Peggy with "such a rotundity in front as to disqualify her from working her passage,"[4] instructing Chief Factor John Rowand to forward her with the brigades back to Norway House or York Factory and eventually to Fort Alexander, where she could be reunited with Jordie, who turned two in February, as well as with her mother and sister, whose husband in the manner of the country, Chief Factor John Stuart, Simpson knew would provide for her and bill the costs to his account.

Though ailing, Simpson continued his frenetic pace, crashing east across country from Fort Carleton to Fort Pelly on the Upper Assiniboine River and on to Fort Garry, where he tended to the business of the Selkirk colony for almost a week. Since he had been here the last time, his old friend *bois brûlé*[5] leader Cuthbert Grant had been awarded the title of Warden of the Plains, in an effort to dignify his authority among the Métis and to see if his influence could help stem the violence and unrest among lingering HBC and NWC factions and the people of Aboriginal descent in what is now southern Manitoba. These groups had been fighting over territory and trading opportunities almost since the Selkirk settlers had first set foot in Assiniboia. Grant had impressed Simpson on his first Inner Circle Tour, and since then had been a powerful ally for Simpson in the social complexities of the Selkirk settlement. But there was no time to linger, as Simpson knew that if he was ever to make good his plan to get back to the United Kingdom to court and marry, he would have to fight his way to Norway House and York Factory, convene the Council of the Northern Department, travel again to Moose Factory, convene the Council of the Southern Department and check up on measures of economy put in place the previous year, before returning to Lachine and New York to catch the packet back to Liverpool.

It must have been with some measure of relief that Simpson met up with his young cousin Thomas Simpson, who had had a change of heart since turning down the Governor's offer of work in the HBC instead of continuing his studies at King's College in Aberdeen. Perhaps he had been swayed by letters from his stepbrother Aemilius, or by communications from his younger brother, Alexander, who had also been lured by his cousin George's "highly coloured descriptions of adventure to be encountered, and wealth to be won, in this ungenial region"[6] when Simpson was home in 1825 and who was now working as a clerk in the company's establishment at Lachine. As a bright and literate man of twenty-one years, Thomas had said no to his cousin with a view to becoming either a doctor or a minister. But since the invitation had first been proffered, he had learned that getting a medical education was more than he could afford, and that following the church might leave him "little chance of obtaining a living" because of his inability to speak Gaelic in a parish where that was the vernacular tongue.

In a letter to Aemilius, Thomas wrote, "These considerations ... combined with a strong though hitherto latent desire to travel, have induced me to take a step which, be it for my good or for my ill, has cast my lot, for some years at least, in the wilds of the New World." When George Simpson arrived at Norway House on June 18, 1829, Cousin Thomas was waiting for him with pen and journal book in hand, ready to become his secretary and amanuensis. Thomas had no idea of the nasty end this career turn would bring nor of the power of his cousin the Governor, who could flick his fingers and make almost anything happen.

In the short term, Thomas was a quick study, and he seems to have adapted well to life on the trail, because Simpson seemed to rally after meeting him. One of Thomas's first assignments might well have been—regardless of what he might have thought of the propriety of such a manoeuvre—to draft most of the brief and perfunctory resolutions for the Northern Council before the meetings actually took place. A touch wide-eyed as he was at everything that had happened to him since leaving home, the sheer diversity and volume of the facts, figures and trade minutiae in his cousin's head must have baffled Thomas Simpson. In these early days, he had nothing but admiration for the Governor and seemed well pleased with his decision to leave the granite arches, leaded glass, libraries and clipped green campus of King's College for the cedar curves, grimy smoke-stained windows and heath of the tundra and forest floor—although he would surely have noticed, or even seen for himself, that the finest library in Rupert's Land was in the confines of York Factory, built up through 150 years of privileged boredom on the ice-bound coast of Hudson Bay.

Had Thomas been particularly perceptive as he recorded the minutes of the Northern Council and dined with some of the characters who were present that year—Colin Robertson, J.G. McTavish, John Clarke, John Stuart, John Rowand, James McMillan—he might have developed an inkling that his cousin and the York Factory bourgeois were hatching a plan for their time in the UK that autumn. McTavish was going on furlough, taking his eldest daughter, Anne, and leaving Matooskie at York Factory. In taking dictation from Simpson, Thomas would have heard about plans to introduce McTavish to the London Committee (along with Chief Factor McMillan and Chief Trader Alexander Ross, who were also going on leave that year), but had he listened to the chatter between the lines when Simpson and McTavish were together at Norway House and York Factory, he would have heard conversation with a slightly more conspiratorial tone.

McTavish went to England from York Factory on one of the ships of the season, while George and Thomas Simpson continued on through Fort Alexander (where Peggy Taylor was about to give birth) to Lac la Pluie, Fort William, Pic River, Michipicoten, Brunswick House and Moose Factory. After that, continuing southward in an express canoe, they visited Abitibi, then Timiskaming, Lac des Allumettes, Fort Coulonge and Chats Falls on the Ottawa River before gliding down past Bytown, on to Lake of Two Mountains and home to Lachine. Thomas settled in to spend the winter with his stepbrother Alexander, while the peripatetic governor changed his clothes, repacked, maybe saw for the first time his ten-month-old daughter Ann (about the same time Peggy was giving birth to John Mackenzie Simpson, on August 29), crossed the river and made his way down to Lake Champlain to catch the Hudson River steamer to New York.

After a steady decline in health on his last run to and from Columbia, he took such a buffetting as a passenger on the packet ship *William Burns* that people in Liverpool barely recognized the near-invalid who disembarked and feebly called for a carriage to take him to Fenchurch Street in London town. His condition was not constant, but it was totally debilitating; on occasion he felt a renewed surge of energy, then acute lassitude would return. His physicians could not diagnose his condition, though they thought it might be apoplexy. His vulnerability to seizures was no doubt increased by the extreme tension under which he laboured. More than anything, the constant apprehension about becoming old and ill at thirty-eight drained him emotionally.[7]

The quiet vigour of Simpson's constitution that kept him going through difficult times at this juncture in his life is revealed in a letter written to Simpson nearly twenty years later by William Todd, the physician at Assiniboia:

> I have only to remind you, of your state of health when you came out in 1830, labouring under constant apprehension of Apoplexy which had preyed on your mind to such a degree as to make you at times quite miserable, how often on these occasions when fearing an attack have you sent for me to bleed you, your arm bared up and ready for the operation a more subservient man would doubtless have met your wishes, even against his own Judgement, and probably brought you to the brink if not the grave itself, I declined bleedings being of the opinion depletion had been carried too far already. I knew the struggle would be severe and the success doubtful, but depended greatly on your naturally good constitution.[8]

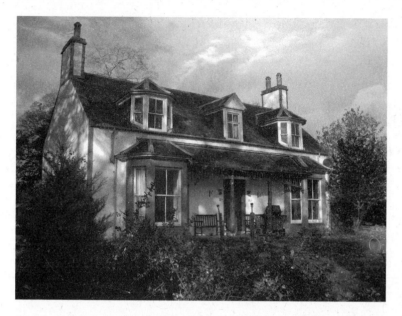

Simpson's base in Scotland when he returned home was Bellevue, his uncle Duncan's home on the Beauly Firth. Although very much diminished from its glory days as a gentleman's country estate, Bellevue still stands, looking out over the walled garden toward Inverness. The guest room, from which Simpson appreciated that view, was to the right above the front door.

In spite of needing regular bloodlettings and leechings to reduce the pressure of blood on the brain, Simpson had far too much at stake to let ill health keep him from his mission. He rallied and introduced McTavish and the others to the London Committee and, with the full blessing of members who were pleased to hear he was finally going to take a rest, went to Scotland to recuperate properly with his uncle Duncan at Bellevue. It wasn't long before the roguish George Simpson was sitting at the secretary desk on the landing at the top of the wide curved stairs of Bellevue, soaking up the sun streaming through the dormer over the salt marshes of the Beauly Firth, writing to McTavish about their plan.

They had talked about it laughingly for years, Simpson more so than McTavish. The old dog was intent on marrying an English woman and, in a letter written to him before he'd left London for Scotland, Simpson observed, "I see you are something like myself, shy with the fair, we should not be so much with the Browns. You have no good excuse & therefore must muster courage, 'a faint heart never won a fair lady'"—adding, on another page, "Let me know if you have any fair cousin likely to suit an invalid like me."[9] And in a later letter, he encouraged McTavish with his own success: "Would you believe it I am in love—how I may get rid of it tis probable I may know tonight, but I trust in the proper Legitimate way.—Do my Dear Fellow muster courage and attack some fair one, if Settlements are talked of say . . . 'I shall settle my B——ks in her.'"[10]

And then, having recovered slightly from his apoplexy, he wrote to McTavish about matters of his own plans for English "settlement" of his desires:

Before I left London I had been feeling my way in your fashion, a cousin under 18 is the fair one, you have seen her, she stands N° 2 on the list at Grove House and the preliminary arrgts [arrangements] are adjusted but cannot be brought to a close until my return from America in the autumn of the year—for which purpose I mean to apply for Leave of Absence. You now have the whole secret, it is still a secret to all *except the fair one, her Father + Mother, myself* and you and I do not mean to say any thing about it until about starting for New York. You will of course bring your Lady in to London in the course of next Month when myself and Friends shall be delighted to see you and her.[11]

By the end of January he was back in London writing to McTavish again about a shift in plans, keen to know what was happening with his old co-conspirator:

I am most anxious to know how your Matrimonial Scheme succeeds and sincerely hope it goes on well; if not the disappointment will to me be great, to my intended better half awful and to your own serious injury and discomfort. When I left London for Scotland it was settled that I should return to England next Year (Fall) for the purpose of getting married but on my arrival the other Day I pressed our immediately union so warmly and seriously that the Father & Mother gave way; with the Lady I had little difficulty as she was as anxious about it as myself. —I merely await Your & McMillan's arrival to get spliced; the Lady understands that she is to have the happiness of Mrs. McTavish and Mrs McMillan's Society during the passage: we proceed from Montreal [stopping] at Red River in going. She accompanies me to York and in the autumn to Red River where we shall pass the Winter; we take a Maid Servant from here with us and a man and maid servant go by the Ship to join us with our heavy baggage at York. —You now have my plans, Mantua Makers and Milliners are at Work, the Parson will be in request in about 3 Weeks time & then the important duties devolve on myself. —Pray muster courage—do not be diffident "a faint heart never won fair Lady." If Miss B knew you as well as I do she would not be so squeamish, but if you do go to work with your wonted energy Sure am I that you will come off succ[essfully].[12]

Strange though it sounds, the hefty McTavish (by all accounts, inactivity and the good life at York Factory had ramped his weight up to nearly three hundred pounds), who had been married *à la façon du pays* for seventeen years to a woman with whom he had had five or six daughters (one of whom was with him on this wife-hunting expedition), was on the hustle. Though his courtship skills were rusty, he tried to woo one debutante. Eventually, he charmed his way into the tentative embraces of a woman less than half his age, one unsuspecting Catherine A. Turner. He wrote to tell Simpson that he had finally made good on his end of the arrangement. He too had nuptials in the works and would like the Governor to attend. Simpson wrote back to say well done but, because his own plans were proceeding, he was unable to attend:

It is a curious circumstance that we are both to be made happy the same Day as at 11 o'clock A.M. of the 22nd [*sic*] I likewise lose my liberty. I am vexed beyond measure that you cannot be present and had our arrangements not been too far advanced to be delayed now I should certainly have deferred it until your arrival. From church we return to my uncle's where a few Friends will meet us at "Dejeune a la Fourchet" as the Frenchmen call it and about 2 P.M. I and my Spouse start off for Tunbridge Wells where we shall have a Day or two to ourselves & be back about the 25th and on the 26th we must make the Ladies known to each other. I shall leave a line for you with our friend Scott at Tower S^t before Starting. —We go by the Packet of the 8th and I shall write to L'pool in a few days to secure passages. —I shall take a maid Servant who with your man George will be all the attendants we shall require as the women will do all the Ladies will require on the passage & the latter answer our purpose. —I shall endeavour to secure the whole of the Ladies' Cabin for ourselves by which means we keep all interlopers out & stop wth our wives which is desirable.[13]

In the manner of a man choosing socks from a selection limited by his own reluctance to open another drawer or walk to a haberdasher's shop, George Simpson looked only as far as his cousin Frances, who, on his first trip home from Rupert's Land, had been a gawky young girl but who now was a pretty and available eighteen-year-old living in her bedroom down the hall from his guest room in New Grove House, Bromley. Applying Simpsonian "smoothing" in full flight to her parents, he soon sealed the deal. The urgency of the proposal was driven by convenience—call it "oeconomy" in human affairs—and by ambition.

George Simpson was burdened with drive to succeed, to break the stigma of his bastard birth and to arrive socially in his lifetime. After his harrowing second trip to Columbia, in which his health had failed noticeably, perhaps he was in even more of a hurry to marry than he might otherwise have been because he thought he was starting to die. Clearly he felt no particular attachment to any of the five women we

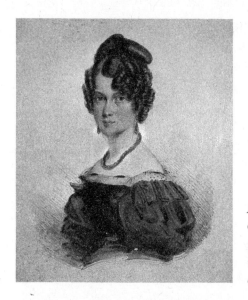

Frances Ramsay Simpson, George's first cousin, was twenty years his junior when she became his wife on February 24, 1830.

know of who had borne his children up to this point, because he was able to move forward with his hasty wedding plans knowing full well that Peggy, with newborn John Mackenzie at her breast and two-year-old Jordie at her side at Fort Alexander, was counting the days to his return: a letter from Chief Factor John Stuart confirmed that. "A little ago," wrote Stuart, "when at supper I was telling Geordie that in two months and ten days he would see his father. [His mother] smiled and remarked to her sister [Stuart's wife] that seventy days was a long time and [she] wished it was over."[14]

With a rush of final adjustments to fancy Regency dresses, suits and the appropriate hats for the occasion, banns were read at St. Mary's Church in Bromley St. Leonard, Middlesex, and on February 24, 1830, the following entry was written: "George Simpson of the Parish of Saint Dunstan in East London a Bachelor and Frances Ramsay Simpson of this Parish Spinster a Minor were married in this Church by Licence with Consent of Geddes Mackenzie Simpson, the natural and lawful Father of the said Minor . . . By me Rodk. MacLeod D.D. Rector of St. Anne Westminster in the presence of Geddes M. Simpson, James Webster,

Jas. W. Simpson, Willm. Scott, James McMillan and W. Simpson."[15] This was a very proper occasion, witnessed by family and friends, including Chief Factor James McMillan, Simpson's trusted associate who had accompanied him on his first trip to Columbia and who, until his brand-new wife fell deathly ill and couldn't travel with him back to Rupert's Land, had been enjoying the same furlough/wedding caper as McTavish and Simpson. The name one would have hoped to see on this list of witnesses besides the father of the bride was G. Simpson, George's father and the bride's eldest uncle. Even with the hasty arrangements, his absence from this event is noticeable.[16]

Time was short between February 24 and the departure of the packet from Liverpool in early March, but Simpson wanted to consummate the marriage in the most auspicious British circumstances; hence, as he had confided to McTavish by letter, the newlyweds made their way southeast from London into the unspoiled heart of the Kent County weald, to a spa town called Tunbridge Wells, which was *the* place to see and be seen among royalty and the British high gentry. The Governor could behave as a perfect gentleman when he chose to do so, just as he could raise his voice and swing his fists with the best of the rough traders. What it was like for delicate young Frances, leaving town with her burly new husband, one can only imagine.

Frances Simpson returned to New Grove House with "Mr. Simpson" after two days and nights at Tunbridge Wells, perhaps with a fuller appreciation of just how little they had in common besides their common immediate ancestry. With an ache in her heart and more than a little doubt about what she had agreed to do, she repacked for a transatlantic crossing and for the lengthy journey by canoe that would be the real honeymoon. It would be an experience from which she would never really recover. Saying yes to George Simpson meant saying yes to wild adventure in Rupert's Land, but it also meant saying yes to a life of partial truths.

Because Simpson's eldest two children, Maria and Isabella, had lived in London and were living at Bellevue with her father's brother Duncan,

Frances probably knew of them—she may even have known one or both of their mothers and the circumstances of the girls' births. But she knew nothing—although she later suspected and actively asked not to hear— of her husband's other family improvisations in North America before and after the wedding. Marrying George Simpson meant embarking on a life that would, for whatever joy she found living with him in Rupert's Land and without him when she returned to England to await his semi-annual return to New Grove House, end with sadness and regret in her fortieth year.

—

Glimmers of that life in North America as it began, and of the character of the semi-maniacal cousin she married, are contained in a four-by-six-inch ruled honeymoon journal from Blight & Burrup Stationers on Lombard Street in London that Frances kept "in order to amuse myself and likewise to refresh my memory on subjects connected with this voyage at a future point."[17]

The journal opens with a clear understanding that embarking for North America was her first time leaving home. Although this departure was difficult for her in the extreme, she seemed able to summon some of the optimism she felt in saying yes to her venturing cousin's proposal: "I arose from my bed at 5 A.M. for the first time in my life with an aching heart, and a mind agitated by the various emotions of Grief, Fear & Hope. Grief at parting from my beloved Parents and a large & united family of Brothers & Sisters from whom I had never been separated. —Fear for the changes which might take place among them during my absence. And Hope, which in the midst of my distress diffused its soothing influence, and acting as a panacea, seemed to point to the home of my infancy, as the goal at which some future period, however distant, I should at length arrive."

After a tearful goodbye to her mother and sisters at New Grove House that left her "with feelings . . . I cannot attempt to describe,"[18] Frances and "Mr. Simpson" were driven into London by her father and eldest brother, to meet up with McTavish and his new bride at the Swan and Two Necks pub. Never one with much patience for women in a wailing frame of mind, the Governor likely bit his lip or looked away as his new bride took her last farewell with her "beloved Father, who was equally overcome at the first parting from one of his children." Perhaps in deference to Frances, though, Simpson's normal practice of bulling through from London to Liverpool was amended to include an overnight stop at the Swan Inn in Birmingham as well as two nights at the Waterloo Inn in Liverpool to get accustomed to those climes before boarding the *William Byrne*.

Simpson had been successful in booking the entire ladies' cabin on the packet for Frances, Catherine and their two travelling maidservants. From details in Frances's journal that her husband never thought to mention in his reports or correspondence, we get some idea of the grandeur of these fine old clipper ships: "[The ship had] a very pretty appearance [with] the Wainscot being formed of the Curly Maple, highly polished and bearing a strong similarity to the finest Satinwood. This ornamental work however was more for show than comfort as the carved partitions were constructed so as to slide backwards and forwards with every motion of the vessel, accompanied by the most tiresome and distressing noise, sometimes so loud as to render the exertion of talking quite painful."

When the *William Byrne* slipped from the Liverpool wharf and headed directly into a gale in the Irish Sea, Frances reported seeing a rainbow "dancing before my eyes" before she went below decks to avoid the weather; and it was there she stayed, so instantly incapacitated with motion sickness in the ensuing storm that Simpson thought she might never recover from exhaustion and lack of nutrition. Frances reported that in the dark of night her husband visited the captain (who was bound by the policies of the Black Ball Line not to deviate from his appointed schedule) to see if he couldn't be persuaded to stop for an hour to land Frances in Ireland so that she might somehow find her way home and so that he might continue to New York to continue his important work for the HBC. The "bribe," as she referred to Simpson's offer to the captain, amounted to five thousand American dollars, enough to sway the master "although going into Port except when the safety of the Ship [was] concerned was contrary to his instructions." The story continues in her lovely cursive script: "The attempt . . . was made, but the darkness of the night and the stormy state of the weather rendered it dangerous to approach the land. This attempt had nearly proved fatal to us all, as the wind shifted in the course of the night, and the utmost exertion was necessary to prevent the ship from drifting ashore. —From that time I began gradually to recover after having experienced the distressing effects of Sea Sickness to such a degree, that I felt at times perfectly indifferent as to whether I lived or died."

In New York they bypassed Mechanics Hall for a suite of private apartments at Mrs. Mann's Boarding House, where the newlyweds were "called upon by many of the first people in the City who were very polite . . . in their invitations, especially Mr. [Charles] Wilkes, President of the Bank, and Mr. Astor, founder of the settlement of 'Astoria' since rendered famous in story by Washington Irving." Astor, whom Simpson had missed on his previous trip through, was very much taken by the Simpsons and invited them to his country house at Hockham, but "the limited time at our disposal was received as an ample excuse for declining visits."

After a trip up the Hudson on the steamer *Commerce* and a comfortable stagecoach ride to La Prairie, during which Frances made note of the houses, farms and scenery along the way, they arrived in Montreal, where they were received even more warmly than they had been in New York. It is clear from Frances's account of crossing the St. Lawrence River by boat that she had worked through the terrible beginnings of her journey and was actually starting to enjoy herself: "The first appearance of Montreal from the water is striking in the extreme. All the buildings are roofed with tin, which causes it to glitter in the sun, like a city of silver."

And by her continuing account of the journey, it would seem that Simpson's advance work in Montreal, perhaps aided and organized by

Chief Factor James Keith, who was in charge of the HBC establishment there, had done wonders to surround them with people at the wharf, and during their evenings in the next few days, that may have allowed Frances to appreciate for an instant that North America was more civilized than she'd ever imagined. They were treated to a fancy luncheon on arrival, and would have attended a grand military ball that evening had not fatigue from the journey overtaken them. Instead they boarded a carriage with Keith and made their way nine miles upriver to Lachine, where they remained, Frances and Catherine entertaining themselves with letter writing and visiting and heading in and out of Montreal while Simpson and McTavish went about HBC business, for eight gloriously stationary days.

During that week in Lower Canada, Frances Simpson would have appreciated something of the stature her new husband occupied in the culture of the fur trade but also something of how rare it was for an officer of the HBC to be contemplating companionship of a non-Native woman on his travels to the wintering grounds west of Fort William. "Speaking of this voyage," she wrote, "I must observe that it was regarded as a wonder, was the constant subject of conversation, and seemed to excite general interest—being the first ever undertaken by Ladies and one which has always been considered as fraught with danger." She had no idea. She would survive the canoeing, but their husbands' taking of "ladies" into the country would change forever the social fabric of the trade.

The journey itself was relatively uneventful compared to Simpson's previous canoe adventures, and Frances's unique journal offers a ladylike view into the details of the travel process. They left Lachine at a lazy 4 a.m. on May 2, 1830, later than Simpson might have departed alone. Frances wrote:

> Our canoe, a most beautiful craft, airy and elegant beyond description, was 35 feet in length, the lading consisted of 2 waterproof trunks, known by the name of Cassets, containing our clothes. One basket for holding cold meat, knives and forks, towels &c. One egg basket, a

travelling case [probably the same one Margaret Taylor had carried the previous season] ... 6 wine bottles, cups and saucers, tea pot, sugar basin, spoons, cruets [for condiments], glasses and tumblers, fishing apparatus, tea, sugar, salt ... also a bag of biscuits, a bale of hams, a keg of butter ... [and] a keg of liquor, called a Dutchman, from which the people are drammed three or four times a day according to the state of the weather.

Given Simpson's earlier objections to John Clarke—or any other company employee, for that matter—taking up room in company canoes with their country wives, one might have thought he would have shown at least a modicum of restraint in creating an entire expedition to take his new young wife into the country. That was certainly not the case. Indeed, instead of express *canots du nord*, with eight or nine paddlers, he opted for thirty-five-foot *canots du maître*, each manned by fifteen paddlers. In one sat the McTavishes side by side, with their two maidservants behind them; in the other were Simpson and Frances, one servant and "Messers Keith and Gale, who kindly volunteered to favour us with their company for a day or two." In charge was Jean Baptiste Bernard, who was by now Simpson's favourite guide and who would spend almost the remainder of his career as head of the band of hard-working rogues who ported the Governor around North America. And with them as well was Felix Tomma, "our principal vocalist [who sang] 'La Belle Rosier' and other sweet voyageur's airs."

There was a certain gentility to the travel, or perhaps the travel was described by Frances in a more genteel manner. When the water was too shallow to allow the big canoes to touch the bank, for example, she describes herself and Mrs. McTavish being carried ashore in the arms of "sturdy Canadians." What is a bit surprising, however, is to learn that the gentlemen too were carried ashore, on the backs rather than in the arms of same sturdy voyageurs. Meals were rather more civilized as well. She describes their guide Bernard kindling a breakfast fire with flint and steel, a small piece of birchbark and touchwood from his travelling "fire

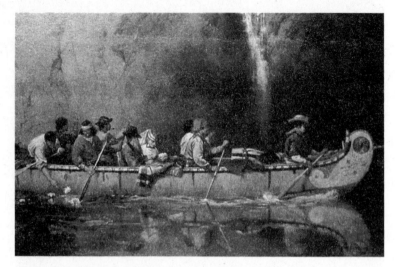

For their honeymoon, the Simpsons travelled from Lachine by canoe, in a manner similar to that depicted by the artist Frances Anne Hopkins in 1869.

bag" before setting up on a tripod a large kettle of pork and biscuits for the men and then laying out a lovely picnic for the gentry: "The cloth was laid on the grass, and spread with cold meat, fowls, ham, eggs, bread and butter, everyone sat down in the position found most convenient, and each made the most of the time afforded."

Nights in the tent were a slightly less dignified affair, on beds made of cloaks and a few blankets laid on the ground, surrounded by the sonorous grunts and nocturnal flatulations of a score of dog-tired men. But before either of the ladies could become bed weary, having retired at nine or ten, Simpson did his best to impress them daily by rising first at one or two, or on one occasion at midnight, and awakening the men by bawling in French slang, "*Lève, lève, star lève*" (meaning "*c'est l'heure pour lever*"), before he would splash into watery darkness to rinse his loins and kick-start the day.

With a pace such as this, and with some new paddlers in the ranks, we should not be surprised that several of the men deserted on the way up the Ottawa; yet, as was his wont, Simpson led unequivocally from the front. On May 6, a day when one of the crew went missing, they made a cursory sweep of the nearby woods but came up with no sign of him, so the Governor ordered the rest on, ignoring their muttering about the additional work this would make. Later that day tempers flared and Simpson took action. Mrs. Simpson recorded the perturbation in this way:

> The morning was cold and disagreeable after the incessant rain of yesterday but neither that, nor the fatigue of the forced march we were making, served to depress the spirits of our voyageurs who paddled, sung, laughed, and joked as if on an excursion of pleasure, until one of them who seemed to feel the force of a joke, which his neighbours indulged in, at his expense, returned it upon him in a still more forcible manner by a blow, which gave rise to a battle in the canoe.—Mr. Simpson was asleep at the time but the noise awoke him and put him into nearly as great a passion as the combatants upon whom he bestowed a shower of blows with a paddle which lay at hand and brought about an immediate cessation of hostilities.

And so the honeymoon went. They turned west to ascend the Mattawa River from the Ottawa, the guide this time arousing them at 1 a.m. to execute Portage La Vase, a muddy seven-mile stretch of ponds and portages over the height of land between the headwaters of the Mattawa River and Lake Nipissing. Frances remarked drolly, "The walking would have been bad in broad daylight but the darkness of the morning rendered it almost impassable as it partly lay in a morass knee deep and blocked up with wind-fallen timber. We contrived however to wade and scramble our way to the other end, where a fire was immediately lighted for the purpose of warming ourselves and drying our clothes," sometime before sunrise. Such was travel with the restless governor.

Arriving at Michipicoten Post with the crews of both canoes singing "La Belle Rosier at the highest pitch of their voices," the ladies were introduced to everyone present, who had gathered for the annual Council of the Southern Department. That night, they dined in the officers' mess at the post but retired early to their tents "anticipating with pleasure the prospect of remaining in bed until 4 instead of rising at 2 o'clock." While the meetings were going on, McTavish and Simpson appear to have simply left the women and their maids to their own devices. "Nothing worthy of notice occurred during these three days [May 18–20]," she wrote. "The Gentlemen were so busily engaged with matters of business that we saw very little of them except at meals—the servants were occupied in washing, cooking[19] and other necessary arrangements for a continuation of our voyage, and I contrived to kill time by reading, drawing, writing, and chatting with Mrs. McTavish who amuses herself principally in the study of 'Meg Doors on Cookery' from which we benefited by some delicious cake she succeeded in making." After the Southern Department Council, the newlywed couples parted company. The McTavishes went up the Michipicoten River and down the Missinaibi to Moose Factory, where McTavish has been posted following leave, and the Simpsons carried on west, through Lake Superior, over the divide and on to Red River, Norway House and York Factory, and back to Red River for their first winter together in the country.

Although Frances Simpson's journal was never published and she did not continue with her writing, her experiences predate by two years those recorded in the famously published characterizations of life in wilderness Canada by sisters Catharine Parr Traill (*The Backwoods of Canada*, 1836, and *Canadian Crusoes*, 1852) and Susanna Moodie (*Roughing It in the Bush*, 1852, and *Life in the Clearings*, 1853), who emigrated to North America two years after Mrs. Simpson. Frances's work is much less well known but equally trenchant and illuminating in its revelations about travelling through Lower and Upper Canada and west, over the Arctic Divide, into Rupert's Land. Her journal, of course, is coloured by her position as the naive wife of Governor George Simpson. People and events float politely in and out of her honeymoon experience leaving her blissfully unaware of the sometimes dark and difficult history they represent.[20]

At Norway House, Simpson's crew raced Clarke's crew, and Frances witnessed the smug satisfaction her new husband took in beating his old nemesis at his own game even with such skewed odds—better craft, better paddlers, a conspicuous empty place reserved for his white wife, and maybe even a word on the sly to the other team that said, "If you beat us, I'll fire you." At Knee Lake, having encountered other canoes heading in both directions on the Hayes River route, Frances was introduced to some of these new people from York Factory and feted with a ceremony of the trail:

The following morning before we embarked, the voyageurs agreed among themselves to cut a "May Pole" or "Lobbed Stick" for me; which is a tall Pine tree capped of all its branches excepting those at the top which are cut in a round bunch. It is then barked and mine being a memorable one was honoured with a red feather, and streamers of purple ribbons tied to a pole and fastened to the top of the tree, so as to be seen above every other object. The surrounding trees were then cut down in order to leave it open to the lake. Bernard then presented me with a gun, the contents of which I discharged against the tree and Mr. Miles engraved my name and the date on the trunk, so that my "Lopped Stick" will be conspicuous as long as it stands among the number of those to be seen along the banks of the different lakes and rivers.

Unknown to Frances, this same Mr. Miles not ten years before had taken Betsy Sinclair and her baby by George Simpson off the Governor's hands.

The most poignant moment of all was Frances's weary bemusement at Simpson as they crashed down the Lower Winnipeg River toward Lake Winnipeg. Under the guise of wanting to get to Fort Garry as quickly as possible, Simpson had been waking the crews at midnight or 1 a.m. after only two or three (as opposed to three or four) hours of precious sleep. On June 2, having been delayed the previous day when their canoe had hit a rock and nearly sunk, they mustered at midnight. Frances, who by this time was totally exhausted, fell back to sleep in the canoe and awoke only when a wave washed over her as they were shooting a rapid in the dark before breakfast. Not surprisingly, there was not time for a proper inspection stop at Fort Alexander at the mouth of the Winnipeg River. Their accounts say very little about this portion of the journey, but their cousin Thomas gives the impression of a very quick hello: "We arrived at Bas de la Riviere [Fort Alexander] on the 5th of June. The Governor and Lady started the same evening for Red River."[21] There was no time to stop—they camped on the shore below Fort Alexander. After rising again at midnight, and in spite of the fact that the wind was "[blowing] very hard, occasioning a heavy swell on Lake Winnipeg," they embarked and surfed their way down one of the most treacherous pieces of shoreline in all of fur country. In the rush to move on to Fort Garry there was no time at Fort Alexander to meet for the first time his new son John Mackenzie Simpson, or to pick up in his arms George Stewart Simpson, or to introduce his unsuspecting English wife to his half-Chipewyan wife, who had been counting the days until his return—the one he had left pregnant at Fort Edmonton fifteen months earlier because she just couldn't keep up. And Peggy Taylor was not the only woman in fur country with Simpsonian freight to bear.

CHAPTER XIII

DARK DAYS
IN RED RIVER

George Simpson's official correspondence was excruciatingly precise and, at times, mind-numbingly detailed when it came to the particulars of the trade. But these accounts were assiduously crafted as well, with information included or carefully excluded. Simpson had learned early, perhaps during his days in the sugar trade, that with only rare exceptions, the perception of London-based overseers of operations happening oceans away was shaped totally by these dispatches.

From his first words written at Fort Wedderburn onward, Simpson realized that great power came with the opportunity to write the history of a business enterprise with which its readers had no personal experience. Not discussed in his public correspondence, to the point that one might think the man was bereft of emotion, conscience or friends, were the machinations of his personal affairs. Archibald McDonald's careful treatment of Peggy Taylor's participation in Simpson's second trip to Columbia suggests Simpson's considerable sway over his underlings and he could extend this deliberate blackout of news to other accounts as well.

With his marriage to Frances and subsequent return with her to Rupert's Land, on what should have been the start of a trajectory to happiness, Simpson instead began a slide into the darkest days of his life. His health was failing, his eyesight was getting dim and his fragile young wife's well-being was starting to fail too. Life at Red River, where he'd chosen to situate them,[1] thinking this might be a suitable place for Frances and himself to raise a family, turned out to be more depressing than he had ever imagined. Astute observers have drawn hints of the Governor's unrest and unhappiness from between the lines of his official dispatches, though a casual observer, reading the annual resolutions of the Northern and Southern Councils or checking the bottom line of HBC operations in North America—which got healthier by the day under Simpson's leadership—would gain no inkling of his mounting personal distress.

Simpson, however, did have a confidant, his friend from the salon of the *James Monroe*, John George McTavish. In the ten years they had known each other, McTavish had become closer to him than anyone else in the trade. And it was in private correspondence to McTavish that Simpson poured out his heart and soul, taking the precaution in almost every letter to encourage McTavish to burn the evidence when he was done and to be prudent in the extreme with the often malicious content. In the end, George Simpson trusted only himself completely, but he was more revealing and more vulnerable in these letters to J.G. McTavish than he was to any other person, including his wife.

McTavish's side of the epistolic exchange was always much briefer than Simpson would have hoped, and he often chided the old Nor'Wester for the paucity and reticence of his replies; the Governor's own letters go on and on with what in many cases amounts to nothing more than the juiciest gossip of the trade. By Christmas of 1830, when the McTavishes were installed at Moose Factory and the Simpsons were ensconced in a four-room house in the Red River settlement, looking forward to the day when they might move into more suitable housing at the new limestone establishment being built downriver, news of the arrival of two white wives had crackled like lightning through the trade. And this news did not sit at all well with those traders who thought these two men, especially McTavish, had done their country wives a grievous wrong.

John Stuart at Fort Alexander, where both Peggy Taylor and her two boys as well as Nancy McKenzie and her brood of girls had ended up, had joined with former Nor'Wester (and Nancy McKenzie's uncle) Donald McKenzie at Red River, and together they mounted a vigorous campaign to discredit McTavish. They had the good sense to distinguish between McTavish's abandonment of his country wife of many years with their six daughters and Simpson's abandonment of his Aboriginal mistress with whom he had only sired two children—and who would heap upon them the wrath of God should they speak ill of the Governor's infelicities—but the two of them nevertheless did their utmost to make McTavish, at least, atone for his callous act. Meanwhile, at Red River, Simpson did what he could to speak up for his friend and to tell him so in monthly letters. This issue, as Simpson's revealing letters show, eventually blew over, to be replaced by other emotional matters.

In this first letter, Simpson starts with an admonishment for unacceptable brevity:

Private
Red River Settlement
3 January 1831

My Dear Sir:
  I believe it is my turn now to complain of silence, as by the two opportunities you have had of writing you have only given me about 20 widely penned lines whereas by every opportunity which has been within my reach I have given you volumes: but my Friend, I do not complain, as I know well your kind feelings toward me and have had too much experience of your steady & solid regard to fancy

the possibility of its being shaken and I should in like manner trust
you know mine towards You to be too firmly rooted in my heart to
experience blight or diminution by time or distance. As regards me
rest assured you have not a more steady & sterling Friend either in
Rupert's Land or out of it nor one who would go greater lengths to
render you a benefit and I trust I am not mistaken in my opinion of
your Sentiments towards me when I say that I would calculate more
on Your Friendship than that of any man in the country in any matter
of serious moment. Having disposed of this important point let us
have a peep into domestic matters. I am truly delighted to hear that
Mrs. McTavish is well and likes Moose; you may if you chose be the
happiest fellow on the face of the Earth (myself always excepted) as
you have the best wife I ever knew (my own in like manner excepted).
I wish from the bottom of my heart we were situated near each
other and my wife re-echoes this wish every Day of her life. We have
thousands of Society but none that we care much about. Donald
[McKenzie, chief factor at Fort Garry, where Simpson was living] and
I are very good Friends but not over thick; his Wife is a poor Stupid
good creature, but there is nothing in her. The Parson's wife is pass-
able but she is 3 miles distant and we see little of her and Cockran's
Wife had been a "Dollymop" or some such thing who can pray &
cook & look demure and Eat and say Yes & No. But if our better
halves were near each other they would both keep themselves and us
alive. I have really serious thoughts of passing next or the following
Winter with you at Moose—say how you could accommodate us the
following Winter . . . The old man [Chief Factor John Stuart, who
regularly visited Fort Garry from up the lake at Fort Alexander] and
Donald are constantly knocking their heads together about your concerns [about abandoning "Madam" for a white wife]. I have had some
sharp words with both on that subject which led to a little coolness
with the latter and high words from the former; the object seemed to
be to Bully you through me to make a fixed Settlement for Life on the

268

old one . . . The old Lady [Nancy McKenzie] does not seem disposed
to take another Husband but by giving her a little time I have no
doubt she will come round. I have sounded Leblanc and two or three
others but the bait does not take. Dond. and Stuart are very anxious
to make an [exception] of her by sending her to Red River to which I
said I had no objection providing they could do at £30 [per annum]
covering all charges of Cloathing Board &c &c. I mean unless you
give directions to the contrary to make that Sum cover your charge
for her this Year. She & her Children are quite well and still at Bas de
la Riviere. In your communications with Stuart do not use my name
further in the business than that I have your instructions regarding
the advances to be made to her and should he write you volumes on
the subject I think the less you say in reply thereon the better. My old
concern [Peggy] & yours are Barrack & Mess Mates they have each
two Children and the same allowance say £30 will be made to each
until disposed of. I am looking out for a Husband for my own but cannot fall on one to my mind.[2]

A week after completing this letter, and before it was placed in the
satchel of a solitary packeteer who would convey it to Moose Factory
(or at least to a post where another winter courier would take it with his
packet to Moose Factory), Simpson was able to tell McTavish that he
had "nailed Leblanc for your old concern." Pierre Leblanc was a skilled
carpenter who had been renovating Simpson's rooms at Fort Garry. No
doubt, a serious dose of smoothing was being applied to the unsuspecting Leblanc, between projects. Until he saw the object of Simpson's
approach, he may have marvelled momentarily at his good fortune to
have the Governor's complete and undivided attention. Yet for the good
of the team, and for a dower of four times his annual salary, he agreed to
marry McTavish's "old concern," and signed a letter to that effect, which
Simpson drafted for him on the spot and included with his January 3
dispatch to J.G.:

George Simpson Esq.

R R S 10 Jany 1831

Sir:

I hereby bind and oblige myself to marry Nancy McKenzie the Woman lately living with John George McTavish Esq. within Three Months from this Date providing she accepts my proposals to that effect, it being undertaken by you on behalf of the said John George McTavish Esq., that I shall receive as a Dower with her the Sum of Two Hundred Pounds Sterling by D[ra]ft on England immediately after the marriage shall be solemnized . . .

Always one for precision in fiscal matters, Simpson also included his written reply to Leblanc, by way of receipt:

Mr. Leblanc

R R S

10 Jany 1831

Sir:

In the event of your marrying Nancy McKenzie the Woman lately living with John George McTavish Esq., within Three Months from this Date I do hereby bind and oblige myself on behalf of the said J G McTavish Esq. to give you a Dower with her of Two Hundred Pounds Sterling by D[ra]ft on England

I am Sir Your mo: obed. St.

Geo. Simpson[3]

The following day, Simpson wrote another addendum to his letter of the previous week. But in the meantime, he had heard rumours of an insulting letter, written by Stuart but never sent, which, thanks to John Clarke, who would take any chance to get back at Simpson, was provid-

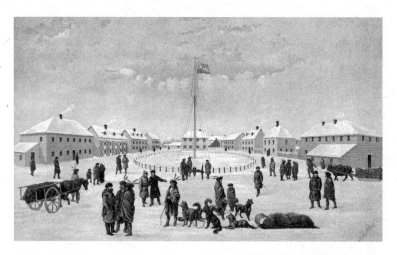

George Simpson was intent on creating a suitable place for his new bride to live and was eager to move to Lower Fort Garry. But during their first winter, he had to live in these less exclusive surroundings upriver at Fort Garry.

ing much winter merriment around the trade at McTavish's expense. In telling his friend about the pending arrangement for his country wife, and knowing McTavish's temper and likely response to a personal attack, Simpson couldn't resist advising him to lie low and stay out of the line of fire, lest he be "threatened into [settlement] terms" by his two indignant colleagues:

11th Jany

This arrangement I communicated to McKenzie and Stuart last night without letting them know anything about the money part of it and closed it with Leblanc without their knowing that the subject was on the carpet; the object was to prevent them saying [any]thing about terms as both seemed determined to have a Thousand Pounds out of you. McKenzie applied to me this morning to know the particulars of the Settlement but in short terms I said I had nothing to do with him therein and would therefore give no information but that he might

apply to Leblanc if he chose, in short I am nearly at hot war with
both these Worthies about it and they, finding I have stolen a march
upon them, are quite enraged. Leblanc is to have a week's leave of
absence in the course of a few days to go down to Bas de la Riviere
to make love, tis possible I think that Stuart may dissuade him but if
he does I shall have a letter & Leblanc in waiting at the bottom of the
River for Sandy Stuart who will overrule objections. McKenzie &
Stuart have both behaved exceedingly ill in this business in my opinion, they talk of compulsion and Stuart has read to several people
a letter which he says he wrote to you but which I feel satisfied he
did not choose to forward; this letter I understand was most insulting, he read it to Clarke in passant at Bas de la Riviere & Clarke has
blazed the contents at Lac la Pluie & along the communication. I do
not mean to advise but were I in your situation I would never put
pen to paper to either and certainly not allow myself to be threatened
into terms.[4]

Leblanc made good on his promise. He duly snowshoed sixty miles
up to Fort Alexander and managed to convince the beleaguered Nancy
McKenzie that she and her daughters would be best continuing their
connection to the HBC but with a slight shift in status. Simpson knew
that in order to make this work, he needed to dot the last *i* and cross the
last *t* on the deal:

Private [J.G. McTavish]
Red River Settlement
8 February 1831

My Dear Sir,
    Agreeably to the authority given me in your letter of 19th May 1830
[written at the end of the Southern Department Council meeting
and just before the McTavishes and Simpson parted company on

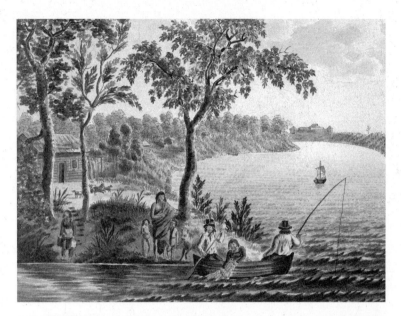

Life at Red River, at the junction of the Red and Assiniboine rivers, in the centre of what is now the city of Winnipeg, was nice enough in the summer months. But in winter, with the north wind blowing in across open prairie, it was much bleaker.

their honeymoon trip] to pay "One Hundred or even Two Hundred Pounds" "to induce some decent man to marry" Nancy McKenzie the Woman who lately lived under your protection, I have paid the latter sum to Pierre Leblanc (to whom she was yesterday married) by my Draft as Your Attorney of this Date at 60 Days sight on the Honble Compy, with an authority to pay the same on my private account in the event of there being no funds at your credit with the Compy as p. the enclosed copy of my Dft., and I have taken Leblanc's rec[eipt] for the same in duplicate, copy of which is likewise enclosed also Mr. Harper's certificate that the marriage was duly solemnized by him. In the event of your not having funds in the Compy's hands to meet the Dft the amount can be repaid me at your convenience.[5]

By April 1831, McTavish had written back to Simpson, apparently incensed by the gossip and by Simpson's intervention on his behalf. But he was 750 miles away on the coast of James Bay. Simpson did his best to placate his friend:

Private
Red River Settlement
10 April 1831

My Dear Sir . . .
   I am truly sorry to find that the substance of my communications . . . wounded your feelings so deeply. If I had command of time, I should probably have smoothed down and qualified my report of the abominably malignant aspersions with which my ears were assailed out of delicacy to your feelings; but with the pressure of business on my hands in the absence of your Friendly council and able support to which I have been long accustomed, I could barely note down in brief what was passing, far less set myself down regularly to the rounding of periods. Suffice it now to say, that all is blown over, and that none even of your bitterest enemies believes one hundredth part of what was said of you.[6]

To make McTavish feel better, he deviated to other subjects (including tangential reference to the fact that both their young wives were pregnant and quite sick). Then, as if to show McTavish that all was settling in the most idyllic domestic way, he added some detail about the actual wedding and the well-being of the Nor'Wester's daughters.

By May, the furor over McTavish's callous move was over. It is noteworthy that through all of this discussion of McTavish's situation, Simpson made only one vague reference to the "other widow," starring the term in the letter and adding in a note at the bottom of the page that "That Widow is now Madame Hogue," with no further details. Although Stuart and McKenzie were too smart to cast aspersions on the Governor, one company officer could not resist a snipe in a letter to one of his friends in the trade: "The Govrs little tit bit Peggy Taylor is . . . Married to Amable Hogue . . . what a downfall is here, particularly in the latter from Governess to Sow."[7]

Simpson, ever the politician, was clearly much better able to manage the nasty consequences of his summary dismissal of his own country wife than was his friend McTavish. With that issue finally behind them, attention turned to their young wives, who both continued to suffer in pregnancy. While Catherine McTavish seemed on the road to recovery, Frances Simpson had needed almost constant care from the Red River physician, Dr. William Todd. Simpson's spirits were sagging. Spring was late. His wife was bedridden. He was feeling fed up and confined at Red River and worried how Frances would fare as he did his rounds of summer Councils:

Red River Settlement
20th May 1831

My Dear Sir . . .
We are very anxious about Mrs. McTavish but I trust she has long ere now recovered her Wonted health and spirits. Mrs. Simpson still continues a great invalid, the greater part of her time in Bed and her symptoms by no means favourable. Tod is in constant attendance and I think I must keep him during the summer as Hamlyn goes off wt the first crafts, if our calculations be right she will be in the Straw [deliver the baby] about the middle of Septemb. which is a most awkward time for me as I can scarcely get back from York so early . . . I should like to pass the Winter of 1832 or 1833 wt you, can you make room for us. My better half is constantly on that subject. We are both heartily tired of our Red River quarters and Society . . . I expect to hear from you fully . . . both publickly & privately. All your communications have been more brief formal & reserved since we last Saw each other than usual or than I could have wished or expected. From

York, I shall have this pleasure again in the course of the Summer
and at greater length. Pray remember me in the kindest manner to
Mrs. McTavish. Mrs. Simpson has already written her and now again
desires her Warmest regards to you both.

Believe me Ever,
My Dear Sir,
Yours very Sincerely,
Geo. Simpson[8]

A month later, Frances's condition worsened and Simpson made
good on his idea to have Dr. Todd live with her while he was away at
the Northern Council. He congratulated McTavish on the arrival of his
first child with Catherine—his ninth on record.[9] But, ever comfortable
with contradictions between what he did and what he chastised others
for doing, he couldn't resist poking fun at his old nemesis John Clarke,
who was looking to ease out of the trade with a comfortable post in the
St. Lawrence River valley. While his prose was the picture of restraint,
Simpson was obviously peeved that Clarke, having gotten nowhere with
the Governor, had gone over his head directly to the London Committee
to negotiate his exit from the trade:

Red River Settlement
8th June 1831

My Dear Sir . . .

   Accept and convey to Mrs. McTavish the warmest congratulations
of my better half and Self on the late addition to your household, we
sincerely trust that both Mother and child continue to do well and
hope in due course to show that we also have not been idle altho you
have got the start on us. My poor wife you'll be sorry to learn is very
ill indeed, almost entirely confined to her Bedroom and altho not in

an immediately dangerous state much worse than Women generally are while in such situations. Under such circumstances it really breaks my heart to part with her and she poor Dear girl is if possible more distressed at the separation than myself. I shall Tomorrow bring and leave Tod with her, my stay shall not be so long as usual at York, indeed I have almost made up my mind to start from there by the 1st of Augt. so as to be here by the 15 or 18 . . .

Our friend Clarke has had his trips to England for nothing, the committee treated him with the contempt he deserved and he is in high dudgeon. When he reached Canada a letter from me was put into his hand which perfectly amazed him & drove him stark mad. He is gone to [the HBC post] at Mingan [in the Gulf of St. Lawrence]. I transcribe an extract of one of his letters to the committee which will make you laugh "To the joint efforts of Mr. Robertson & myself are the HB Coy in a great measure indebted for the splendour & importance of their rank & standing in the Great Commercial World". Well done John! Pray say to Mrs. McTavish with my spouse's kindest regards that she was delighted by the rec[eip]t of her letter & intelligence it contained; and that she will have the pleasure of replying to it when she is able to sit up. She has been closely confined to Bed for several Days past. Do me the favour likewise to present to her my warmest wishes—wt a kiss to little Miss—accept the former both from the good Wife & myself & believe me Ever wt sincere regard

> Yours most truly,
> Geo. Simpson[10]

Simpson rushed up to York Factory, probably with a York boat crew who silently cursed his name the whole way for his driving schedule, and managed to conduct the business of the season in record time. He penned a quick note to McTavish while there, mentioning again his wife's alarmingly bad health, but in his casual chit-chat of things running through his mind he also mentioned an apparent role he had been filling for various chief factors, including McTavish, in advising them on investments in stock and property both in Canada and back in the United Kingdom. In McTavish's case, Simpson discussed the pros and cons of keeping or selling a farm he owned on the Ottawa River. Simpson seemed keenly aware of developing settlement in Upper Canada and of the increasing value of land close to civilization, advising his friend to "keep it by all means [as] it will be a fortune to whoever inherits it and is the best bargain that ever was made in Canada."[11]

Good to his word, Simpson was back at his wife's bedside in Red River by mid-August, admitting that working around the clock at York Factory had left him "so unwell in consequence that not only Hamlyn but myself and the Gentlemen who were there became alarmed about me." In passing, he mentioned his disgust that his old nemesis Colin Robertson had brought his Aboriginal lover with him to Red River earlier in the season "in hopes that she would pick up a few English manners before visiting the civilized world."[12]

Robertson, who perhaps better than anyone knew of Simpson's long and chequered history of liaisons with Aboriginal women, frequently having them share his quarters at posts across the land, was dumbstruck at the double standard and, as politely as he could, told the Governor so. To McTavish, Simpson wrote, "I told him distinctly that the thing [having his country wife stay with him at Red River] was impossible which mortified him exceedingly," adding "he is without exception the most trifling frivolous man I ever saw,"[13] before going on to take another swipe at John Clarke and closing the letter.

On September 2, 1831, Frances Simpson, who had never really gotten over the shock of marrying a man more than twice her age and moving halfway around the world to a place like nothing she had ever experienced during her eighteen years as a child of the mercantile elite, gave birth to a baby boy—George Geddes Simpson—whose health was worse than his mother's. Simpson's pace of correspondence to McTavish

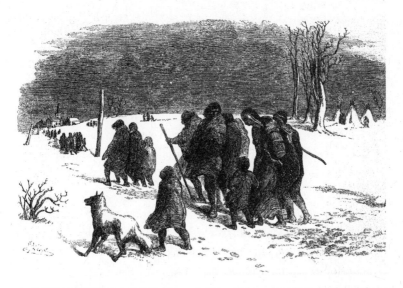

At Red River, Métis and Indian people from the surrounding area intermingled with HBC personnel and settlers of European extraction. Simpson and his new English wife never felt at home there.

slowed during the autumn, but a letter in the new year confirmed that all was not well in Assiniboia:

Red River Settlement
3rd Jany 1832

My Dear Sir . . .

My poor Wife had the most narrow escape imaginable; during the whole 9 months previous to her confinement she was in extreme ill health and so much reduced & weakened that at the crisis, she was more Dead than alive; her recovery was exceedingly slow, 6 weeks in Bed and she is still very thin and by no means strong. Our little Boy was for a time ailing and delicate, but he is now picking up and promises well.[14]

By May the unimaginable had happened:

Red River Settlement
1st May 1832

My Dear Sir,

I am sure your kind warm heart and that of your amiable Lady will sympathize with us in our present affliction which is greater than I have the power to describe. It pleased the Almighty to take to himself our Darling our beloved Boy on the 22nd Ulto [April]; he was ailing a little for some time previous but we had no apprehension of danger and on the morning of that Day my poor Wife went to Church it being Easter Sunday, leaving the Child tolerably well; at her particular request I remained at Home to have an Eye over him as it was Death to her when we were both absent, but she had scarcely got seated on her Saddle when he was seized wt violent retching on my knee, soon after became convulsed and breathed his last as she was in the act of crossing the threshold after pouring forth her prayers for him at the Lord's Table. This awful visitation has quite distracted us and broken our Hearts; the mournful duty of consigning his Earthly remains to the Grave devolved on me on the 25th; The violent transports of grief have given way to fixed & deep melancholy and I much fear it will be long very long ere my poor wife will recover from the Shock which has already made sad ravages on her Health & spirits. This poor Child was the Idol of our Hearts, we doted upon him, we lived but for him, he was the constant subject of our thoughts & conversation and without one moment's preparation he was torn from us. I am sure, I am very sure, My Dear Friend you will pity, you will commiserate wt us from the very bottom of your kind & feeling Heart.[15]

Simpson had shown only passing interest in his numerous children by other women, but George Geddes had been born in Christian wedlock and would have been a socially acceptable heir. Still, the Governor's uncharacteristically maudlin tone in these letters to McTavish suggests conventional posturing as much as genuine grief.

Simpson was turning forty in 1832 and had serious health problems. The promise of marriage to a woman half his age, which should have brought joy, hope and new life, had gone horribly wrong with Frances's sickness during pregnancy and the subsequent death of their first child together. And although his work on behalf of the Hudson's Bay Company had impressed his London overseers, the adventure of his first year in the wilds of Athabasca had given way to explorations by canoe that, over the passing years, had become almost routine. He knew the ropes. He knew all of the major players in the trade. And, living now among the Métis and underlings of the trade at Fort Garry, he was more immersed in the petty politics of settlement living than he ever cared to be. There was nothing glamorous about life at Red River.

A letter written to McTavish on a brief visit to York Factory to conduct the business of the season gives a stark indication of Simpson's flagging health and spirits: "I was so very unwell the Evening previous to the departure of the people wt my packet for Red River that I could not look at the papers after Miles had copied them nor Sign the Despatch which will account for some inaccuracies I have since discovered on looking over the original Drafts. Since then I have been ailing more or less and my nerves are so much affected that when overpressed wt business I can with difficulty put pen to paper—in fact I feel that my best Days are gone and that it is drawing near the time when I must withdraw from this harassing Service."[16]

He went on in the same letter with a candid revelation that in spite of making a fat salary relative to all other HBC employees, he had been spending to support his creature comforts in the trade and on risky investments in England to the point that he felt that the only way to stay solvent was to remain in the trade for at least several more years. Simpson complained: "Since I last wrote to you I find myself a poorer man than I was two years ago, having within the past 12 months got a wipe to the tune of nearly £4000. This you can keep to yourself, as I do not choose to have my misfortunes baited all over the Country & this will in some degree account for my taking another 2 years Lease of the country of which I am sick and tired."[17] And in a later letter he returned to the same theme, leaving one to wonder what he was spending these significant sums of money on: "I believe I wrote to you that I got in a pinch in money matters of late. I shall endeavour to be more cautious in future . . . although I allow Hundreds and Sometimes thousands Slip through my fingers, I am very particular about odd pounds, Shillings & pence or in other words am like many greater Men penny wise & pound foolish." That he would confide this to McTavish is curious given Simpson's normal reluctance to expose himself publicly, and all the more insensitive given that McTavish, an even more lavish spender, was in worse financial circumstances at Moose Factory.[18]

By December 1832 Frances was better, but she was still depressed and in fragile health. The pair of them were thoroughly fed up with life at Red River. Cousin Thomas, who was with them that winter as Simpson's personal secretary, noticed the Governor's failing fettle—in fact, there is an edge to his correspondence with his brother Alexander that indicates not only Simpson's continued slide but growing enmity between the young university-educated clerk and his rough-edged boss: "His firmness and decision of mind are much impaired: both in great and small matters, he has become wavering, capricious, and changeable; in household affairs (for he is his own butler and housekeeper) the very cook says openly, that he is like a weathercock. He has grown painfully nervous and crabbed, and is guilty of many little meannesses at Table that are quite beneath a gentleman."[19]

On the second of the month, now apparently more or less inconsolable, Simpson wrote to McTavish: "I myself am become so melancholy & low spirited that I scarcely know what enjoyment is, in the fact I am from Year's end to Year's end in the blues and feel that my Health & strength are falling off rapidly. I am most anxious to get away from the Country of which I am Sick and tired but my means do not enable me to shake off the Harness."[20]

A reader of this correspondence might think that Simpson was baring his soul in letters that began with felicitations such as "My Dear Sir, Your very kind & soothing letter . . . filled my heart wt gratitude & my Eyes with Tears: I wish to God my Dear Fellow that I had it in my power to show how much I value your Friendship and how high you stand in my regard,"[21] but the real Simpson was still lurking beneath. The shrewd businessman had embarked on a secret project in which, among other things, a less charitable image of his "dear" friend McTavish was being etched.

During these dark months in Red River, Simpson had occupied himself in reading the assessments of company personnel that had been part of the improved record-keeping system since his entry into Rupert's Land in 1820. Over the years, notes on clerks in particular had made their way to London in Simpson's correspondence, and some of these had made it into lists compiled by London Committee secretary William Smith. But Simpson also knew that rumour and innuendo concerning the character of HBC operatives throughout Rupert's Land had been filtering back through the moccasin telegraph. He decided to discontinue sending any information about his employees to London, as "the information, which was intended to be strictly confidential [found] its way back to the interior [and led] . . . as may be readily imagined, to personal difficulties and other inconvenient results."[22] But unbeknownst to anyone until long after his death,[23] Simpson committed to paper, using a number-coding system for each officer, his own candid assessments of each of the 25 chief factors, 25 chief traders, 88 clerks and 19 postmasters under his command, in what he called his "Character Book."

On those he liked, Simpson heaped high praise. About James Keith, for example, the chief factor who ran HBC affairs at Lachine, he wrote, "A scrupulously correct honourable man of a serious turn of mind, who would not to save life or fortune, do what he considered an improper thing . . . withall I consider him the most faultless member of the Fur Trade."[24] About John Rowand at Fort Edmonton, Simpson wrote, "Of fiery disposition and as bold as a Lion. An excellent Trader who has the

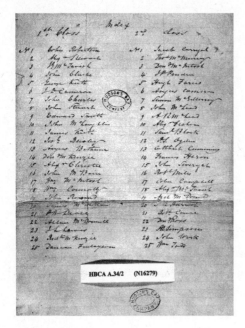

The secrets to Simpson's coded comments in his Character Book, written in the winter of 1831–32, were not unlocked until 1935, when archivist Leveson Gower found this key on a single sheet of paper buried among Simpson's papers.

peculiar talent of attracting the fiercest Indians to him while he rules them with a Rod of Iron . . . has likewise a Wonderful influence over his people."25

Of those he disliked, Simpson's summary dismissals were entertainingly swift and decisive. Colin Robertson, "a frothy trifling conceited man."26 John Clarke, "a boasting, ignorant low fellow . . . a disgrace to the Fur Trade."27 Of John Stuart and Donald McKenzie, McTavish's nemeses at Fort Alexander and Red River, Simpson wrote respectively, "worse than useless being a cloy upon the concern . . . may be considered in his dotage and has of late become disgustingly indecent in regard to women"28 and "he is one of the worst and most dangerous men I ever was acquainted with. My presence alone keeps him Sober, but when left to himself he will assuredly become a confirmed Drunkard."29

John George McTavish, his closest friend, receives surprisingly faint praise. McTavish's entry, "No. 3" in the Character Book, reads as follows:

Was the most finished man of business we had in the Country, well Educated, respectably connected and more of the Man of the World in his conversation and address than any of his colleagues. A good hearted Man and generous to extravagance, but unnecessarily digni-fied and high minded which leads to frequent difficulties with his associates by whom he is considered a "Shylock" and upon many of whom he looks down; rather strong in his prejudices against, and partialities for individuals, which frequently influences his judge-ment, so that his opinions on men and things must be listened to with caution; is about 54 Years of Age, has of late Years become very heavy, unwieldy and inactive; over fond of good living and I must fear is get-ting into habits of conviviality and intemperance.[30]

Through the winter and spring of 1833, as Simpson did his best to improve his young wife's disconsolate constitution in time for her twenty-first birthday, his spirits were definitely on the ebb. On May 20, while standing in the doorway of his Red River home talking to visit-ing London Committee member Henry Hulse Berens and Assiniboia governor Alexander Christie, Simpson finally collapsed from "a sud-den attack of determination of blood to the Head approaching to apo-plexy"—a mild stroke. Subsequent bleeding to relieve pressure on the brain left him too weak and disoriented to walk without assistance. It was quickly determined that there was no way he would be going to Norway House or York Factory that season—indeed, it looked doubtful at times that he would even make it home to England—so meetings were rescheduled for Red River.

On sheer willpower, Simpson saw himself through those meetings and packed up Frances in an express canoe as soon as they were able to move. With the strong and willing arms of the voyageurs who had borne him to and fro across the continent, Simpson and his wife, now preg-nant again, were carried to Lachine. They travelled through the Catskill Mountains down the Hudson River to New York and, via the Black Ball Line packet, back to England. Simpson, amazingly, rallied yet again to return the following year, but Frances stayed, delivered a healthy baby girl that December, and for the next five years slowly recuperated in her childhood home from this cruel matrimonial adventure.

—

CHAPTER XIV

MERCHANT EMPEROR

O n the packet back to England in 1833, Simpson could barely
walk, and Frances, having never really recovered from the
birth and death of her first child and pregnant again, moving into her second trimester, was not steady on her feet either. The
only small mercy was that the journey took place this time in summer,
not winter. The North Atlantic Ocean is nevertheless a cold, rough and
forbidding body of water to cross. The pair of them were confined by ill
health to their cabin for the bulk of the month-long voyage. Frances was
even more seasick than on the first crossing, but this time they didn't try
to bribe the captain to drop her off in Ireland. All they wanted to do was
get home. On arrival, the poor woman collapsed into her mother's arms
at New Grove House. The family noticed too that Simpson was not in
much better shape than their daughter.

The England to which they returned was thrumming with the engines
of the Industrial Revolution. Canal mania had given rise to the age of
steam. London was noticeably busier and the air sootier, if that was possible. Although there had been improvements in civic sanitation, sewage
still ran in the streets and, for all the material improvements in lifestyle,
life expectancy had not risen nor the likelihood of death by water-borne

diseases like cholera diminished. The science of medicine was still in its infancy.

The ailment from which Simpson suffered had been first described by Hippocrates, who characterized unexplained sudden paralysis or changes in consciousness or well-being as "apoplexy," meaning "struck down by violence." A more common term today would be stroke or "brain attack," which we now know is brought about by bleeding or blockage in the tiny blood vessels of the brain. By the 1830s, physicians had known for more than a century that this condition was caused by lack of blood flow in the brain, but little more; besides leeching and the barbaric practice of bloodletting by mechanical means, George Simpson's caregivers in Rupert's Land and the United Kingdom had no treatment. Modern medicine now lists the causes of stroke as a complex interaction of genetic predisposition, diet, weight, age, blood pressure and occupational stress levels. Any one or a combination of these may have contributed to Simpson's health problems. The most common type of stroke, and the one most effectively ameliorated by the lowering of blood pressure or volume through leeching or bleeding, is that caused by blockage, as opposed to by the rupture of blood vessels in the brain. Whatever the physiology or pathology of the Governor's malaise, no permanent or major damage was done, at least in these early years; after a few months of rest and relaxation in England, he appears to have made a full recovery.

By now, just about everyone in Rupert's Land, from chief factor to lowly *engagé*, was in awe of Simpson's omniscient grasp of the people and the trade as well as of his ability to get from place to place, to appear and disappear, like a genie in a bark canoe, demanding efficiencies and rattling lives. Some were convinced that Simpson was "in league with the Prince of the Power of the Air."[1] He had so thoroughly learned the trade and made such an impression that many bent to their tasks in his absence, knowing that if the Governor didn't know what was happening right now, he would sooner or later, and when he did there would be hell to pay. For the moment, then, Simpson could carry on his supervision

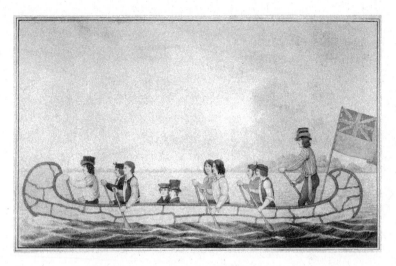

The Governor of Red River travelling in a light canoe.

and management duties through correspondence and by chain of command. Still, carrying that level of responsibility for his far-flung multifactorial business enterprise while he was ill must have been wearing in the extreme.

And then there was the matter of balancing his productive family life with everything else that was going on. It is not clear if he ever actually told Frances about any of his children with other women—likely not— although, having met the McTavishes, Frances would have had tangible suspicions. Adding to the complexities of arriving back in England and moving in with his wife's parents, Simpson had to think about his two daughters in Scotland. Maria, who turned eighteen (and who was only three years younger than Frances, her would-be stepmother) in 1833, had been thriving in and around the Beauly Firth and was to be married to a young Inverness solicitor called Donald Mactavish. Although he was most certainly invited, for reasons of propriety or health Simpson appears not to have attended the wedding on October 25, but he did quietly pay Mactavish a dowry of £500 (Simpson's salary that year, not including expense allowances, was £1,800) to allow the newlyweds to emigrate to Canada and purchase property in Haldimand Township in Upper Canada.

At year's end, however, all was eclipsed when Frances delivered, on December 30, 1833, her second child, a thriving baby girl they named Frances Webster Simpson. The mixture of relief and joy that attended this birth was amplified by the attention showered on the new mother by her family. The baby also added a new focus to her mother's life that helped quell her Rupert's Land experience. Heading into the new year, with Frances occupied with the baby and his own health improbably restored, Simpson turned again to business, travelling back and forth from New Grove House to meet with Andrew Colvile and the other members of the Committee at Hudson's Bay House on Fenchurch Street and, at some point, purchasing a future house for his family at 5 Trinity Square, overlooking the Tower of London and the Thames.

By February 1834 he was itchy to travel again. Motion was for Simpson a salve for the rub of insecurity he often felt. By March or April he was on a return packet ship to North America, landing on the east coast and trundling once again overland to Montreal. And, as soon as the ice was out at Lachine, he was back in a canoe headed for a May Southern Council meeting (and reunion with J.G. McTavish) at Moose Factory and a June Northern Council at York Factory. With his wife and daughter safely ensconced with her parents in London, he was free again to engage the trade—and life within the trade—with a vigour it hadn't seen from him for nearly five years. Simpson was quick to say that he never felt better than when he was in a canoe.

———

And so the pattern developed: travelling quickly around Rupert's Land when the lakes and rivers were open, wintering in London with his family, except for the first winter, which he spent back at Red River, in the brand-new quarters at Lower Fort Garry, where he once again connected with his younger cousin Thomas.

Although, in keeping with the prevailing attitudes of HBC managers

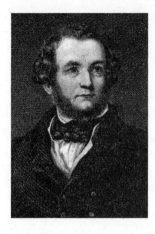

Thomas Simpson, George's first cousin.

of the time, Simpson often had little good to say about Aboriginal people
and only slightly higher regard for "half-breeds" (though he had sired
a number of children in this category), he had earned the respect, if not
the admiration, of many non-whites. Simpson was a company man who
knew that the increasingly contested royal charter on which the whole
HBC operation was founded required that these North American First
Nations be looked after properly. He tended not to accept the prejudg-
ments of others with respect to the character of his colleagues and
would-be Aboriginal partners in the trade, preferring to trust his own
judgment. The Governor was supremely confident in his ability to look
another man in the eye and talk him into almost anything. In fact, having
travelled in the company of Native people for thousands of miles over
more than a dozen years, Simpson ironically may have been inclined
to conciliation more with Métis and Indian people than with his own,
where more Machiavellian leadership, bolstered by the tyranny of rank
in a hierarchical management structure, could prevail.

His cousin, in contrast, would earn nothing but contempt from the
non-white population. And for this, he would have to pay dearly.

After serving with the Governor on entering HBC service, and again
as his clerk at Red River during the disastrous matrimonial winters,
Thomas Simpson had been given a position of added responsibility at

Red River that put him in charge of a fractious rump of discontented Métis who lived beside the equally unhappy, though less rebellious, Selkirk settlers and HBC traders.

Unlike his more manipulative cousin George, Thomas could not hide his racist views. That, combined with arrogance and condescension, alienated him from the Red River rank and file. Unfortunately, Thomas ended up beating a Métis employee who had come to him for an advance on his pay. Thomas's brother Alexander, who was also in the trade, described what happened in late December 1834 this way:

I had the delight of again meeting with my beloved brother on the last day of the year, 1834. Dissatisfied with the prospect which I saw before me, of a monotonous winter's residence at Moose Factory . . . I "took my foot in my hand," started from that place in October, and reached Red River on the 31st of December, after a journey of no little hazard, fatigue, and privation.

I found the colony in high excitement. Rapid increase in numbers, from a continual influx of retired servants with their native families, had caused the half-breed class of the population to become mutinous and insolent. This class has ever entertained a deep hatred against the whites—a feeling in which the pure aborigines of but very few tribes participate.

This rancourous feeling, at all times existent, had recently been roused to increased bitterness, by some trivial changes in the mode of transacting business; and there wanted only a slight cause to call it into action.

That cause had been found two days before I arrived. A young Canadian, half-breed, had come half drunk into my brother's office, and insisted upon having money for his holiday diversions. He had, already, received in advance a considerable part of his pay for the succeeding summer, and was refused any further advances. The fellow, who had been my brother's voyaging servant, grew insolent; he was ordered out; refused to obey, and my brother proceeded to eject him;

he resisted, and got the worst of the scuffle, coming off with a black eye and a bloody nose.

This very trivial affair was magnified into a *class* affront, the half-breeds assembled in great numbers, and in high excitement. Even those of the colonists, who had only a sixteenth part of Indian blood in their veins, some of them educated in the civilized world, linked themselves with the Canadian *Bois Brûlés.* The storm was not met with spirit and promptitude on the part of Governor Simpson. Instead of putting on a bold front, which would soon have cowed these blusterers, he entered into negotiations with them—receiving their deputies and sending missions to their meetings . . .

Even the demand made by them, that my brother should expiate his imputed or imagined offence by receiving a public flogging, could not rouse this vacillating plausible man, to a resolution of defiance, which everyone knew might, with the utmost safety, have been given. His only step was a tampering negotiation with a neighbouring Indian chief, which being an attempt to set class against class, excited the half-breeds still more; and finally he succumbed so much to their menaces, as to give them a barrel of rum, and a sum of money as an expiation. He moreover intimated his intention of removing my brother from the colony.[2]

And that is exactly what Simpson did, in good time. He shipped his cousin off with Peter Warren Dease on an Arctic expedition.

This incident shows George Simpson at his best. The highest good in the situation was not his impetuous cousin's well-being or standing in the community, but maintaining a working relationship with the *bois brûlés*, or "burnt-wood," people who ruled Assiniboia south and west of Fort Garry and did great service in keeping the Sioux and other Plains Indians, as well as the Americans, in check in their advances against HBC interests.

That summer, Simpson finished the first (and only) gubernatorial sweep of the entire operation of the Hudson's Bay Company's interests in North America with a tour of the installations downriver on the St. Lawrence—the so-called King's Posts—that had come into HBC purview when the two fur companies had amalgamated. In September he headed across the Atlantic, clearly back on top of his game. He travelled with James Keith, chief factor of the HBC head office in Lachine, and when the two of them presented themselves to the London Committee, William Smith, Secretary, noted in a letter to J.G. McTavish that "our friends the Governor with Chief Factor J. Keith made their appearance this morning via Liverpool by the Packet of the 1st [of October 1835] . . . The former has grown blooming again and looks ten years younger than when he left London Spring 1834."

With operations in Rupert's Land running more or less smoothly on their own, Simpson now had time to extend his personal and corporate bases both in North America and on the world stage. His biannual sojourns in Lachine, where he stayed in handsome Hudson's Bay House, the largest mansion in the tiny town, situated opposite the old stone NWC depot from which, for decades, laden canoes had come and gone, allowed him to continue his integration into the political and social life of Montreal, nine miles downriver. Of course, as the settlements of Upper and Lower Canada had grown and matured, with them blossomed a diversity of opinion about how things should be run. Without doubt, as Simpson sipped fine wines and discussed the politics of the day with other Montreal businessmen at the reorganized Beaver Club or at any other of a number of institutions and establishments, such as the Beef-Steak Club, of which Adam Thom, a Montreal newspaper editor, was secretary, he was able to wheedle advantages for HBC affairs as well as to advance his own social and financial agendas. In London, even with the growing influence of the mercantile class, peerage and family roots were everything, whereas in Montreal, status was unofficially awarded on the basis of other qualifications, such as business success. Simpson had money and corporate heft, and he had made a number of shrewd investments and strategic associations in Montreal that would see him become an integral member of the Canadian business elite.

Upper and Lower Canada were the scene of much political ferment during the 1830s. William Lyon Mackenzie, one of the legendary rabble-rousers of this era, was first expelled from the assembly of Upper Canada in 1831 for criticizing the government and would be twice more removed from that same house before famously marching down Yonge Street with a band of rebels in December of 1837, and fleeing south of the border for sanctuary when the coup failed. In Lower Canada during the same period, in a conflict based as much on language and ethnicity as on politics, Louis-Joseph Papineau led a patriot movement that culminated in his also ultimately unsuccessful declaration of independence for French Lower Canada in October of 1837. As he had done in the trade, George Simpson seemed to be able to mute his opinions when it mattered and to voice them as required; he remained on good terms both with conservatives siding with the governments and with restless liberals agitating for reform.

On the government side, Simpson befriended leading Upper Canadian politician Francis Hincks, who made several decisions as a cabinet member and premier that were advantageous to the HBC. As Simpson biographer John Galbraith noted, Hincks "assigned responsibility for making government payments to Indians in the Lake Huron area to the company's trading posts, thus keeping them attached to the company rather than having them travel to central distribution points where they would come in contact with influences which might seduce them from their roles as fur hunters."[3] Simpson, as the unofficial official for the British government almost everywhere else in northern North America, would have stressed to Hincks the advantages of an alliance between the HBC and the ruling party.

On the other side of the political spectrum, Simpson befriended a smart, outspoken and irascible character whom he may well have met first at a dinner meeting of the Beef-Steak Club in Montreal. Adam Thom was another Highland Scot, from Brechin on Tayside, south of Aberdeen. His anarchical spirit and his literate if racist rants against Papineau and his followers on the one hand and the government on the other (for kowtowing to the French) appealed to Simpson, who'd had a soft spot for radicals since he was young. Ten years younger than the Governor, Thom had emigrated in 1832 and started work as a lawyer but within months had assumed the editorship of the *British, Irish and Canadian Gazette*. Polemical rants in this periodical, also called *The Settler*, soon earned the paper and its vociferous editor the nicknames "Slop Pail" and "Dr. Slop."

Thom lasted only a year in this incarnation before moving on to other teaching and editorial jobs in Montreal, including the editorship of the *Montreal Herald*, where he continued propagating his anti-government, anti-French views until the Rebellion of 1837 confirmed his fears and he got better offers to move on in his career. One of those offers came in 1838 in the form of a contract to write about better government for Lower Canada from newly installed governor general Lord Durham, who had been charged with the task of sorting out a solution to the separation of Upper and Lower Canada. The other offer came, surprisingly, from George Simpson, who invited Thom to fill the newly created post of "recorder of Rupert's Land," which was essentially an opportunity to reorganize and rebuild the laws and administration of justice in Assiniboia.

To Simpson's delight, Thom accepted and moved to Red River. This was the beginning of an important association with the HBC that would see Thom ghostwrite prose for the Governor that would eventually land Simpson in almost as much hot water with the British parliament as Thom himself had been in with the government of Lower Canada.

———

The machinery of the trade running smoothly, though still very much under the synoptic view of his eagle eye, Simpson could afford to pay more attention to the geopolitical stage in which the HBC drama was being enacted. In truth, the politics of an emerging Canada had less impact on the affairs of the HBC in North America than did the politics of the United States and Russia as they collided with company interests in the Pacific.

Border issues with the Americans in lands east of Assiniboia were much clearer than they were west of that land grant, although since 1818 there had been an agreement that the border would travel from "the North Western Point of the Lake of the Woods, along the forty ninth parallel of north latitude,"[4] at least as far as the Rockies. But on the ground west and south of the Red River settlement, in the absence of laws or anyone to police them, there was constant and often lethal bickering over who was hunting and fishing where, and who was trading what commodities with whom.

In 1831, President Andrew Jackson and the American Congress, increasingly alarmed by British influence south of the border, conducted hearings spurred on by John Jacob Astor and any number of other owners of fur-related businesses in the American west. Testimony by flamboyant American soldier-trader General William H. Ashley, who had led a party into fur country to reconnoitre the situation, estimated that activity by the HBC and its allies north of the border cost the Americans in the order of a million dollars a year, alleging further that these same interests were "exciting our own Indians against us."[5]

Through his periodic visits to the United States, through a network of contacts in New York, Boston and even Washington, DC, made largely through business connections and his frequent use of the Quaker packet ships, Simpson knew many of the principal players on the American scene. Quietly, in his own inimitable style, Simpson offered Ramsay Crooks, the general manager of the American Fur Company, an annual payment of three hundred pounds in return for a promise that the Americans would not interfere with Indians or the Indian trade to the north or west of Lake Superior, which was about as close as the firebrand Scot could come to saying he was sorry. But with John McLoughlin, Peter Skene Ogden, James Douglas and other good men on the ground in the far west, and with the Oregon situation in abeyance—the parties having agreed to disagree and to share the contested lands for ten years in the 1818 agreement, though the matter was still far from settled—Simpson realized that of equal or perhaps greater concern to HBC interests in the Pacific was Russia. Czar Alexander I's famous *ukase* (proclamation) of 1821 had unilaterally declared ownership of everything north of fifty-one degrees north latitude. As with everything else he set out to manage, Simpson knew that the only way to work things out with the Russians was to speak to them directly. There was no point negotiating with the men who were doing the work in Russian posts on the northwest coast. Simpson knew he needed to face the top management of the Russian-American Company directly.

Competition with the Russians in the Pacific northwest was as much about territory as it was about business. The Russians had been there first, since 1745, and therefore for much longer than either the British or the Americans, and they had developed a robust business with the Chinese in trade of sea otter pelts. But there were also the First Nations of the coastal areas—Aleuts in the archipelago; Tlingit; Haida in the Queen Charlotte Islands; Tsimshian, Heiltsuk and Nuu-chah-nulth farther south along Vancouver Island—who had furs to sell as well as material needs to be supplied with European goods. A Russian move to the south, onto the mainland, meant reduced opportunities for the HBC to move north. Simpson's original assessment, made during his trips to Columbia, was that the company should retain maximum business potential and flexibility by developing trade based in coastal vessels. He also knew that the Russians' supply lines to the Pacific northwest were long and expensive to maintain. He understood that if the HBC could provision the Russians at Sitka more cheaply than they themselves could by shipping goods from home, this would be a lever of control on Russian affairs as well as a profit point for the Company of Adventurers.

Chief Factor John McLoughlin, on the ground, had a very different perspective. He felt that creating a string of coastal establishments was the best way to secure an economic and geographic foothold against the Russians and, after Fort Langley had been created at the mouth of the

Fraser River in 1827, he moved quickly, in 1831, to build Fort Simpson at the mouth of the Nass River (named after Simpson's cousin Aemilius, who had died suddenly in the process of establishing the post), Fort Nisqually in 1833 on Puget Sound and Fort McLoughlin west of Bella Coola, also in 1833. After his success in trapping out the Snake River District, thereby creating an almost fur-free buffer zone south of the Columbia River, Peter Skene Ogden had been dispatched north to explore the lower valley of the Stikine River for trading possibilities there. This outreach transgressed into effectively Russian territory at the mouth of the Stikine and, before the HBC could establish a post there, the Russians seized the opportunity and hurriedly constructed a fort called the Redoubt St. Dionysius on the Stikine estuary, with the fourteen-gun brig *Chichagoff* anchored just off shore.

Discussions with the Russians conducted by Simpson when he was on the west coast in the winter of 1825 had left open the possibility for a British installation upriver on the Stikine, but the Russians may have divined at that time that Simpson was more interested in an itinerant ship-based trading system. Eight years later, however, when Chief Factor McLoughlin dispatched a small vessel called the *Dryad* to the Stikine River with the intention of moving upriver and establishing a post, it appeared that the Russians had had a change of heart. No shots were fired, but the *Dryad* was turned south again without achieving its goal. When word of the incident filtered east into Rupert's Land and thence to London, it was clear that there were fences to be mended with the Russians.

But Simpson, who may have dealt with Russian buyers in Europe during his days in the sugar trade, knew that if any kind of deal was to be hammered out, it would have to be negotiated either at the HBC office in Germany, to which representatives of the Russian-American Company could be invited, or on Russian soil, perhaps at St. Petersburg on the Gulf of Finland, next to the Baltic Sea.

Business liaisons between the British and the Russians were nothing new. As early as 1695, the HBC had appointed a former company agent in Hamburg, Charles Goodfellow, to open a Russian office to oversee sales of 50,000-plus beaver skins into that market. In fact, with a head start in the fur business, the Russians had been in the European market longer than the Hudson's Bay Company and had developed superior techniques and technologies for the preparation of pelts. For the first century or so of the Hudson's Bay Company's procurement of beaver furs in North America, for example, skins that had not been worn by the Indians prior to trading and that still had the long coarse guard hairs in the fur (wearing the furs caused the guard hairs to be shed, leaving the valuable underfur available for manufacturing) had to be shipped first to the Russians, who alone had an industrial process for separating the two types of fibre. And once the domestic markets in their respective countries were exhausted, the Russians and British competed head to head in the sale of both raw furs and derivative manufactured goods such as hats and fashion garments in the markets of Europe.

Chief Factor McLoughlin was livid over the *Dryad* incident, demanding that the Russians pay £22,150 in damages for the injury to British trade caused by the HBC's failure to establish a Stikine River post. But Simpson and the London Committee knew that there was more to this than mercantile squabbling between two fur companies. The HBC was, in a very real sense, acting for Britain in these matters, and the RAC was acting more or less on behalf of the czar. Both knew that these lands had potential value for settlement and territorial expansion that far exceeded the commerce of trade.

The situation was of such importance that for the first time in eighteen years—for the first time since he had joined the HBC—George Simpson forwent his annual canoe trip in North America, opting instead to stay with his family in London through the spring and to accompany John Henry Pelly, governor of the London Committee, on a journey to Russia from July to September 1838 to try to negotiate a new working arrangement.

Simpson's 1838 trip to Russia is of particular interest because he documented the travel in a journal, written in his own confident scrawl, for the benefit of Frances. The diary reveals perhaps a more poised or relaxed Simpson, insofar as he took risks in revealing details of his personal life and dealings that heretofore had not turned up in his correspondence or personal papers. One of the things we learn, for example, is that the private Simpson was a man for nicknames, referring to three-and-a-half-year-old little Frances as "Ded" or "Deddy" and to his wife as "Decky" or "Little Mole." And although he is still far from effusive in his prose, there is almost a tenderness in this journal written, perhaps, by a man who was mellowing with age. In St. Petersburg he wrote, "Wednesday, August 29—Up at 6"—a very late sleep in for Simpson—"good night & better. Dreamt of Deck and Deddy & when I awoke and wished myself back with them. Wrote a letter to my little Charmer & forwarded it to [British chargé d'affaires] Mr. Milbanke for the purpose of being sent by his Foreign Office Courier." Later that day, he tossed in another entry: "Got my Hair cut by a French Barber who said a Toupee would become me exceedingly."[6]

Having left 5 Trinity Square on July 17, Simpson and Pelly travelled by ship from London northwest through the North Sea to Kristiansand, Norway, through the Skagerrak and south around the horn of Denmark and the toe of Sweden into the Baltic Sea—variously wined and dined by merchants and politicians at ports along the way—before heading northwest again up the Baltic coast and east up the Gulf of Finland past Kronstadt to St. Petersburg, arriving Monday, August 27, 1838. There they were met with apparent indifference on the part of the Russians, who had no particular urgency to meet with the visiting merchants. Britain's man on the ground in Russia, John Ralph Milbanke, who worked daily on matters of trade with the Russians, held out no hope at all of bringing them to any kind of resolution of the Stikine River affair, much less to any larger agreement on cooperation in the Pacific northwest of North America. But the sheer force of Simpson's personality seems to have changed all.

Pelly and Simpson had to cool their heels in St. Petersburg for nearly two weeks, getting their proposal to the Russian-American Company

translated, going to the theatre, visiting parks, state buildings and libraries (at one of which Simpson was nonplussed to see a fresh copy of
his cousin Thomas's report, written with Peter Warren Dease, of their
Northern Discovery Expedition)—essentially waiting until they could
connect with the people they had come to see. No matter where he went
or what he did, Simpson always seemed to make a point of noting the
pretty women he encountered, from the "dark-Eyed Parisienne" actress,
to the pretty women passing in and out of their carriages at the Vapour
Baths, or the ones he encountered when window shopping with Pelly
along Regent Street in St. Petersburg's imposing central business district.
Eight days after their arrival, they finally connected with Mr. Savarine,
the chairman of the Russian-American Company, who explained (by
way of excuse) that they had been waiting for the arrival of their main
man from the field, Baron von Wrangel, who was due in another day or
two. At that point, the tenor of the visit warmed considerably.

On the evening of Thursday, September 6, they were asked to dress
formally, and a carriage sent to their hotel whisked them to Baron
Studleozs's dacha outside of town. Simpson seemed most impressed
with what transpired that evening:

> The company continued to pour in till ½ past 6 when we sat down
> 50 in number to the most Splendid Banquet I ever beheld . . . The
> old Baron sat at the middle of the Table, the British Minister on his
> Right, Mr. Pelly on his left, then General Wilson on the one side &
> Admiral Record on the other then my self & corresponding with
> me Count Somebody . . . The Baron's Iced Champagne Punch was
> the most delicious thing I ever tasted. The Table [was] set out with
> ornamental plate & glass & beautiful Silver Stands with Flowers a
> Tumbler & 5 beautifully cut glasses of different sizes, plate, napkin &
> Bread for each Sitter. Two soups handed round on each side the table,
> afterwards . . . Larded Beef, afterwards Artichokes, afterwards 2 kinds
> of fish, afterwards Game Pie, afterwards Venison Steaks, afterwards
> Vegetables of some kind, afterwards double Snapes[7], afterwards Iced

Champagne Punch, afterwards Iced Creams, afterwards other Sweets, afterwards Peaches, Apricots, Pineapples . . . Then a general move to the Drawing Room. Coffee . . . Then Liqueurs. Then cards, then Tea and at 12 o'Clock adieus & breakup. In going one of our Horses got the Staggers & on wheeling round came in contact with the chariot of 4 of Milbanke & the Dutch minister: knocked off the lamp & broke the carriage glasses, down came our Horse. The Dutch Minister's open carriage light driving after Milbankes picked up. Gave the Driver 5 Rubles. The ambassadors laughed heartily & so did we having the best joke which only cost 5 Rubles whereas to the Diplomatists it must have cost 100 in Broken Lamp & glasses . . .

Friday, September 7—Got up with a head Ache . . .[8]

Later that day Pelly and Simpson attended a meeting at Russian-American House to discuss peace in the Pacific northwest. There, among other company officials, they finally encountered the illustrious Baron von Wrangel. Simpson, on first blush, was not impressed: "At 12 went to the Russian American House, found Baron Wrangel there, an extraordinary looking ferret eyed, Red Whiskered & moustachioed little creature in full Regimentals . . . very thin, weak & delicate but evidently a sharp clever little creature . . . stupid to a degree."[9]

Simpson and von Wrangel not only had obvious physical similarities, they were already known to each other. These two highly placed field operatives for their respective fur companies had been corresponding for more than a decade, since Simpson's first trip to Columbia. Both were curious and adventuresome characters who, after what may have been for both a bad first face-to-face impression, struck up an instant friendship. Almost immediately, von Wrangel spoke of his interest in Dease and Thomas Simpson's findings. Governor Simpson (in spite of being insanely jealous of his ne'er-do-well cousin's book) took the opportunity to give von Wrangel a copy of their narrative that he had brought with him, along with an Arrowsmith map of the HBC posts in

North America. A week later, it was clear that any reservations Simpson might have had about von Wrangel had vanished. He wrote: "Wrangel and I very thick, a nice intelligent clever little man, regret much we have not seen much of each other."[10]

The upshot of this chemistry between Simpson and von Wrangel was that the British chargé's prediction was proved wrong and the rudiments of a comprehensive and mutually beneficial deal (which turned out to be much better for the HBC than for the RAC) were worked out. The terms were not sufficiently advanced for them to sign the agreement before they headed back to London, but the following winter, keen to meet up again, both men travelled to Hamburg, where the deal was finally concluded. The Russians gave the HBC a ten-year lease on all contested territories in the northwest, in return for two thousand seasoned land otter skins, and also committed to allow the HBC to furnish food and other supplies needed by its installations in North America, at a profit. [11]

Perhaps the event most emblematic of the fact that Simpson had in eighteen short years mastered domestic trade and gone beyond the role of a mere business operative was a state dinner that was held in Christiania (now Oslo), Norway, in honour of his and John Henry Pelly's visit. It was here that the overseas governor (not Pelly, his boss) was feted as the "head of the most extended Dominions in the known world the Emperor of Russia the Queen of England and the President of the United States excepted." By 1838, Simpson the statesman had taken centre stage.

Not long after arriving home in London, although he had been running Caledonia, Columbia, the King's Posts and the Northern and Southern Departments of HBC operations in North America on his own for some time, he received from the Committee a formal commission as president of Council and governor in chief of Rupert's Land. Strangely, by that time the promotion seemed somehow inconsequential.

CHAPTER XV

GEORGE SIMPSON, MURDERER?

After the Russian experience and a summer away from the North American trade, Simpson returned to Rupert's Land with renewed vigour. Crossing the Atlantic, as he had done by now more times than he could readily count, he dashed to Hudson's Bay House at Lachine, then on across Canada to meetings at Norway House and York Factory, via the Red River settlement. From there, with exhausting successions of eighteen- and twenty-hour days, borne in the arms of his proud coterie of tireless Mohawk voyageurs, he doubled back to see McTavish at Moose Factory and continued on south and east through Abitibi, Timiskaming, Mattawa, Lac des Allumettes, Fort Coulonge and Lake of Two Mountains to Lachine. Changing his kit at Hudson's Bay House and shifting from canoe to riverboat, the Governor charged down the St. Lawrence in September, for his second visit to the King's Posts at Quebec, Tadoussac, Chicoutimi and Lac St. Jean in September, before returning to Lachine and heading down through the Catskills to catch a Hudson River steamer for New York, leaving New York harbour aboard the packet ship *Mediator* on October 1. On the surface, all was right as right could be.

That summer of 1839, adding currency to the successes of the St. Petersburg trip, his underlings in the trade decided to congratulate him in a special way. A plan to mark the occasion was circulated by the senior officers among themselves at Norway House in a secret memo:

24th June, 1839
To the Chief Factors and Chief Traders
of the Honble. H. Bay Compy.

Gentlemen,

The unexampled prosperity of the British Fur Trade during a period of nearly twenty years under the direction of Governor Simpson, to whose masterly arrangements that prosperity is mainly owing, has called for the admiration of every person interested in its affairs, while that Gentleman's active habits of business, conciliating disposition and address have been productive of the happiest effects in diffusing a spirit of enterprise and harmonious co-operation through the wilds of British North America unequalled perhaps in any other part of the world.

These considerations forcibly present themselves at this particular time, when entering on a remodelled constitution under the most flattering auspices and embarking in new and important branches of business, chiefly brought into view through the unremitting exertions of that Gentleman which renders the present a fitting opportunity for marking our sense of his management in such a manner as we trust may not be disagreeable to him, while we feel assured it will be most gratifying to every member of the Fur Trade.

We therefore, the Commissioned Gentlemen now assembled at Norway House, forming ourselves into a Committee of management, beg to propose that each Chief Factor subscribe £50.-.-. and each Chief Trader £25.-.-. in order to create a fund for the purchase of a service or piece of Plate, to be presented to Governor Simpson as a small token of our respect and regard, with a vote of thanks for his valuable and important services to the Fur Trade, which will shed lustre on his government while that Trade exists.[1]

This gesture resulted in the presentation of a lavish silver six-light-standard candelabrum with feathered bowl above and three Aboriginal figures (in almost Greco-Roman drapes) on guard on a tri-cornered base.[2] The trophy was an affirmation of Simpson's success as a business leader and manager of widely dispersed and disparate men. The levy raised was in excess of £1,200, and the subscribers, who were named on the trophy, included every chief factor and chief trader in the land. Funds in excess of the cost of the candelabrum were given to Simpson in cash with the wish that they be used to build "a residence to be named Beaver Lodge," which they thought Simpson might want to construct for himself and his family in Lachine. (Simpson eventually did build a summer house on an island in the St. Lawrence River, and may in fact have used the funds given to him on this occasion to do just that, but the catchy name suggested by the Commissioned Gentlemen in 1839 did not stick.)

What is most interesting about this gesture is that, in the fullness of time, it revealed something less than unanimity among the rank and file. It turned out that whether you adored or feared the Governor, you had ample reason to contribute to a conspicuous gesture of support for his leadership.

A famously cranky senior HBC officer named John McLean had this to say in his memoirs about the presentation:

This circumstance may be adduced by Sir George's friends, with every appearance of reason, as a proof of his popularity; but the matter is easily explained. Some two or three persons who share Sir George's favour, determine among themselves to present him with some token of their gratitude. They address a circular on the subject to all the Company's officers, well knowing that none dare refuse in the face of the whole country to subscribe their name. The same cogent reasons that suppress the utterance of discontent compelled the Company's servants to subscribe to this testimonial; and the subscription list accordingly exhibits, with few exceptions, the names of every commissioned gentleman in the service; while two-thirds of them would much rather have withheld their signatures.[3]

John McLean had lived out one of Simpson's bad ideas and, for his trouble, had been overlooked repeatedly for promotion. In the early 1830s, the Governor had heard from traders passing through missions established on the Labrador coast by the Moravians, a Protestant sect from Saxony, that the fur potential was strong and well worth investigating in Labrador and the Ungava region of what is now the province of Quebec. Simpson had sent McLean, who had shown great promise as a company man in HBC posts in the Ottawa Valley and Caledonia, to proceed to a new post called Fort Chimo at the base of Ungava Bay, established in 1831 by traders from Moose Factory. From there, McLean was to move overland into Labrador, which he did, travelling from Fort Chimo down the entire spine of Labrador to Hamilton Inlet (and along the way discovering the Great Falls of Labrador—now the site of the Churchill Falls power development). The ambitious clerk's understanding was that if all went well in Ungava and Labrador, he would be rewarded with a promotion to chief trader.

Ultimately, over the next decade, efforts to develop a fur trade in the Labrador interior failed: beavers were all but absent from the country, and it cost a fortune to operate the posts. McLean was relieved of his duties at Fort Chimo but did eventually get his promotion and went on leave. Hungry for a new charge, he returned and became acting head of the HBC operations at Fort Simpson, at the confluence of the Liard and Mackenzie rivers, thinking that it was only a formality until he would be placed officially in charge of the Mackenzie River District. But that was not to be. Instead McLean was commissioned to convene an expedition led by scientist John Henry Lefroy to make observations in the northwest that the company hoped would triangulate the position of the magnetic North Pole.

McLean, while he played along with organizing the Lefroy expedition, was vexed in the extreme that Simpson had done him out of his more significant command, and in the summer of 1844 he finally exploded. He wrote to Simpson as no one had written to Simpson before:

Sir—I have the honour to acknowledge your several favours from Lachine and Red River, and am mortified to learn by them you should think me so stupid as not to understand your letters on the subject of my appointment to the charge of the district; your language being so clear, in fact, as to admit of no other construction than the one I put upon it . . .

When in 1837, I was congratulated by every member of Council then present at Norway House on the prospect of my immediate promotion (having all voted for me), your authority was interposed, and I was, as a matter of course, rejected. You were then candid enough to tell me that I should not have your interest until the two candidates you then had in view were provided for, and that it would then be my turn. With this assurance from you I cheerfully prepared for my exile to Ungava. My turn only came, however, after seven other promotions had been made, and I found myself the last on the list of three gentlemen who were promoted at the same time.

You are pleased to jest with the hardships I experienced while battling the watch with opposition in the Montreal department [traders who, like McLean, objected to the Ungava/Labrador experiment], and the privations I afterwards endured . . . Surely, Sir, you ought to have considered it sufficient to have made me your dupe, and not to add insult to oppression. While in the Montreal department I have your handwriting to show your approval of my "meritorious conduct", the course I was pursuing being "the direct road to preferment"; and your intention, even then, "to recommend me to the favourable notice of the Governor and Committee"—promises in which I placed implicit confidence at the time, being as yet a stranger to the ways of the world.—The result of these promises, however, was that the moment opposition had ceased, I was ordered to resign my situation to another, and march to enjoy the "delectable scenery" of New Caledonia; from thence you sent me to Ungava, where you say you are not aware I experienced any particular hardship or privation.

You are aware of the circumstances in which I found myself when I arrived there: that consideration was not allowed to interpose between me and my duty, however; and I accordingly traversed that desolate country in the depth of winter,—a journey that nearly cost myself and my companions our lives. I then continued to explore the country during the entire period of my command, and finally succeeded in discovering a practicable communication with Esquimaux Bay [Labrador], and in determining the question so long involved in uncertainty as to the riches the interior possessed, and by so doing saved an enormous expense to the concern. The Hon. Committee are aware of my exertions in that quarter, themselves, as I had the honour of being in direct communication with them while there.

> I have the honour, &c.
> (Signed) "John McLean"

The "&c." of McLean's closing was not published until several years later, after he had resigned his commission. He wrote: "In no colony subject to the British Crown is there to be found an authority so despotic as is at this day exercised in the mercantile Colony of Rupert's Land; an authority combining the despotism of military rule with the strict surveillance and mean parsimony of the avaricious trader. From Labrador to Nootka Sound the unchecked, uncontrolled will of a single individual gives law to the land."[4]

Principal among McLean's many concerns was the illusion of democracy that surrounded Simpson's interpretation and enactment of the deed poll, which called for participation by chief traders and chief factors in the decision making of the trade. On the occasion of his parting of ways with the HBC and its "despotic" governor, McLean wrote,

As to the nominal Council which is yearly convoked for form's sake, the few individuals who compose it know better than to offer advice where none would be accepted; they know full well that the Governor has already determined on his own measures before one of them appears in his presence. Their assent is all that is expected of them, and that they never hesitate to give ... Some years ago, I happened to be at [Norway House] where a "Council" was about to be held. On inquiring of his Excellency's Secretary what subject of moment he thought would first engage their attention—"Engage their attention!" he replied; "bless your heart, man! the minutes of Council were all drawn out before we arrived here; I have them in my pocket."

Clothed with a power so unlimited, it is not to be wondered at that a man who rose from a humble situation should in the end forget what he was and play the tyrant. Let others, if they will, submit to be so ruled with a rod of iron. I at least shall not.[5]

John McLean was certainly not alone in his enmity for George Simpson, but he was one of the very few who had the courage to vent directly to the Governor. McLean knew that had he not resigned on his own volition after writing this letter, Simpson would have found ways to see him summarily out of the trade. As quickly as word spread through Rupert's Land about the 1849 publication of McLean's discontent, in a book called *Notes of a Twenty-Five Years' Service in the Hudson's Bay Territory*, people scrambled to distance themselves from the man. To this day, the copy of McLean's book in the library of the grand provincial legislature in Victoria, British Columbia, contains a hand-written caveat scribed in a margin by McLean's trader colleague in New Caledonia, Alexander Caulfield Anderson (grandson of Scottish botanist Dr. James Anderson), who felt compelled to write: "As regards the remarks generally of the author upon the H.B.C. and the system pursued in the Indian Country I shall make no comment on them. There is no one who has travelled through the country who could not contradict most of the statements made. The animus that inspired the whole is obvious ... I have

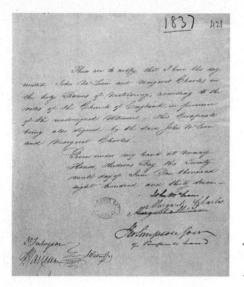

John McLean and Margaret Charles's wedding certificate, signed by the Governor.

always had a high respect for the author, with whom indeed I have been in correspondence until very recently; and I feel assured that on reconsideration he would at this day wish much of what has evidently been written under feelings of anger and disappointment, were unwritten."[6]

Whatever the veracity of McLean's particular complaints, his public denunciation of Simpson points to the Governor's almost absolute control and authority in Rupert's Land and the west. Simpson alone was head of a large international company covering a vast territory. He was proxy for the British government for much of that territory. He was even proxy for the Church of England in some places, having officiated at, among other events, the marriage of one John McLean to a Métis woman named Margaret Charles, at a quasi-religious ceremony at Norway House on June 20, 1837. People didn't flinch at referring to the balding little spark plug as "Your Excellency." George Simpson had the power to change the course of history and the trajectories of people's lives. As important as his absolute hold on people in Rupert's Land was his control of information flow within that milieu. Perception was everything, and no one knew that better than George Simpson.

With Simpson's changes for good the record is well stocked—much of it written or dictated by the man himself, or by those afraid of retribution. Of darker influences, of the man's deepest drives and insecurities, there has been murmured speculation over the years, but very little of this has been committed to the printed page. Yet there is one incident—one unsolved mystery—arising from the untimely and unexplained death of Simpson's cousin Thomas, which raises questions of conspiracy and, worse, murder.

———

Simpson's departure from his childhood home was coincident with the 1808 birth to his principal caregiver, Mary Simpson, of Thomas. Even though Thomas, many years later, at first shunned his cousin's overtures to join the HBC, Simpson's impressions of him as a young adult were on the whole quite good. After he enticed Thomas to join him in the trade, those feelings developed into an easy respect, even admiration, for the young scholar's industry and intellect. In his 1832 Character Book, for instance, Simpson characterized his cousin-cum-clerk as follows: "A Scotchman 3 years in the Service 24 Years of Age; Was considered one of the most finished Scholars in Aberdeen College: is hardy & active and will in due time if he goes on as he promises be one of the most complete men of business in the country; acts as my Secty and Confidential Clerk during the busy Season and in the capacities as Shopman, Accountant & Trader at Red River Settlement during the Winter. Perfectly correct in regard to personal conduct & character."[7]

That view, sadly, gradually faded, especially after the Red River incident in 1832 when Simpson was left to quiet a storm among the Métis brought about by his cousin's temper and management foibles. Thomas's ego and arrogance began to rub people, including his cousin, the wrong way. Indeed, if Simpson had gotten wind of his cousin's letters to his brother Alexander, written from Red River one winter when the Governor was in the UK (which he may well have, through his long-established gossip channels or from sycophants on the dark

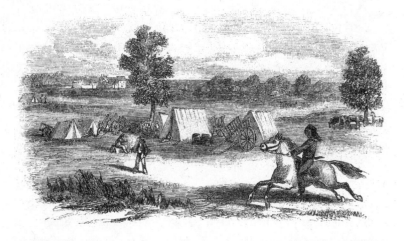

Land in the upper Red River valley, between St. Paul, Minnesota, and the Red River settlement, was contested ground, occupied by various Aboriginal tribes and groups of Métis who were able to liaise with Americans and others not directly affiliated with Red River to work around the HBC's monopoly on trade.

side wishing to curry favour), he would have been even less impressed. Thomas had convinced his brother that "when the Governorship of the country became vacant, he himself would be the person best adapted to fill it,"[8] an impression buoyed regularly in letters with comments like this: "You would, perhaps, like to know how we have been going on this season—exceedingly well; far less bustle and as good and rapid work as if the Governor himself were on the ground. Entre nous, I have often remarked, that his Excellency miscalculates when he expects to get more out of people by sheer driving; it only puts everyone in ill humour."[9] Or this: "If the Governor does not come out again, I have no idea who will step into his shoes. Old Keith [at Lachine] is a dried spider: good heavens! what a Governor! I wish I were five years older: in every other respect, without vanity, I feel myself perfectly competent to the situation; and, with one or two exceptions, hold the abilities of our wigs in utter contempt. This season I have been intimate with many of them—have in the Governor's absence, had much to do with the general business, and see how easily these men can be led."[10] In December 1834, when Thomas nearly caused a Métis rout at the Red River settlement, Simpson was forced to remove him from authority with breathtaking speed.

In many respects, Simpson's decision to appoint Thomas second-in-command on an expedition to the Arctic led by the old hand Peter Warren Dease made sense. In anticipation of future assignments, and inspired by his relative Alexander Mackenzie and David Thompson, Thomas, on his own volition, had studied astronomy and surveying in Scotland, Canada and Red River with exactly this kind of challenge in mind. The expedition itself, to chart the unexplored coastline of Rupert's Land, honoured one of the covenants of the HBC's original charter—a prudent move in the mid-1830s, a time when an increasingly influential merchant class in the UK was agitating against government-sponsored monopolies. And to team up a bright young officer with a seasoned hand like Peter Warren Dease, who had been with Captain John Franklin on his second overland expedition, was also a smart move. But where the whole plan to extricate Thomas from trouble in Red River by sending him to the hinterland went horribly wrong was that Dease and Simpson achieved success and acclaim in their northern travels. Simpson was enraged that his upstart cousin's achievements might somehow eclipse his own ambitions in Rupert's Land.

What Thomas achieved in 1837, in the first of three summer expeditions, was to chart the 150-mile connection between Return Reef, the westernmost point reached by Sir John Franklin's 1826 expedition, and Point Barrow, the easternmost point reached in 1826 by a party from HMS *Blossom* sailing up and over from the Bering Strait, thereby completing the western end of the Northwest Passage. It was the report of these findings that George Simpson found in a Russian library and that he proudly took with him—perhaps hoping that people would see and celebrate his role in commissioning the voyage—to give to Baron von Wrangel. Had Thomas stopped his explorations there, he might have survived longer than he did.

Encouraged by their success, Dease and Simpson wintered at Fort Confidence, a post they built on the northeast shore of Great Bear Lake, and pushed down the Coppermine and the other way, east, the following summer, to try to make a similar connection on the eastern side of the Northwest Passage. That summer, 1838, they were turned back by ice. In 1839, they did not connect eastern exploration points, as they had done in 1837, but they came close enough to think that establishing the geography of the Boothia Peninsula (named after the founder of Booth's gin, who had funded the original discovery expedition) and completing the charting of the Northwest Passage was not only possible, but within their grasp—at least within Thomas's grasp. Fifty-year-old Dease's eyesight was failing, and he was plagued by family troubles as well; by 1839, he had decided to leave continuance in Simpson's hands. At this juncture, Thomas wrote to his cousin the Governor for permission and funding to extend the project another year, which he was certain would see him claim discovery of the Northwest Passage. It was at this point that Simpson determined to make absolutely sure that no such discovery would be made, at least not by Thomas Simpson.

In a classic Simpsonian letter, sent to Fort Simpson, where Thomas was making preparations for a fourth and final triumphant push to conclude his exploration between Hudson Bay and the mouth of the Great Fish (Back) River and finally to chart the Northwest Passage, the Governor dashed his cousin's aspirations:

> We observe that, whether successful or otherwise, in accomplishing the survey to Great Fish River, you are not prepared to continue the operations of the expedition next year, which is to be regretted, as we were in hopes that, after that section of the coast had been surveyed, you would have been in a condition to push your discoveries to the Straits of Fury and Hecla [between Baffin Island and the Melville

Peninsula]. That, however, we find cannot be done under any circumstances; you may therefore repair to the depôt [Fort Garry] and take a winter's leave of absence if agreeable to you, by way of recreating after your severe and hazardous labours; during which I have no doubt plans will be matured for completing this very difficult and interesting service, which cannot be allowed to fall to the ground while a shadow of hope remains that there is a possibility of accomplishing it.[11]

Thomas was livid. Until now in his reporting on their joint expeditions, he had soft-pedalled the fact that Dease, as nominal leader of the expedition, had not pulled his weight. He himself had stepped into the breach at key times—walking, for example, the final 150 miles from Return Reef to Point Barrow while Dease languished in a tent. But no more would that kind of discretion be exercised. In prose that John McLean might have appreciated, breaking ptarmigan quill pens as he dipped and scrawled, Thomas Simpson first went above his cousin's head and sent a request for permission and support directly to the London Committee. Then he scratched out a reply to his cousin, "whose jealousy of his rising name was not but ill disguised":[12]

Fort Simpson, October 25, 1839

. . . So far from wishing to avail myself of the leave of absence you have so kindly offered unasked, it gives me great uneasiness that a whole year will probably elapse before the final expedition can be set on foot that is destined to accomplish this North-east, as my excursion to Point Barrow in 1837 achieved the North-west Passage.

Probably you considered the discretion I solicited in my letter of the 31st of January too great, at least I infer so from your silence on that head . . .

As for what remains to be done, I am so far from seeking to convert it to my future advantage, that, with my life, I hereby place at your disposal, towards meeting the expenses of the new expedition, should there be any obstacle, the sum of five hundred pounds, being every shilling I am worth at this moment, beside all the future proceeds of my double commission, til the whole charge of the said expedition shall be redeemed.

Fame I will have, but it must be mine alone. My worthy colleague on the late expedition frankly acknowledges his having been a perfect supernumerary; and to the extravagant and profligate habits of half-breed families I have an insuperable aversion.[13]

Consumed by his anger, and with possibly a winter to wait before he would receive any kind of reply to his missives, Thomas packed up his notes and maps in a satchel, pulled on his well-worn woollen blanket capote, laced new moosehide mukluks made by the Dehcho people of Fort Simpson and stomped southeast on snowshoes. Averaging a phenomenal 30-plus miles per day, probably with dog carriole support, he left Fort Simpson on December 2, 1839, and covered the 1,910 miles from the Mackenzie River to Fort Garry in a scant 61 days.[14]

By this time, of course, the Governor was comfortably ensconced with Frances Sr. and Jr. in London but, with his well-established control over people and information flow on both sides of the Atlantic and his deep roots in both the white and Métis communities at Red River, and surmising that Thomas would sooner or later find his way there, he had any number of ways to circumvent his angry cousin's drive for recognition. A quiet word here or touching the palms of a person there with money was all it would have taken.

In London, the Governor's first tactic was to delay letters to Thomas[15] containing the Committee's endorsement of the fourth expedition, plus a second dispatch to Thomas with news that he had been awarded the Royal Geographical Society's Gold Medal for his 1837 discoveries as well as, for both Dease and Simpson, a government pension of £100 per annum. Simpson would have known that if he slipped into the transit room in the quayside warehouse and stowed these dispatches in canvas mail bags destined eventually for York Factory, instead of in express mail bags that went back and forth on the year-round monthly packet ships out of Liverpool, this news would reach Thomas at best in mid-summer, stalling his plans for at least another year.

In Red River, Thomas waited until the arrival of the express canoes from Lachine on June 2, 1840, to see if there might be a note of congratulation for his achievements or, more important, a reply to his request to the Committee. These never came. Thomas Simpson would be dead before his letters would arrive.

Intent on getting to London to speak directly to the Committee, Thomas left Fort Garry in early June 1840, headed south for St. Paul, Minnesota. This was the much-contested territory of the Sioux Indians, so it was customary for travellers linking to east–west transportation options in St. Paul to be armed and on their guard. Several days south of Fort Garry, Thomas Simpson died of a mysterious gunshot wound, probably to the head.

That Thomas Simpson died on the bald prairie between Fort Garry and St. Paul is an indisputable fact. How Thomas Simpson died remains a contentious and much-debated subject. Various accounts put him in the company of four other men, all Métis, travelling with a larger group of settlers heading south: John Bird, a relation of the George Bird who had travelled with Simpson back from Columbia and who had gotten lost for three weeks with Tom Taylor; Antoine Legros and his son, Antoine Junior, who had worked off and on for the HBC; and Red River labourer and hunter James Bruce.

Keen to move faster than the main party, on or about the ninth day south of Red River these five galloped ahead and started making camp on their own. One long summer evening on the sun-soaked plains somewhere south of the forty-ninth parallel, a skirmish happened and, deposed witnesses agree, Thomas Simpson shot dead John Bird and mortally wounded Legros Sr. It is possible Simpson was wounded as well, though how this injury was inflicted unclear. Some versions of the story have Legros Sr. appealing to Simpson to let his son go free but not before kissing him one last time. Whether or not that happened, Legros Jr. and James Bruce apparently scrambled onto their mounts and rode back through the night to the main group of settlers, whereupon a posse from the larger group came south to the shooting scene. There they found Legros Sr. and Bird dead and Thomas Simpson down but very much alive. During the drama that played out in the next few minutes, Thomas Simpson died of a gunshot, which everyone later agreed, based on the depositions of James Bruce and of Robert Logan Jr. and James Flett, two of the settlers who participated in events on the second day, was self-inflicted. The official explanation of Thomas Simpson's death was that he "committed suicide while of unsound mind, after murdering two of his four Métis (half-breed) companions."[16]

The circumstances of Thomas Simpson's death have been debated almost from the day it happened. James Bruce claimed that after Simpson had shot Bird and Legros, while they were putting up the tent, he told Bruce that his life was not in danger and that he had shot the other two "because they had intended to murder him on that night for his papers."[17] Why Métis frontiersmen who probably couldn't read would want such documents, unless they were acting on instruction or with the understanding that these might be sold for some consideration, is a mystery. That these men, given the fracas at Red River in December 1834, might want to kill Simpson is not surprising; indeed, given the mutual enmity between Thomas Simpson and the Métis community, it is a wonder that these men were with him at all, even for generous pay. How two presumably skilled hunters could be killed by an Englishman with a double-barrelled shotgun in two different shots without either of them fighting back is more curious. It is also odd that by these accounts Thomas Simpson lay more or less beside his two supposed victims through the night before allegedly shooting at the party that arrived the next morning, and before putting the shotgun between his knees and blowing off his own head. There are many questions.

The first thorough treatment of the matter appeared in a paper by amateur historian Alexander McArthur, read before the Historical and Scientific Society of Manitoba in 1887. In a detailed and engaging treatment of both facts and conjecture, set up as a report on a trial of Thomas

Simpson for the crimes of murder and suicide (which was as much a criminal act as a moral infelicity in those times), McArthur concluded his monograph as follows: "I have performed my task imperfectly if I have not convinced you that at least a verdict of 'Not proven' would be returned to the charges of murder and suicide. To my own mind the evidence carries the conviction which would justify me in giving the much stronger verdict of 'Not guilty.' The contrary nature of the evidence; the fact that no report of his death was carried back to Fort Garry; the apathy of the participants in the events; the careful procrastination of the company; the carelessness of the investigation, if such it could be called, all point to a dread of other revelations."[18]

Almost every other writer since who has considered the strange death of Thomas Simpson[19] has, in one way or another, broached the obvious "other revelation" in all of this speculation—that George Simpson was involved in, indeed could have engineered, his cousin's premature death. Historian Marjory Harper, for one, writes, "A more intriguing (if somewhat fanciful) version of the murder theory implicates George Simpson himself in his cousin's death."[20]

The venerable Arctic explorer and writer Vilhjalmur Stefansson, in his consideration of the strange death of Thomas Simpson, is less speculative, suggesting that besides good old-fashioned jealousy, there might have been a more pragmatic reason for the Governor to suppress his cousin's discoveries: "Then, too, there has been talk that the murder was instigated by George Simpson, through jealousy of the fame that was to be his cousin's, or, more plausibly, to hinder the development of the Northwest Passage as a route of commerce and thus to delay the settlement of the Fur Lands by agriculturalists and the loss of the Company's trade monopoly."[21] But he too eventually backs away from the idea: "We have, as said, no evidence to support the idea that Sir George, in his long career, ever plotted with anyone to kill anyone. We have no evidence, either, to prove that he did not go that far in a passionate loyalty to the Company which, unless it be murder, seems to have had no other limit."[22]

Simpson's connection to these events certainly merits another look. Since his first winter journey around the inner circle of posts through Rupert's Land, when he met, travelled with and was much impressed by Métis leader Cuthbert Grant, through his other various travelling parties, which often included Métis, like George Bird, and up to his siding with the *bois brûlé* community in the December 1834 debacle with his cousin Thomas, Simpson was well-connected with this community. Simpson had personally chosen and recruited Montreal lawyer and writer Adam Thom to reorganize and administer the justice system in Red River, and by the time Thomas died, Thom was firmly in control of all things legal in Assiniboia. If Simpson had wanted a full and impartial investigation of his cousin's death, all it would have taken would have been a letter to his friend Adam Thom. Why did Thom not, on his own volition, take more interest in the Simpson death? Perhaps he was discouraged from doing so by any number of influential people with vested interests in advancing the murder-suicide version of the story.

And then there are the other things that Simpson did and did not do in relation to this case. Three years after the death, when it became evident that the shallow grave in which Bird, Legros and Simpson had been buried where they died had been disrupted by wild animals, Thomas's body was then taken to Red River. That the body of his kin was not better treated—dumped in a grave with those he was supposed to have murdered—is astonishing. What is even more surprising is this: on the Governor's instruction to Pierre Leblanc, the carpenter at Red River (who had willingly, on Simpson's request, consented to marry Nancy McKenzie when she was cast aside by J.G. McTavish), Thomas Simpson was given an outcast's burial and interred in an unmarked grave on the outskirts of the settlement.

There is also the matter of the diary, maps, letters and other papers Thomas was carrying on the day that he died. If these were part of a Métis motive for killing him, they were not stolen or sold but were duti-fully turned over to HBC officials at Red River, who directed them to the Governor. Simpson did not actually receive them until May 17, 1841, but he certainly knew of their existence, that they were on their way to him and what he was planning to do with them, because on February 25 of that year he wrote to his friend HBC London governor Pelly with the following news: "His [Thomas's] Journals and Narrative I should, if you have no objection, wish to be reserved for myself, to be embodied in a work which, if I live to return [from his planned round-the-world journey] and command a little leisure time, I have it in contemplation to publish."[23]

Simpson, of course, never did publish anything based on his cousin's papers. In fact, three years later, when Thomas's papers were finally turned over by Simpson to his cousin Alexander, Thomas's younger brother, the diary and all correspondence from the Governor to Thomas were absent from the dossier (the diary has never surfaced). This fact could lead one to surmise that the Governor had no intention of letting his cousin's achievements ever see the light of day.

Did Simpson give the quiet instruction to kill Thomas and make it look like a suicide? We can never know. But a direct consequence of the suicide was that when Thomas's brother Alexander placed in the Dingwall parish church an alabaster stone tablet celebrating Thomas's achievements, it had to be quickly removed to a less controversial location in the Dingwall Town Hall, "on the grounds that a man who had committed the crime of suicide should not be commemorated in a church."[24] To this day the tablet, which remains in old Dingwall Town Hall (now a museum), erroneously but nevertheless conspicuously heralds Thomas as "the discoverer of the long sought North West Passage."[25] By virtue of this claim, people in Dingwall know all about the town's explorer son, Thomas Simpson.

The ultimate irony is this: When asked about another Dingwall man, who was once feted as "head of the most extended Dominions in the known world the Emperor of Russia the Queen of England and the President of the United States excepted"—a man described as one who "combined the widest range of authority with the widest range of territory and the longest tenure of power ever enjoyed by one man in North America"[26]—the people of Dingwall reply, "George who?"

—

PART III

SIR GEORGE AT LAST

CHAPTER XVI

AROUND THE WORLD

The most important outcome of Thomas Simpson's northern explorations was the role they played in ensuring the renewal of the company's licence for exclusive trade in North America for another twenty-one years. The Hudson's Bay Company's monopoly had been affirmed earlier, in 1821, following the amalgamation of the North West Company and the HBC on terms set out in the deed poll signed the same year. The British government now, in the latter 1830s, had its hands full in Upper and Lower Canada and was well aware of the important role the HBC, led by George Simpson, was playing in exercising its national interests elsewhere in North America, notably on the Pacific coast. So when the HBC moved early and somewhat preemptively to secure renewal of the licence, the government was inclined to look favourably on the request from an applicant that was doing in a vast territory what Whitehall had neither the resources nor the political drive to attempt. But with critics and detractors watching its every move in monopoly trade situations, Parliament had to demonstrate that the applicant was upholding its end of the bargain, including conditions that custodial care of Aboriginal peoples be exercised, that attempts at colonization be brought forward and that the company be seen to be

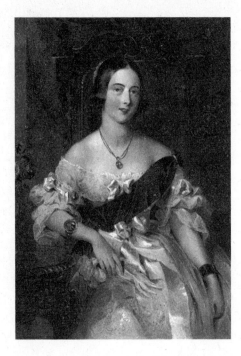

A young Queen Victoria as she looked about the time she knighted John Henry Pelly and George Simpson at Buckingham Palace.

contributing to the knowledge of North American geography through exploration. Pensions for Peter Warren Dease and Thomas Simpson were one conspicuous way to let the public know of the government's approval of HBC activities. But an even more conspicuous message was a correct manipulation of London levers to see to it that senior HBC officers who had supported the explorations were knighted by the Queen.

For Simpson, who hungered for recognition, the good news came in a letter from Lord John Russell in July 1840, written just two weeks after Thomas Simpson's untimely death. John Henry Pelly was to be made a baronet, Simpson a knight bachelor.

It must have been at best a pyrrhic victory with Thomas dead. But, having written the letter of commission to Dease and Simpson and engineered the logistical support for the expeditions, Simpson felt he deserved the recognition. Still, he must have been frustrated that the well-stationed chair of the London Committee, who had really contributed very little compared to Simpson, was being given a higher honour than the man who had done all the work.

In the hierarchy of chivalrous orders, baronet was a hereditary honour, meaning the title "Sir" could be passed on to the bearer's son (though no title passed to a daughter). The more common title of knight bachelor conferred a non-transferable honour to its recipient. Pelly got his honour in July 1840, and Simpson made plans to attend his own ceremony at Buckingham Palace in January 1841.

In the trenches there were those who celebrated Simpson's rise in status and accompanying new honorific and those who thought the whole thing was a sham. Among the detractors was John McLean, who felt about the "bauble" as he did about the piece of plate given to Simpson when he had become governor in Rupert's Land:

> Sir George owes his ribbon to the successful issue of the Arctic
> expedition conducted by Messrs. Dease and Simpson. His share of
> the merit consisted of drawing out instructions for those gentlemen,
> which occupied about half-an-hour of his time at the desk. It is quite
> certain that the expedition owed none of its success to those instruc-
> tions. The chief of the party, Mr. Dease, was at least as well qualified
> to give as to receive instructions; and Sir George is well aware of
> the fact. He knows, too, that Mr. Dease was engaged in the Arctic
> expedition under Sir J. Franklin, where he acquired that experience
> which brought this important yet hazardous undertaking to a success-
> ful issue; he knows also that in an enterprise of this kind a thousand
> contingencies may arise, which must be left entirely to the judgement
> of those engaged in it to provide against . . . Sir George's administra-
> tion, it is granted, has been a successful one; yet his friends will admit
> that much of his success must be ascribed to his good fortune rather
> than to his talents.[1]

McLean's legitimate complaints about Sir George notwithstanding, the disgruntled trader's assessment of the source of Simpson's success

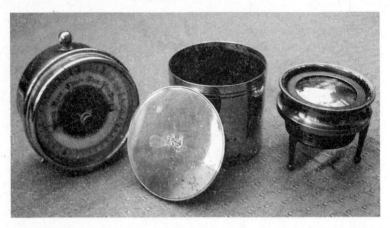

Sir George's travelling aneroid barometer and a hand lens, used to keep track of his correspondence as his eyesight was failing, are two of a few of his treasures that remain with the Haddon family in Peebleshire, Scotland.

could not be more inaccurate. Once Simpson entered the trade—and there was a certain measure of serendipity in that—he had his share of luck, certainly, but much of his success was entirely of his own making. He was keenly observant of people and circumstance, he had a phenomenal memory and he was a strategic player with a hot temper to get things done on the spot and the patience of Job in assembling complex plans and waiting for them to come to fruition. And in his pending knighthood, he saw a potent opportunity that could not be missed.

Between June of 1840 and his date with the young queen in January of the following year, Simpson wrote the necessary letters and did what was required to put in place the necessary ingredients of a crowning achievement that, in the absence of boasts about family pedigree, would befit his entry in Dod's *Peerage*: he would circumnavigate the globe, going overland when possible, as no one had done before, employing his now absolute command of HBC resources from London to Labrador across to Columbia, California and the Sandwich Islands, and, prevailing on his new-found friendship with Baron von Wrangel, over northern Asia, across the vast territories of Siberia and Russia, back to St. Petersburg and finally across the sea route he already knew home to London. And he would write (or have written for him) a book about this venture that would put the name George Simpson on the map, along with Mackenzie, Kelsey, Henday and Hearne, as a literary gentleman, an explorer, a man of courage and character—a knight of the titled classes.

Of the actual ceremony we know little, except that it happened in the throne room of Buckingham Palace on January 25, 1841. Simpson would have been dressed to the nines in topper and tails, with ample heels on his hand-stitched patent-leather shoes under pearl grey spats that would have brought him to a full five foot seven inches. On his arm, stepping from a fine carriage provided by the HBC, would have been a frail and pale Frances, his wife of almost eleven years now, in the rocky first trimester of her third pregnancy after having recovered from a bout of smallpox in the fall, and not yet thirty years old. But she too would have been splendidly attired in new garb for the occasion, in crinolines, lace and whalebone corset. Unlike her husband, Frances was schooled by breeding and knew the protocols for entering the palace and making their way to the throne room to velvet chairs placed beneath the pear-shaped crystal chandelier that dominated the centre of the grand hall.

Young Princess Victoria had ascended to the throne four years earlier on the death of her childless uncle, William IV. She had married her German cousin Albert nearly a year before. The Prince Consort would have been present for the ceremony as well, sitting to one side of his bride under a proscenium arch over the dais supported by two winged figures of victory holding garlands above the throne. But none of this would have stopped Simpson from a quick sizing up of the twenty-year-old queen as he knelt before her sword.

A month following the ceremony, on March 3, 1841, Sir George left London to begin his world tour. With him was twenty-year-old Edward Martin Hopkins, a talented young journalist whom Simpson had plucked from the London press corps to be his amanuensis. Hopkins could make up for the Governor's failing eyesight and, with shorthand for dictation and an excellent grasp of English, help Simpson with the all-important task of journal keeping on the journey. Hopkins's father, Martin, was a London ship and insurance broker who had an office in Cornhill, not far from Fenchurch Street, but the connection to the HBC may have been through John Henry Pelly, who attended the same church as Hopkins in West Ham parish. Soon, Simpson and Hopkins, during their transatlantic passage on the steam packet *Caledonia*, would meet the engaging, Gaelic-speaking young Mr. McIntyre who, on a whim, was invited to accompany them for the rest of the journey.

Stopping at Boston on March 20,[2] and travelling overland on the now very familiar road to Lachine, Simpson, Hopkins and McIntyre arrived at Hudson's Bay House on March 25. There the newcomers were shown to spare bedrooms in the spacious accommodations of the main house, and Simpson fell immediately back into the life of a bachelor emperor, tending to the business of the HBC, as guided by Chief Factor Keith, and pacing the hardwood floors of his office at Hudson's Bay House, dictating to his new secretary.

There were still the outfits and indents to reconcile and the efficiencies of each post to measure and assess. Farming and retail operations in Assiniboia, Columbia and Caledonia all required scrutiny; figures had to be matched against anecdotal accountings of success and failures. And, of course, there was incoming correspondence on every matter under the sun, from disciplinary problems that had made their way up to the boss to matters of international diplomacy with the Russians and the Americans in the Pacific.

Despite his comings and goings, Simpson was well integrated into the society of Montreal and Lower Canada, never missing opportunities for making or building strategic alliances for the company or for himself in social, political and even military circles. Simpson allowed selected members of the British forces stationed in the St. Lawrence Valley to accompany him on his journeys west into Rupert's Land. In the summer of 1839, a Colonel Fowler from the Coldstream Guard, the oldest British regiment, stationed at Quebec City, was among a select number of military officers who travelled with Simpson and his canoe-borne entourage from Lachine to Fort Garry. In the spring of 1841, a similar arrangement was struck with two young nobles also serving in the British army in North America: George Augustus Phipps, the earl of Mulgrave, and James du Pre Alexander, the earl of Caledon. They were to travel westward with Simpson on this next leg of his round-the-world tour.

Lord Caledon was twenty-nine at the time, but there was boyish enthusiasm in a letter to his mother back in Ireland written that spring:

Quebec April 9 1841

My dear Mother . . .

I entirely forget whether I told you of my projected trip with Simpson in my last letter. I am going for 3 months to shoot in the neighbourhood of Red River and returning with the next party. I have leave till the first of August. I may be back before that time if I am bored but not much if I find that I like it I daresay I shall remain a little longer. Two of our officers went the year before last and they liked the trip but found the constant paddling rather monotonous, but I shall never have another opportunity of seeing the country so well . . .

I shall go to Montreal and visit Mr. George Simpson before starting from where I shall write after which I have any opportunity, I shall send letters to you but unless there is a party leaving Red River the instant we get there I shall be back nearly as soon as any letter can come . . .

I believe we are to travel in great state with about 20 voyageurs in each canoe. There is no great difficulty in the voyage as our old Colonel Fowler who is near 60 went the year before last . . . I shall be glad to get a little recreation as I have been nearly 10 months at work here . . .

Your affectionate son,
Caledon[3]

The advantage to historians of Lord Caledon's participation in the canoe journey west that year is that he, as well as Sir George, kept a journal of the voyage. And although Caledon's notes are much less detailed than Simpson's (or Simpson's as dictated to Hopkins in the long canoe hours as the voyageurs paddled from before dawn to after sunset), an engaging image emerges of Simpson as an old Rupert's Land hand and storyteller.

Having been up and down the route from Lachine to Red River many times over more than two decades, Simpson had stories for almost every rapid, every portage and every Indian band they encountered and, by Caledon's account, relished the chance to retell these to a rapt audience. At Lake of a Thousand Islands (now Lac des Mille Lacs), for example, Caledon recounts Simpson's telling the young officers of getting lost for four days on a previous trip, nearly starving and finding their way west "only by a mere chance."[4] Simpson may not have told the young lords about a small insurrection that had taken place near that very spot, where one of his voyageurs, utterly fed up with the boss's noisy petulance, pitched the raging little emperor into the lake and hauled him out again before he knew what was happening.

Caledon appears to have taken all this in stride as a grand adventure, with the possible exception of Simpson's penchant for early starts. As usual, "sleeping in" meant going to bed at dark and sleeping until 1:30 or 2:00 a.m. "Getting up early" meant rising almost on the same day the men had gone to bed. "So sleepy, I lost my gun," Caledon wrote on May 17 after getting up at 12:30 a.m. and stumbling around in the dark to gather his things quickly lest Simpson leave without him.

At one point in the journal, Caledon noted an audience between Simpson and a large group of Salteaux Indians near Fort Frances, the post on Lac la Pluie named after the Governor's young English wife. The Indians were vexed and perplexed that the old traders in the area (the NWC or possibly the Americans) had promised them liquor "as long as the rivers flowed." The rivers were still flowing, but since the HBC had become the principal trader in the area the rum had stopped,

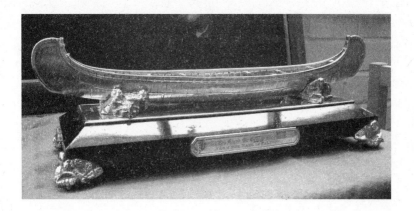

As a thank-you for taking him west to hunt buffalo in Assiniboia, James du Pre Alexander, the young earl of Caledon who was an officer of the Coldstream Guard in Quebec City, commissioned from Garrard of London a sterling silver replica of Sir George's express canoe. This exquisite piece of Canadiana, on loan from the Haddon family in Peebleshire, Scotland, was exhibited at the Canadian Canoe Museum in Peterborough, Ontario, beginning in autumn 2007.

and they wanted to speak to Governor Simpson about reopening the tap. Caledon wrote, "The nut was cracked and some presents were given them. Dressed in the Sergeant Major's coat. Most of the men were painted, smoked with them . . . toasts to chiefs past."[5]

What Caledon's journal fails to mention is that there were actually a hundred or more Salteaux warriors in full regalia, who had been drumming and dancing and getting more and more restless by the day as they awaited the Governor's arrival. Nor does it mention that Simpson, for his part, knowing his party was seriously outnumbered, called for all of the pomp and ceremony he and his party could muster.

In his narrative of the event, Simpson recounts "invit[ing] my children to attend me at four in the morning" after having spent a sleepless night inside the fort with the Salteaux outside the palisade "pelting away at me with their incantations." He mentions asking Mulgrave and Caledon to put on their best regimental dress. The rest of the party, "not to be outdone in magnificence . . . , equipped ourselves like so many mandarins in our dressing gowns, which luckily happened to be of rather showy patterns and hues." The account of proceedings from that moment on in the stand-off, with the Governor in his silk dressing gown and beaver topper listening intently to all that was being said, shows diplomacy and a sense of superiority:

> All these preliminaries being concluded, the spokesman of the party stepped forward; and, first ostentatiously displaying a valuable present of sundry packs of furs, he commenced his harangue, in a bold and manly voice, with great fluency and animation. After a tedious prelude, which I was obliged to cut short, about the creation, the flood, &c.,—the object probably being to show how and why and when the Great Spirit had made one race red and another white,—he plunged at once from this transcendental height into the practical vulgarities of rum, complaining that we had stopped their liquor, though we, or at least our predecessors, had promised to furnish it "as long as the waters flowed down the rapids." "Now," said he, in allusion to our empty casks, "if I crack a nut, will water run from it?" In reply I explained to the Indians that spirits had been withdrawn, not to save expense to us but to benefit them. I then pointed out the advantages of temperance, promising them, however, a small gift of rum every autumn, not as a luxury but as a medicine. In thanking them for their present of furs, I told them that, besides receiving a suitable present in return, they would be paid the usual price for every skin. In conclusion, there was another shaking of hands; and then this grand council between the English and Chippeways broke up about six o'clock, to the satisfaction of both nations.[6]

But behind these daily events on Simpson's journey west in the spring of 1841 are darker issues that Caledon touches on unwittingly in his journal. When they arrived at Fort Garry, for example, the two young noblemen were to head off on a hunting trip with Cuthbert Grant while Simpson was to continue west on horseback with Fort Edmonton chief

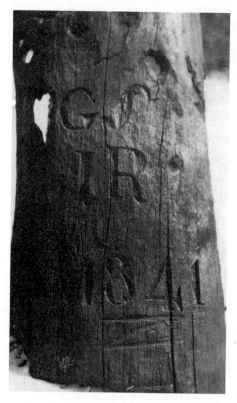

In a great piece of detective work, amateur historian Jim Brewster, of Banff, took two years to find the tree on which John Rowand etched his initials and those of George Simpson when they became the first non-Aboriginal people to travel through Simpson Pass. He finally found it in 1912: a conifer about sixteen inches in diameter that had fallen with the initials down. It is thought that pine pitch, which migrated into the wood on the lower side of the tree, preserved the initials for posterity.

factor John Rowand. But Grant represented a community that not a year previously had participated in a lethal encounter with Simpson's cousin Thomas.

Caledon's journal now adds another strange coincidence to the list.[7] Of all the people in Red River to whom he might have turned to purchase a horse for his hunting trip with Cuthbert Grant, the one he was directed to he described as "Mrs. Bird, widow of the man shot by Simpson's nephew." Why was George Simpson—or any member of his party—anywhere near Mrs. Bird? Was it some sort of compensation?

Interestingly, until Caledon's account of Simpson's 1841 cross-country journal surfaced during the research for this book, historians have pointed to another event on the Lachine-Red River portion of the trip to suggest guilt on the part of the Governor. As they were moving north from Sault Ste. Marie up the north coast of Lake Superior, they were stopped by ice and fog on the lake. While they were camped waiting for travel conditions to improve, an express canoe from the HBC post at the Sault caught up with them and, among other mail, handed the Governor a satchel of his cousin's effects. Given the fact that the man had recently come to a tragic end and that Simpson had just been knighted, in part, on the strength of what was contained in the dispatch that arrived at their little campfire, one wonders why Simpson chose not to say anything worthy of the young officer's mention. In his own account of the journey, Simpson wrote, "A boat from our establishment brought me the journal and other papers of my late lamented relative, Mr. Thomas Simpson, whose successful exertions in arctic discovery and whose untimely end had excited so much interest in the public mind. By the same conveyance we got a supply of white fish. This fish, which is peculiar to North America, is one of the most delicious of the finny tribe, having the appearance and somewhat the flavour of trout." In his book *Unsolved Mysteries of the Arctic*, Vilhjalmur Stefansson is quite sure that there is something decidedly fishy in this notation: "The real affection of the Governor for Thomas, and the approximate depth of his sorrow for his death, we gauge through [this] paragraph from the Governor's book."[8]

Obviously awed by his experience with the illustrious governor, as his letters home illustrate, Caledon had the time of his life on this journey. After this grand canoe adventure, he headed west with Cuthbert Grant, had various encounters with the Sioux and other Indians, and hunted with abandon on the prairie south and west of Red River, killing with his Métis companions "2 to 300 buffalo a day (before breakfast)."[9]

Lord Caledon, after retiring from the army, continued making regular hunting trips to almost every corner of North America for the rest of his life. As a mark of his esteem for Simpson and the way in which this first canoe journey had whetted his appetite for adventure, he commissioned Garrard of London, the Queen's silversmith, to fashion of pure silver an exquisite 1:25 scale likeness of a birchbark *canot du maître* on an ebony base with an inscription plate that reads, "To his friend Sir George Simpson from the Earl of Caledon." It remains one of the very few of Simpson's personal effects identified today.[10]

At Fort Garry, Simpson joined Chief Factor John Rowand, who was heading for Fort Edmonton by horse and cart instead of by canoe. Even though they were able to travel the six hundred miles from Fort Garry to Fort Carleton along the North Saskatchewan this way in just under two weeks, Simpson was frustrated by the fact that they had to stop to allow the horses time to graze enough to give them food sufficient for another day on the trail. This was difficult for the Governor, "inasmuch as the horses could not eat, like the voyageurs, as fast as ourselves."

Interestingly, when he eventually got to the west, boasting of "having performed a land journey of about 1900 miles in 41 days," the equine travel seemed like a cakewalk, with a scant eleven or twelve hours a day in the saddle, as compared to eighteen and twenty hours a day in the saddle of his far-ranging bark canoes. Horses or canoes—as long as he was moving, and as long as there was some measure of adventure and excitement in what he was doing and where he was going, Simpson seemed satisfied. But in spite of his fur trader's heart, there was satisfaction from another source that had not been present on his earlier journeys to the west: out of Fort Carleton they encountered a mile-long straggle of livestock and Red River carts carrying twenty-three families from Assiniboia who were making their way west to try their luck homesteading in Oregon Country. Simpson noted in his journal, "The emigrants were all healthy and happy, living in the greatest abundance and enjoying the journey with the highest relish."[11]

Proof of the man's indomitable pioneering spirit was etched yet again in his chosen route west through the mountains from Fort Edmonton. Instead of heading west and north up the North Saskatchewan to Fort Assiniboine and on over either of the other two passes through which he had travelled previously to the coast (probably because conventional wisdom said that the rivers on the other side would be in flood), Simpson continued west and south on horseback, and by a much more direct but untravelled line (at least by Europeans) through Devil's Gap, by Lake Minnewanka,[12] and on up the Bow River to the present-day site of Banff, Alberta. Whether he had intelligence from his sources in the Aboriginal community to stay away from canoes on this journey or whether he was acting on other information from his network of contacts throughout the trade, in August 1841 Simpson, with twenty-two men and forty-five horses, became the first European to push up Healy Creek, past a mountain with a large crater in its side now known as the Goat's Eye and on to the height of land at 6,914 feet above sea level between Arctic and Pacific waters. There he left his initials and the date carved in a tree at the zenith of Simpson Pass.[13] Back on the Pacific slope, but this time on horseback, Simpson followed an old Indian trail along what are now the Simpson and Vermillion rivers to the Kootenay River Valley, Kootenay Lake, Fort Colvile and eventually Fort Vancouver, where he reconnected, for the first time since 1829, with Chief Factor John McLoughlin—and re-entered the internecine politics of HBC affairs in the Pacific.

In his Character Book of 1832, Simpson appeared to appreciate at least some of Dr. John McLoughlin's qualities as a person, calling him "a good-hearted man and a pleasant companion," but it was evident, even then, that from the moment he had overtaken the "proud giant"[14] and his disorganized crew on the way west in 1824 (remembering that McLoughlin and his party had had a three-week head start), the Governor had more or less dismissed the old Nor'Wester's business acumen. McLoughlin, he wrote, "has not the talent of managing the few associates & clerks under his authority . . . very anxious to lead among his colleagues with whom he has not much influence owing to his ungovernable Violent temper and turbulent disposition . . . altogether a disagreeable man to do business with as it is impossible to go with him in all things and a difference of opinion almost amounts to a declaration of hostilities."[15] So whether Simpson walked into Fort Vancouver with the express intention of picking a fight with McLoughlin or whether he was right that the chief factor's thin skin would turn constructive criticism into a war, the Governor's arrival in Columbia in August 1841 marked the beginning of the end of John McLoughlin's long career in the trade.

Simpson's first move was to start immediately for an inspection tour of HBC installations in the Columbia River valley and northward, checking for himself the state of the western union. Just as the presence of settlers working their way west on the Saskatchewan prairie had indicated the progress of development in the east, so had HBC ambition left its mark on the west coast. With Chief Factor James Douglas at his side, Simpson visited the company's thriving dairy on an island at the mouth of the Willamette River, which was milking a hundred head and feeding a breeding herd two or three times that size. From there, Simpson and his party travelled upriver to another HBC agricultural operation at Cowlitz River, on nearly two square miles of tilled land, which was now producing in a single season 8,000 to 9,000 bushels of wheat, four thousand bushels of oats, and salable quantities of barley, potatoes and root crops. From the Cowlitz farm, they headed back downriver and thence north overland to Puget Sound, where Simpson visited two very successful livestock operations that had been established by the HBC and subsequently turned over to the fledgling Puget Sound Agricultural Company. As summer turned into autumn in 1841, hardworking hands at the Puget Sound farms were husbanding 6,000 sheep and 1,200 cattle, as well as pigs for the table and horses for the mountain trails. Times had certainly changed since Simpson had last been here with his dreams about self-sufficiency for the Columbian operation.

At Puget Sound, Simpson and Douglas boarded the first steamship ever to sail on the west coast, the 101-foot sidewheeler SS *Beaver*, which had been commissioned by the HBC (with Simpson's encouragement), built in England and sailed around Cape Horn to assume trading duties on the northwest coast. The Governor's cousin Aemilius, whom he'd sent to the west to hatch his plan to mount a ship-borne trading operation, had died unexpectedly several years earlier, but his efforts had resulted in a substantial fleet of coastal sailing vessels, the largest of which were the 71-ton *Cadboro*, with its four guns and crew of twelve, and the more imposing 324-ton HBC SS *Vancouver*, with its crew of twenty-four, who muscled, supplied and manned six guns as need be.

The idea of setting up a string of HBC posts along the Pacific coast made sense as long as there was active competition against the Americans and Russians for furs from the northwest-coast First Nations. But since the St. Petersburg agreement, now that the HBC had made a deal to supply their main post at Sitka and to work *with* them instead of against them, there was no longer any real competition from the Russians. And since the purchase of Astoria from the Americans, the application of the "scorched earth" policy by the HBC in the Oregon Country and other anti-American shenanigans executed by Peter Skene Ogden and the Snake River expeditionaries had effectively driven American traders away from the coast and back into the valley of the wide Missouri. As well, for strictly business reasons—meaning he thought it would be more efficient—George Simpson was of the opinion that putting more funds and energy than absolutely necessary into coastal establishments was a waste. His journey north on the *Beaver* in 1841 confirmed that in his mind.

His destination was Sitka, the Russian-American Company outpost on Baranof Island established in 1799, so that he could see how the sole-provider HBC supply arrangement negotiated at St. Petersburg was working out. But on the way north, Simpson stopped at the bucolic Fort Nisqually property, near the present-day city of Tacoma, Washington, on Puget Sound, leaving Edward Hopkins to learn about that operation. From there, he continued north to Fort McLoughlin, near Bella Bella, and eventually to Fort Simpson, built on Russian property on an island in the Nass estuary. At each stop, Simpson called clerks and factors to account and transferred personnel if he thought it in the company's best interest—moves which, in two cases, had lethal consequences. These posts had all been built in the 1830s, with permission from the

London Committee, but they had assumed an importance that contravened Simpson's view that trade should be ship-based. At some point during this voyage on the *Beaver*, Simpson came to the conclusion that it was time to act—time to wind down fixed outpost trading locations in the Pacific.

This move, of course, incensed the old Nor'Wester McLoughlin. To picture a confrontation between these two self-made men is to imagine a study in contrasts. Both men had intelligence and considerable ego, but there the similarities ended. Simpson was a balding little bantam; McLoughlin had a mane of shoulder-length silver hair. Simpson biographer John Galbraith aptly characterized the clash in 1841: "Simpson expected to rule; McLoughlin was accustomed to independence," a spirit which became stronger while he ruled "the remote empire of Columbia."[16] That Simpson would favour a shift away from a constellation of posts that McLoughlin had worked hard to build was bad enough, but this was only the beginning of a conflict that was to intensify over the next few weeks as Simpson continued along the Pacific coast.

The sailing on the *Beaver* forever marked that vessel for McLoughlin as a symbol of all that went wrong with his realm. The two men travelled ninety miles south, to the site of old Fort George, where they switched from steam back to sail, boarding the HBC brig *Cowlitz* with the intent to sail south to check in with the company's outpost in California. But nasty weather and tides played havoc with sailing conditions at the mouth of the Columbia River, and it took eighteen days before the little wooden vessel could clear the shifting esturine sandbars and set sail for Yerba Buena, on the shores of San Francisco Bay. At some point during these rain-soaked miserable December days, beating upriver against tide and buffeting southeasterly winds, George Simpson made another decision contrary to McLoughlin's view of how the Pacific world should work for the HBC. If coastal trade was to be conducted by ship, instead of from fixed posts along the shore, the Honourable Company would require a more predictable supply point for its vessels than the capricious mouth of the Columbia River. That point, in concert with what was now becoming (to Simpson, at least) a foregone conclusion that the border between British and American territory would be extended to the coast along the forty-ninth parallel, so that the Americans would eventually own the land on which Fort Vancouver was situated, led the Governor to conclude that the southern tip of Vancouver Island, across the Strait of Georgia from the mouth of the Fraser River, would be a much better depot for the company.[17] McLoughlin, of course, disagreed but was powerless to countervail.

In Simpson's account of his visit to California, he describes in detail the land and the people (especially the Mexican women whose mysterious lace mantillas and "witchery of manner," "sparkling eyes and glossy hair," "sylph-like forms" and "neatly turned ankles"[18] totally beguiled him), based on stops at Yerba Buena, Monterey and Santa Barbara, but he neglects to say anything about business affairs in this part of the world. The upshot of the visit, however, was another blow to John McLoughlin, who, on the basis of a report from James Douglas (whom he'd sent the previous year to reconnoitre sea otter and other fur potential along the Californian coast), thought the Californian enterprise had great potential for the HBC. But Simpson came to the conclusion that while this outpost had equal chance of falling under American or British rule, it could not and should not be a priority for the HBC. In his analysis, it would never be profitable. Again, McLoughlin disagreed and in due course would be overruled by Simpson.

After a grand party hosted by one of California's leaders, General Mariano Vallejo, the two men parted company in California. McLoughlin caught another HBC supply ship back to Columbia to contemplate packing up and leaving the home he had built and lived in since the day in March 1825 when his little firecracker of a boss had christened the flagstaff with a bottle of good dark Hudson's Bay brand Jamaican rum. Simpson—still driving forward, always in motion—headed out to sea on the *Cowlitz*, destined for the HBC outpost in Hawaii.

Since James Cook's visit to these subtropical islands in the Pacific, Hawaii had been a natural stop for water and fresh food resupply. HBC ships had stopped in since expansion west of the Rockies and eventually, in 1833, had established a post here to take advantage of trading opportunities. But until Simpson arrived on the *Cowlitz* in February 1842, his understanding of commerce with the Hawaiians had been nothing more than lines on ledgers and annual reports about shipments of west-coast timber, salted salmon and flour in return for sugar, molasses, salt and coffee. On-the-ground experience, as a guest of King Kamehameha III, gave the Governor a much better sense of the political complexities of trade at this outpost. With no way of defending against overtures from the French, Spanish, Russian, Americans or British, all of whom had expansionist dreams for strategically situated islands in the Pacific, the King conveyed to Simpson the tenuous nature of his island's independence. Of course, HBC personnel in Hawaii, as well as the British consul stationed there, were all in favour of annexation to protect British interests. But Sir George sided, at least publicly, with his indigenous hosts, arguing that the best option for all concerned was for Hawaii to remain independent. Privately, though, in confidential correspondence with the London Committee, he allowed that "if a private purchase of the islands were concluded a profitable resale to the Russians no doubt could be arranged."[19]

Dining with kings and generals, as quasi-emissary for Her Majesty the Queen, circling the globe playing statesman and diplomat as it suited him, Simpson was clearly in control, on top of the world as he went about his business in the palm splendour of Hawaii. And, though it is difficult to determine what kind of internal reaction he might have felt when mail from England caught up with him here—even homesickness—outwardly he seemed unmoved by the news that his wife had come to term and very nearly lost another baby. In the Hawaiian packet were letters from Frances with this troubling news, as well as a note from a family friend, Sir Augustus d'Este, the baby girl's namesake; but the sweetest and most candid report of September 1841 events at New Grove House was written by his now seven-year-old daughter, the one he had nicknamed "Greyhound":

New Grove House
September 4th

My dearest Papa,

I am very happy to be able to write you a few lines, I cannot write very well but I hope the next letter you receive from me will be better. I am delighted to say that on Tuesday week, Mamma received a little baby, it is a very sweet good-tempered little thing, and no one can put it out, but, I am sorry to say that the poor little dear was born dead, and that Mr. Elliott did not think he could rally it, but I am delighted to tell you that it is quite well now and very like you and me also, it has dark blue eyes, a very fair complexion, and is altogether very pretty. I am sorry to tell you that Mamma has been very ill but Mr. Elliott hopes she will soon be better. I do not go to Mrs. Curtis now, because Mamma was afraid of giving me cold by sending me in the wet weather, but Mrs. Curtis' cousin comes every day to teach me, and Mamma likes that a great deal better. Mamma says if she is well enough she will write you a few lines, if not, I am to write them for her, but I hope she will be able to write them for herself. The garden has looked very pretty this summer. Uncle Webster has been for a trip to Scotland with cousin Alexander, and has enjoyed it very much. Mamma received your kind letter on Monday and told me your message. I will try to be a very good girl and obedient to Mamma. Give my love to Edward Hopkins and Dr. Rowand, and tell him that all the things he gave me are quite safe and I wash my monkey every fortnight. Mamma and all around me unite in kind love and believe me,

> My dearest Papa,
> Your truly affectionate Daughter,
> (Sgd.) Frances Webster Simpson[20]

By now, however, Simpson was a world removed—geographically, emotionally, psychically—from home and family, travelling to advance his company's interests as well as his own. George Simpson was on the world stage, and loving it.

The previous trip to Sitka had confirmed arrangements to sail in the spring to Siberia on a Russian vessel. So from Hawaii, having dispatched Edward Hopkins back to London with the expansive journal he had been keeping—"Herewith I hand you some books and papers made up into a sealed packet, which you will take charge of for me and convey to London, taking special care that they do not get wet . . . The volume of the private journal left out, you will write up, keeping up the narrative until your return to England and not exhibiting either the Journal or the notes to anyone until my arrival"[21]—Simpson reboarded the *Cowlitz* and set sail for return to Baranof Island.

The *Alexander* was not yet ready to sail to Okhotsk, so the Governor decided to improve the shining hour by sailing the short distance south and east to the mainland to finish the inspection tour he had started in the fall. At Fort Durham, all was as expected. But at Fort Stikine, where he had been just months before, flags were at half mast.

To understand the cascade of events that led to the lowering of the colours at Stikine that spring day, it is important to know that leadership in these isolated outposts was critical to their success and that there was not always the talent in their area the HBC would have preferred. So it was common for officers to be moved at a moment's notice either to defuse situations gone wrong or to sort out problems at other posts. Moves were also made regularly for business reasons. Fort Stikine had been run since 1840 by William Glen Rae, Dr. John Rae's brother, who had married one of John McLoughlin's daughters. Second in command was Roderick Finlayson, the young nephew of Duncan Finlayson. McLoughlin's half-breed son and namesake, John McLoughlin Jr., who had had a chequered career to that point both in and out of the employ of the HBC, was assigned to be Rae's assistant. But after only one season at Fort Stikine, William Glen Rae was transferred out. This left second-in-command Roderick Finlayson with McLoughlin Jr. as deputy. But on his inspection tour in the fall of 1841, Simpson had decided that Fort

Stikine was overmanaged and had summarily transferred Finlayson to Fort Simpson. Young McLoughlin was left alone at Stikine with a cadre of undisciplined frontiersmen.

On landing at Stikine for the second time in only a few months, Simpson learned that John McLoughlin Jr. had been shot dead by Urbain Heroux, one of his own Canadian men. Simpson, who was normally an effective judge of character and circumstance, conducted a cursory investigation of the murder, took Heroux into custody for transport to Sitka (because Fort Stikine was a property leased from the Russians), and tossed off a letter to McLoughlin explaining this decision. Historian Willard Ireland describes Simpson's blunder this way:

> After a too hasty examination of evidence, Simpson came to the conclusion that the younger McLoughlin, as a result of drunken excesses and brutality, had driven his men to murder. He consequently sent the suspect to Sitka for investigation but reported to McLoughlin his opinion that it was "justifiable homicide." McLoughlin immediately sprang to the defence of his dead son, and thereafter assiduously collected evidence, all of which was forwarded to London with lengthy explanatory comments. In all fairness, it must be added that McLoughlin was in the right. He established the fact that there was a conspiracy amongst the men against his son [for enforcing company policy on the presence of Aboriginal women in their quarters], that he was not a drunkard or excessively cruel, and that his administration of the post had not been inefficient. The misfortune was that the younger McLoughlin had been left alone at this post by Simpson's withdrawal of Roderick Finlayson. The responsibility for the murder, in McLoughlin's eyes, rested entirely with Simpson, and consequently he did not hesitate to claim that his son "came to an untimely end in consequence of Sir George's most injudicious arrangements."[22]

From that moment on, John McLoughlin could focus on nothing other than revenge on Simpson. He wrote to the London Committee, who closed ranks around Simpson. McLoughlin was told to mend his views about the Governor lest he be forced to retire. Sir George, for his part, simply cut off McLoughlin's five-hundred-pound salary until such time as he might apologize. But McLoughlin was well beyond that and, in fact, wanted to lay a second death at Simpson's feet. He was sure that William Glen Rae's suicide in California, after he'd been sent there from Stikine to run HBC operations, was the direct result of depression brought about by the sudden closure of HBC operations on that front. As Simpson carried on, John McLoughlin became consumed by hatred for the globe-trotting governor. "I have Drunk and am Drinking the cup of Bitterness to the very Dregs," he would later write. In this same letter to HBC London governor John Henry Pelly, he crystallized his anger into one sad postscript:

N.B. I hope you will consider the situation in which I am placed an apology for troubling with these Details—as so Distressed am I at being disgraced and Degraded and which you will admit is natural that though the people are very kind to me if I had my money I would not Remain here if a present was made of it to me—Sir George Simpson's Visit here in 1841 has cost me Dear—taking Mr. Finlayson from Stikine for which there was no necessity and which necessity could hardly Justify led to the murder of my Son, the careless manner he took the Depositions was Ruinous to his character—the Deception practised on Rae by telling him the California Business would be carried on an adequate scale and giving it up when it held such fine prospects Drove Rae to Distraction and because I felt as I ought at his want to Stultify me and make me Believe contrary to the Evidence of facts—and therefore could hold no further private correspondence with him —for which my Salary of five hundred pound p. annum is stopped—I am Deprived of my charge—and called to the other side which will make me lose this property and Ruin me—and which I purchased to prevent the Company Being Despoiled and to manage their business to Better advantage—But my conduct must have been misrepresented—and I trust that the Company will when correctly informed do me justice.[23]

With this discontent swirling in his wake, Simpson dined again as guest of the Russian-American Company in Sitka, boarded the *Alexander* and continued his tour. In the world at large, the Russians had been encroaching on India and Afghanistan with expansionist designs that would eventually lead to the Crimean War. But in Sir George Simpson's world, where Russians and Englishmen of business—"true objects of divine preference,"[24] as he liked to call them—ruled over lesser mortals, the St. Petersburg agreement excluded from possible future theatres of war the entire northwest coast of North America. Simpson's was a world apart. In it, he ruled supreme, regardless of the cost. In the spirit of corporate collusion with his friend von Wrangel, Sir George made his way over land across Siberia to St. Petersburg and on by sea to London.

This epic round-the-world journey had but one purpose, beyond the adventure itself. Six years after his two-volume account of his journey was finally written and published,[25] Simpson was forthcoming with some personal details for Dod's *Peerage* to accompany the entry announcing his knighthood. But instead of family aristocracy, university education, noble affiliation, inventions, discoveries or achievements, Simpson's entry mentions the book and very little else:

SIMPSON, KNT. BACHEL. Creat. 1841.—SIR GEORGE
SIMPSON, governor of the Hudson's Bay company's settlements;
mar. the 2nd dau. of the late Geddes McKenzie Simpson, Esq., of
Great Tower Street, London, and Stamford Hill, Middlesex (she
died 1853); is author of "Narrative of an Overland Journey Round the
World." Residence—LaChine, Montreal, Canada.[26]

Sir George Simpson had returned from his round-the-world journey, but had he "arrived" as he had always dreamed? Probably not.

CHAPTER XVII

PRESIDING AT LACHINE

The village of Lachine to which Sir George Simpson returned after his around-the-world tour was a very different place from the few houses surrounding the NWC depot he had found on his first trip into fur country in 1820. The strategic value of a warehouse and office at the west end of the Island of Montreal was that it was above the first major rapid on the St. Lawrence River and, as such, canoes could be loaded for a long reach of paddling up the Ottawa River before another portage was required. But since that first visit, an 8.5-mile canal had been constructed around Lachine Rapids, and with that had come commercial vessels that could take manufactured goods to settlements up the Ottawa River, to Bytown and, eventually, upriver on the St. Lawrence to places like Toronto, Buffalo, Detroit and Sault Ste. Marie. Coincident with canals and the progress of the Industrial Revolution in North America came a host of steam-powered processing and manufacturing companies, each with an eye on cheap transportation to growing markets in the Great Lakes basin and beyond. What was once a quiet transshipment point on the main highway of the fur trade, nine miles from the City of Montreal, with wafts of wood smoke and manure and echoes of voyageur songs and the gentle bumping of bark canoes, was now a cobbled road and a busy canal awash, when the wind blew from the east, with the smell of eye-stinging coal smoke in the air and the sounds of steamwhistles.

From the biggest house on Rue St. Joseph,[1] looking over the canal to the fur depot beyond, the Emperor of the North presided until his death in 1860. Why Simpson might have chosen Lachine instead of the even more bustling town of Montreal, just nine miles away, might have had something to do with his penchant for hands-on management, for he could sit on the balcony of Hudson's Bay House, or simply look out the tall front window of his office in the southeast corner—or any other window in the house, for that matter—and keep an eye on company operations across the road. Writing in *The Beaver* in 1934, historian Clifford Wilson postulates another reason: "Possibly he felt that residence in Montreal would not bring with it that sense of unchallenged supremacy he so dearly loved."[2]

This is where Simpson held court and from where he ran his empire. The house itself was large by village standards, sixty feet wide, fifty feet deep and two storeys high, with a grand salon on the first floor and bedchambers on the second, which ran the full depth of the house. It had kitchens and a pantry in the back and a full basement for food preparation and storage, as well as attic quarters for domestics. By all accounts the house was finely crafted and well appointed inside, with brass fixtures, generous stairwells and polished wooden floors, banisters, baseboards, wainscotting and sliding panel doors. The Governor's office, with a separate front entrance to the right off the columnar porch that ran across the front of the grey stone facade, was more for show than function, because having been a travelling manager for most of his career, he was able to conduct his business from satchels, paper cassettes and portable writing desks.

It was here in his Lachine office that Simpson surrounded himself with his trail treasures and the personal trappings of success. Among these were ornate pieces of silver he had been given over the years, including Lord Caledon's effervescent silver canoe, given to Sir George as thanks for taking him across the country by canoe in 1841. Also here, for the house help to dust on pain of death should they be damaged or broken, were intricately beaded moccasins from the plains, ornate bark boxes inlaid with weavings of dyed porcupine quills, delicate reed baskets from James Bay, embroidered woollen and moosehide gloves and garments, various paintings and a carved red cedar mask from the west coast. And in a place of prominence was a portrait of Napoleon Bonaparte—the other little emperor.

Simpson's adulation of Napoleon was well known among officers of the trade. Indeed, depending on circumstances and who might have been making the observation, George Simpson embodied any number of maxims variously attributed to the French commander: "I have never found the limit of my capacity for work"; "Impossible is a word to be found only in the dictionary of fools"; "They think I am stern, even hardhearted. So much the better—this makes it unnecessary for me to justify my reputation"; "My motto has always been: A career open to all talents, without distinctions of birth"; "I have recognized the limits of my eyesight and of my legs, but never the limits of my working power"; "I have a taste for founding, not for owning"; "Friendship is only a word, I care for nobody"; "I reign only through the fear I inspire."

And those who came into the inner sanctum of his office at Lachine would have perhaps perched, if invited to do so, on oaken chairs into which Simpson's chosen crest and motto were carved. Sometime after he was knighted, Simpson found or created a heraldic look to associate with his governorship. While this might have had as its central image the lion rampant, like the royal Scottish flag and the heraldry of almost all branches of the Simpson family (sept of the Fraser clan) reaching back into medieval times, Simpson chose instead a falcon volant over a garland of Scottish thistles for his crest, a design that has more than passing similarity to the Napoleonic crest, with its falcon volant over a garland of Nero-esque laurel leaves. And while Napoleon's motto was cast as *Toujours l'attaque*—"always attack"—Simpson chose *Alis nutrior*. This has been interpreted to mean "fed by their wings" or, with

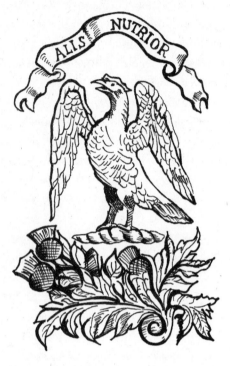

Although he could have chosen a family crest with different totemic elements and iconography, Sir George chose one with a falcon volant and orientation that looked surpringly similar to Napoleon Bonaparte's family crest, which has a right-facing falcon over laurels instead of Scottish thistles.

first-person pronouns, "I am fed by my wings" or, according to one off-beat heraldic scholar's interpretation, "It is sometimes pleasant to act like a madman."[3]

Hudson's Bay House was an effective extension of the Governor's pretensions of grandeur, but it was also a fitting office and residence for a man who had, in a very real sense, rescued a moribund business operation from chaos and near bankruptcy brought on by its battle with the competition, streamlined its personnel and accounting procedures, rebuilt its core business, expanded and diversified its interests, and brought it back for London shareholders to a position of profitability. A combination of good management and strong demand for furs on the British and European markets had produced remarkable profits for the HBC throughout Sir George's decades as governor. In the five years leading up to his round-the-world tour, for example, annual returns on capital investment were never lower than 10 per cent and were once as high as 25 per cent. And to appreciate fully the impact of these dramatic profits one must keep in mind that, as a result of profit sharing written into the deed poll twenty years earlier, HBC officers at isolated posts from sea to sea also saw increases in their annual pay. Without Simpson—or at least without a person with his remarkable and unique combination of intelligence, drive and talent for hands-on business management—the Hudson's Bay Company would most certainly not have thrived as it did during the 1820s and 1830s. This was not lost on the other merchants, politicians and businessmen of Montreal, who, with their wives, business associates and lovers, jumped at the chance to hobnob with the Governor at Lachine.

Hudson's Bay House was the scene of many a grand and occasionally debauched evening of food, drink and lively conversation. Without the limitations of breeding and station that most certainly haunted him in London social circles, George Simpson could preside with the bearing and panache of a viceroy during these meals, standing over crystal and silver settings early in the night to toast the young queen who had knighted him, feasting on fish, fowl and wild meats served on translucent china and crested silver flatware, relaxing with the gentlemen over postprandial brandy while sniffing Upmann's Cuban cigars, or passing fine port from hand to manicured, if unsteady, hand into the wee hours of the morning. Dinner at Hudson's Bay House with the Simpsons was a coveted invitation. Among those who supped with Simpson at Lachine was a young artist called Paul Kane, who, as a result of winning the Governor's admiration, was able to travel across the continent as a guest of the HBC and to produce one of the most venerable collections of sketches and painting documenting life in nineteenth-century Canada.

Simpson had been an influential member of the Montreal elite since his move from Red River in 1828, but it was only after his round-the-world tour, when Frances rejoined him in Canada and they resided mainly at Lachine, that he immersed himself in the freewheeling investment scene of the New World. For these were exciting times. The boom of expansion and technological development that had overtaken Britain during the Industrial Revolution was echoed in North America. Clippers had given way to steamboats. Steel rails had started to wend their way west. Canoes were giving way to canal boats. Worries about impeded commerce between the British and the Americans in North America following the War of 1812 saw the construction of the Erie and Rideau canals, and each of these spurred settlement and investment— neither of which was good for the fur trade, but that seemed not to matter to Sir George. And as the population of Upper Canada, the Upper Great Lakes and the west grew, every new name added to the census increased the drive to open the St. Lawrence for shipping all the way through to Lake Ontario. It was at the Governor's sumptuous dining table, or at the Beaver Club, or at reciprocal meals at other fine households in the growing Montreal community, or at any number of upscale public eating and drinking establishments that George Simpson allied himself with other titans of industry and government, undertaking profitable investments and business dealings, both for the HBC and for himself.

The ventures that seemed to capture Simpson's attention most were railways and canals, both of which were notorious mixtures of private and public money steered by government and individual interests. Montreal merchant and capitalist James Ferrier, for example, involved Simpson in the affairs of the Bank of British North America as a director, and these two, with brewer William Molson, became founding shareholders and directors of the Montreal and Lachine Railroad. This business move came on the heels of an earlier convoluted plan by the North American Colonial Association of Ireland, of which Simpson had also become a director, to speculate on the land on the south side of the St. Lawrence at Beauharnois, owned by former Nor'Wester Edward Ellice. Simpson had watched property values in his own little village of Lachine appreciate steeply with the construction of a canal, and it appeared that the exact same events were about to unfold on the seigneury of Villechauve, where a canal around the second major rapid on

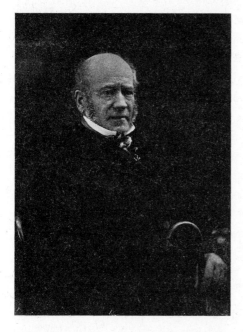

The only photograph of George Simpson in existence is one taken by Montreal photographer William Notman in the late 1850s and printed on silver salts paper using a wet collodion process. Notman's work in photographing the opening of the Victoria Bridge in 1860 earned him the right to be called "Photographer to the Queen."

the St. Lawrence upstream from Montreal would bring prosperity even farther inland.

George Simpson was a shrewd investor, having had some bad experiences early on and having learned from those mistakes. But as he had done earlier for J.G. McTavish and others in the trade, Simpson invested for his officers, and through him, they were building tidy retirement nest eggs for themselves. Among those he convinced to invest in the Montreal and Lachine Railroad (MLR) was Chief Factor John Rowand, of Fort Edmonton renown, whose money was doubled and redoubled when the MLR merged with the Lake St. Louis and Province Line Railway to form the Montreal and New York Railroad. These smaller lines were merged and merged again into bigger and bigger conglomerates, with more and more miles of track and broader and broader reach across the continent, until they were all eventually absorbed into the Grand Trunk Railway system, bringing smiles to Simpson and his fellow fur trader investors.

Since his involvement with Adam Thom and the players in the Rebellion of 1837, Simpson also knew many of the actors in the continuing political upheavals in Upper and Lower Canada, including colonial governors like Charles Metcalfe and Charles Thomson, Lord Sydenham, who championed the union of Upper and Lower Canada—men who, from time to time, were able to help Simpson with his pet projects or with HBC interests that required government intervention.

With the business of running his own empire a full-time occupation, and knowing the value of strategic lobbying—and graft—in the 1840s, Simpson convinced fast-talking adventurer and flim-flam man Stewart Derbishire to be his agent in Montreal society. Simpson saw in the former journalist known for his "excited reporting" (he had taken up the job as Queen's Printer in Montreal) a maven who could wheedle his way into almost any high office in the land, public or private. Just as he knew that the right amount of cash would sway a transatlantic packet captain from his sworn duty not to land anywhere but his destination, Simpson knew that having the right type of persuader in the right place at the right time could work wonders.

Stewart Derbishire was just the man for the job and his assistance to Simpson in the political realm is described by one historian as follows:

Derbishire as a lobbyist was perfectly adapted to Simpson's requirements. He was a good drinking companion [though Simpson was not a big drinker], a gregarious friendly associate who could always be relied upon for the latest gossip. Derbishire came to know legislators intimately, and could assess their virtues and, more particularly, their foibles. He dispensed minor largesse to many politicians as the representative of Simpson, thus enhancing Simpson's reputation as a charming, generous man. Most of the gifts were insignificant enough to avoid any concern about bribery. One favourite present of Simpson was buffalo tongues. When one politician joked that acceptance of this delicacy might cause him to be suspected of taking bribes, Derbishire assured him that "Sir George only pleaded his case with many tongues."[4]

With the Oregon situation ever present in his mind, Simpson persevered as well with his international efforts. In April 1845, having crossed back to Boston on the transatlantic steamer *Caledonia*, the Governor took a side trip to Washington to talk about border issues in the west with American politicians.

Democrat James Polk had been elected president the year before, on a platform of "Fifty-four-forty or fight!" Polk was prepared to take his fellow Americans to war with the British, again, for the territory they had up to that point agreed to share, between the Columbia River and Russian lands bordering fifty-four degrees, forty minutes north latitude, in what is now the northern part of the province of British Columbia. An influx of setters had been sent up the Missouri River to Columbia, and it was well known to Simpson, through his officers, that these people were organizing themselves with a view to setting up a provisional local American government in the west.[5]

While in England, Simpson had written a letter to the London Committee containing his thoughts on how the west might be defended,[6] which was sent by J.H. Pelly to Lord Aberdeen in the British Foreign Office. The result was that Simpson had conferred directly with Sir Robert Peel, the British prime minister. Simpson's trip to Washington was to use his considerable charm and influence to settle the Oregon question peacefully. Acting more or less as the official agent of the British government, he was still very much a company man.

The one thing that Simpson knew for certain was that continued conflict with the Americans would be bad for business. It appears that from the moment he decided to move the company's depot on the south side of the Columbia River to the north side of the river, at Fort Vancouver, he was acting on a premonition that the Americans would eventually "win" and occupy the lower Columbia River basin, at least to the forty-ninth parallel. The premonition must have been even stronger a dozen years later, when he closed the California post and moved the HBC depot yet again, this time to Vancouver Island. But this was still no reason to concede anything to the Americans, and it was one of the reasons why John McLoughlin's toadying to them was so repugnant.

Leaving room for his "low cunning" and "smoothing," his notorious bluster and the other tricks in his repertoire for face-to-face negotiations, Simpson took to these discussions with politicians and officials in Washington in the spring of 1845 the idea that the line of workable compromise with the Americans was the forty-ninth parallel, at least to the Pacific—knowing full well that the site he had chosen for the HBC post on Vancouver Island was half a degree of latitude below that.

When Simpson made his way back north to Lachine that spring and started west by canoe for the annual Council, the British response to Polk's sabre-rattling put two more young British army officers in his entourage. On instruction from the British prime minister, through Lord Aberdeen and Simpson's Montreal friend Lord Metcalfe, now governor of the united Canadas, Lieutenants Henry James Warre and Mervin Vavasour were asked to head to Red River to be briefed by Sir George on the way out and then to continue to Columbia on their own to report on possible defence strategies for the American frontier. Simpson may have known, as he regaled the two young officers with stories to the rhythmic movements of paddles driving a matched pair of six-fathom bark canoes, that whatever plans they came up with would not be required: he certainly knew, on the strength of his visit to Washington, that President Polk had simultaneously picked a fight with the Mexicans for territory on the southern border of his republic—a struggle that was not going well. Even though people had chanted "Fifty-four-forty or fight" during Polk's campaign, a settlement in Oregon Country might be a way to simplify his life. Indeed, on June 15, 1846, the Treaty with Great Britain, in Regard to Limits Westward of the Rocky Mountains (also known as the Anglo-American Treaty, Oregon Treaty or Treaty of Washington) was signed between the Americans and the British, making the border the forty-ninth parallel to the coast and then, continuing to the ocean, on a line moving south and west down the middle of the Juan de Fuca Strait, leaving Victoria and the whole of Vancouver Island—thanks in significant measure to George Simpson, and also to Chief Factor James Douglas, who had actually sited the establishment and was its first commanding officer—under the Union Jack. The first fluttering of the British flag in Victoria was very likely not that flag itself but the red, white and blue of the Union colours in the corner of the HBC ensign.

It was clear to the Americans that the signing of this treaty meant no new British activity in Oregon Country. But what was not clear was the extent of rights that the HBC might have to continue operations south of the new border at its discretion. Also in play were the company's various forts and agricultural properties, including the Cowlitz farm, which was being operated under the auspices of the Puget Sound Agricultural Company. Simpson was adamant that these installations were created for the purposes of trade and that with them came the implicit right to trade. And if the Americans wished to purchase the properties or their attendant rights, then they could do so at fair market value. In the Oregon Treaty, Simpson saw a beaming financial opportunity.

Just as he had teamed up with the illustrious Stewart Derbishire in Montreal, in Washington Simpson affiliated with George M. Sanders, another fast-talking lobbyist and financier familiar with the Democratic back channels in the city. It was Sanders' idea to create a joint-stock company that would float a stock option and buy all of the HBC's assets in Oregon—which Simpson had valued at about £75,000, and in which, presumably, Simpson would have a significant personal interest. They would then turn around and sell at a substantial profit to the American government.

The interplay of private and public interests was something Simpson was getting increasingly familiar with in his high-flying dealings in Montreal. But why stop at canals and railways when the larger financial stage in Washington offered such opportunities?

In his exhaustive two-volume history of the HBC, the normally circumspect E.E. Rich wrote that at this point in the story it is "difficult to avoid the conclusion that Simpson was toying with corruption, unknown to Pelly and the London Committee."[7] If Simpson was toying

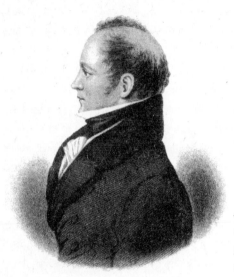

An etching of Sir George commissioned as a frontispiece for his book about the around-the-world journey.

with corruption, bribing politicians through George Sanders or fixing deals for himself independent of his role and duties as an officer of the HBC, it would certainly not be anything he had not done first himself, or with Stewart Derbishire, from the inner sanctum at Lachine. However, George Simpson would be long dead before the matter would finally be settled, in a deal with the Americans that was good for the HBC but from which neither the Governor nor his estate appears to have made appreciable gain.

Inside his private office at Lachine, Simpson sought beyond all else to fulfill his biggest dream: to publish a book about his journey around the world. Edward Hopkins had written the journal for the first portion of the trip, as far as Hawaii, and he had taken this home and handed it off to HBC secretary Dr. Archibald Barclay, who, when Simpson's notes from the second half of the journey were added on his return to London in October 1842, was the first person charged with the responsibility of turning it all into a book. Correspondence between Simpson and Barclay shows the Governor to be anxious about the book, worried that Barclay would be seen to be doing it instead of his work for the company, or that he might leave it lying on his desk at Fenchurch Street for others to see, or that it would not be done properly. After a couple of years of back and forth, Barclay finally wrote to Simpson saying, "Do not be fidgety about your book—it will be all right in good time."[8]

But it was not all right in Simpson's eyes. Soon after Barclay's reprimand he switched ghostwriters, enlisting the assistance of his friend Adam Thom, the "recorder of Rupert's Land." When Thom saw the partially completed manuscript, he was not impressed with the work on it to date. He was concerned about errors of both commission and omission, as well as about the problem of two voices in the text (neither of which would be the person whose byline would be on the title page). Knowing by now something of the Governor's exacting standards and his short fuse, by late 1845 Adam Thom was writing with explanations to Simpson that were as much excuses for delay as they were reports on progress with Sir George's pet project. Through this correspondence, it becomes clear that Simpson's grand vision for this volume went well beyond a day-to-day accounting of where he went and what happened along the way. Here is Adam Thom writing to Simpson in December of that year:

> In one of my latest letters I mentioned that I should be obliged to write
> your California over again in order to incorporate with[in] the journal
> the substance of your historical sketch which Dr. Barclay had altogether
> omitted. This I have done to the extent in all of about 160 pages, equal
> as nearly as possible to Mr. Hopkins's pages, incorporating at the same
> time several historical illustrations of the collateral kind. But I have
> gone farther back than California, partly to get a good point . . . I have
> accordingly taken you up at the moment of your reaching the mouth
> of the Cowlitz on your return from Sitka. To account for the differ-
> ence of style, which a careful reader may be able to detect, without
> involving the appearance of a change of writers, I have taken occasion
> to mark your embarkation on board the Cowlitz as an epoch in your
> journey, as a boundary between all that was familiar on the one side and

all that was new on the other. I have, of course, avoided repetitions; I
have sometimes altered the arrangement of your incidents; and I have
endeavoured to rationalize every particular fact by referring it to some
general principle. I have throughout recollected that I was writing not
for myself but for another, striving to render the work such as you could
yourself have rendered it with an equal command of leisure and an
equal expenditure of application.[9]

Two years later, with the help of yet another contributor to the project,
Edward Hopkins's brother, Manley, who saw the project "through the
press,"[10] the book was finally simultaneously published in the United
Kingdom, by Henry Colburn, and in the United States, by Lea and
Blanchard, giving George Simpson, finally, an accomplishment of suf-
ficient heft to pad his skeletal entry in Dod's *Peerage*.

———

The Simpson that emerged through the 1840s after his investiture as a
knight bachelor and the subsequent publication of "his" book was the
same curious, confident, intelligent and independent operator who had
come as a tenderfoot to the fur trade two decades before, but the accre-
tion of wealth and power over those two decades had distilled those
once possibly endearing characteristics into an impenetrable carapace.
The essential Simpson was still present, but he was less tolerant, quicker
to fly off the handle, more capricious and often more vindictive. An
early view of this character shift came in a letter written by his old nemesis (and the once unofficial keeper of his various first families at Fort
Alexander) John Stuart, who sent a brief sketch of the Governor to his
nephew Donald Smith, who was planning on coming to Canada to seek
employment with the HBC:

> The chief drawback is that you are dependent upon the goodwill and
> caprice of one man, who is a little too much addicted to prejudices, for
> speedy advancement; but this is probably true in many other spheres

of commercial endeavour . . . There is, I may say, no man who is more appreciative of downright hard work coupled with intelligence, or one more intolerant of puppyism, by which I mean carelessness and presumption. It is his foible to exact not only strict obedience, but deference to the point of humility. As long as you pay him in that coin you will quickly get on his sunny side and find yourself in a few years a trader at a congenial post, with promotion in sight.[11]

This new Simpson seemed to project an imposing, even intimidating air. John Henry Lefroy, crossing paths with Simpson in Montreal in 1843 just prior to his cross-country magnetic survey to triangulate the position of the North Pole, described Simpson this way: "Sir Geo. Simpson arrived on Saturday evening and I called on him on Monday; he is the toughest looking old fellow I ever saw, built upon the Egyptian model, height two diameters, or like one of those short square massy pillars one sees in an old country church . . . He is a fellow whom nothing will kill."[12]

What it might have been like to live with such a pompous little stump of a man we can only guess. There is no real record of Simpson's return to his two Franceses after his journey round the world, nor is there any evidence of the father meeting his miracle child "Gussy" for the first time, fourteen months after her rocky entry into the world. For Frances, cloistered much of the time with her family in England, separated from her husband by geographical and often emotional distance, having a man twenty years her senior—one comfortable with power and used to getting his own way—march in and out of her life must have been a trial. But once the Governor was settled in Hudson's Bay House at Lachine, Frances and the children were with him there more often than not, especially during the summer months. In order to keep his wife happy and occupied and to make life in Hudson's Bay House bearable, Simpson also engineered a transfer to Lachine for his old Dingwall chum Duncan Finlayson, who had met and married Frances's sister Isobel in 1838. What the Finlaysons did not know until they moved to Lachine in 1844 was that they were to live in Hudson's Bay House with Sir George and his family—Duncan to assist the Governor, and Isobel to help her sister with her young family. Confiding to his friend James Hargrave, Duncan Finlayson wrote, "The Gov. is coming out bag & baggage, that is wt. wife, bairns, servants &c. & how we are to stow them all here is more than I know. I do not wish to anticipate evils but one thing is to me almost certain—that neither our wives, our servts. nay, even ourselves, must give way. I, therefore, expect to receive notice to quit these quarters, before another year comes round."[13] Simpson was physically removed from the Lachine office for large chunks of time to accommodate his travels and one could understand if Frances hungered for company her own age. Having her sister in the same household would have made life under the high ceilings at Lachine more bearable.

Although actual events may have involved a different would-be suitor, there was a tale that circulated in the trade around this time in which the charming young Donald Smith, John Stuart's nephew, who had been amply forewarned about the possible consequences of such actions, found his way into occasional tête-à-têtes over tea with Mrs. Simpson soon after he arrived in North America in 1838. An article in the Autumn 1978 issue of *The Beaver* speculated, "Once, after the Governor had returned after an absence at Red River, we heard that there had been a scene, and that in consequence young Smith, although innocent of any offence but that of obliging a lady, was in disgrace, one gentleman averring that he had heard the governor, in a highly pitched treble, declare that he was not going to endure any 'upstart, quill-driving apprentices dangling about a parlour reserved to the nobility and gentry.'"[14]

In a slightly more sober and careful recounting of the future Lord Strathcona's early days in the fur trade, historian W.L. Morton concludes that there is no way Smith and Mrs. Simpson could have crossed paths in this way, adding, "Simpson invited caricature, so powerful was his position and his personality, and little said of him is to be taken literally."[15] Yet it is a fact that on Simpson's way through Lachine as he circumnavigated the world in 1841, he transferred Smith from Lachine with just two days' notice to continue his clerk's apprenticeship at the forlorn HBC post at Tadoussac on the lower St. Lawrence. Some thought this a punishment. And, having inspected that post sometime later, Simpson also castigated the young Scotsman for his sloppiness:

> I am aware of your great anxiety to transact the business entrusted
> to your charge in a proper manner, & need not, therefore, advert at
> any great length to the importance of having your business always in
> such a forward state that no delay be occasioned to any of the vessels
> in awaiting either cargo or papers. Your counting house department
> appeared to me in a very slovenly condition, so much so that I could
> make very little sense of any document that came under my notice.
> Your schemes of outposts were really curiously perplexing, & such as
> I trust I may never see again, while letters, invoices and accounts were
> to be found tossing about as wastepaper in almost every room in the
> house. I am aware that during the pressure of summer business, you
> have not much time to devote to the neat arrangement of papers, but
> your winters are very long, with little or no outdoor work to occupy
> your attention, and if you were but to give a few hours a week to the
> arrangement of your papers your business would be in a very different
> state to that in which I found it.[16]

The remarkable aspect to the Governor's life as he presided over his empire from Lachine was that almost without exception he maintained the essential rhythm of his life—his annual summer canoe dashes from Lachine to Council meetings in the heart of Rupert's Land. His trouble with apoplexy came and went, and his eyesight was abysmal (as early as 1838, just before he hired Edward Hopkins to be his stenographer, he lamented in a letter to one officer that "[I] cannot give you a single private line under my own hand").[17] He liked to tell people that he never felt more alive than when in a canoe, but those late nights, early mornings and long, stiff hours on the water exposed to the elements, the insects and the buffoonery of voyageurs who lived brutal, short lives took a toll on George Simpson that did not escape the notice of the London Committee.

Also weighing on the Governor in these peak years of his career was the business itself. It was still running like clockwork in most quarters, but the fur market was changing. On one side of the Atlantic, silk was becoming *de rigueur* in the hat business. On the other side of the Atlantic, throughout North America, the business of settlement was supplanting frontier fur trading. And the old fur traders were dying. His old friend McTavish, who had nearly eaten himself to death at his farm at Chats Falls up the Ottawa River, contracted cholera and died in Montreal on July 20, 1847. In the mid-1840s, Frances, with her already frail constitution, contracted tuberculosis and retreated even more when he was home.

Simpson did his level best to project an image of invincibility, and when he met people face to face, he seemed able to puff himself up accordingly, regardless of how he felt, how long he had been travelling or what was troubling him in business. But there were signs for the London Committee that their man in Rupert's Land was not what he had once been. Although Simpson had total control on information flow to London, instances of questionable business dealings or odd behaviour were conveyed through visitors, and correspondence from HBC employees in Rupert's Land to their families back in Britain fuelled the rumour mills. The London Committee increasingly became concerned. Eventually, in 1849, they acted to shore up their aging Emperor. Although Sir George likely knew better than anyone that he needed help running this vast empire, it must have been a bitter pill for him to swallow to have his old mentor, Andrew Colvile, who was now poised to take the top job on the London Committee (a process that had begun as early as 1812 when he had purchased shares and initiated his retrenchment design for the HBC), pull rank and install his Eton- and Cambridge-educated son Eden as "governor of Rupert's Land," with a mandate to exercise all the powers of Simpson in his absence. The governor in chief, however, had no immediate plans to leave his post.

CHAPTER XVIII

DENOUEMENT

As newly minted governor Eden Colvile and veteran overseas governor, now governor in chief, of Rupert's Land George Simpson made their way west by canoe in the spring of 1849, they were somewhere between La Cloche and Michipicoten when a sure sign of the beginning of the end for the HBC's monopoly in North America unfurled in the General Quarterly Court of Assiniboia. Just as Simpson's hold on his empire was starting to slip, so too was the HBC's unilateral hold on the fur trade, especially in and around the Red River settlement, where, in a manner similar to that of settlers farther west who were starting to organize politically, the Métis nation was asserting its right to self-determination.

The Métis were a cultural by-product of the fur trade and had had a proud tradition of independence long before their affiliates in the North West Company were absorbed into the Hudson's Bay Company in 1821. Throughout the first two decades of George Simpson's reign in Rupert's Land, the *bois brûlé* community had been a powerful and often useful go-between, linking the HBC and the Red River settlers with Aboriginal tribes in the west. They had also been effective players in the commerce of the west, especially in the continuing need for buffalo meat to make pemmican, which fuelled the fur brigades as they made their way east, west and north. As long as the Métis got their supplies and traded with the HBC, all was well, but as settlement and development increased under American auspices south of Assiniboia, American traders, half-breed hunters and trappers increasingly engaged in trade that contravened the HBC's monopoly.

Illicit trade had been the principal reason that Simpson had engaged the services of Cuthbert Grant as "Warden of the Plains." Grant's job, as one who had respect and authority among his Métis peers, was to discourage trade with whites or Aboriginal people south of the border. Indeed, one of the principal reasons for the creation of Adam Thom's post at Red River (when he wasn't engaged in writing and rewriting Simpson's book) was to set up legal machinery that could protect the HBC's charter monopoly on trade. However, as the population grew, rules of conduct and the presence of a courthouse and jail were not enough to quell the growing desire of the settlers and the Métis for self-determination. The settlers felt their options were often constrained by the HBC; the Métis, with familial connections to the Aboriginal groups of the western plains, felt it was their prerogative to trap and hunt where they liked and to sell to the highest bidder.

George Simpson, who was well acquainted with the New Nation, as the Métis called themselves, would often listen to their gripes long after his officers at Red River had cut off communication. In his heart, although Simpson was a company man, he was also a pragmatist and was not convinced that this illicit trade was necessarily a bad thing. The plains around Assiniboia were a dangerous place, and in the end, there were not many sources of supply and even fewer options for trading partners. Even if Red River Métis traded occasionally with the Americans or with Indians south of the border, they would still require supplies, and more and more, they were not actually doing the trapping and hunting themselves. Acting as middlemen in the trade, the Métis needed supplies to get the furs, and these supplies, as likely as not, would come from the HBC. Failing that, the HBC could possibly benefit from the other end of the process, with increased volumes of furs gathered in by an independent network of traders. But while Simpson may have secretly sympathized with the Métis, he knew that they did not require any extra encouragement to organize in their move toward self-government.

Because of his frequent travels through Red River and his intimate knowledge of reports and correspondence from the settlement, Simpson knew that a Catholic missionary at Red River, Father George A. Belcourt, was stirring the pot of independence among the Métis, most of whom, like their French ancestors, were staunch Catholics. This activity went well beyond the kind of ministering a missionary might be expected to do. So Simpson, in his inimitable way, went above Father Belcourt's head to his bishop and secured his recall for reassignment.

For his part, Belcourt, who seemed to have had an equal amount of cunning, complied initially with the request and gave the impression after his audience with Bishop Norbert Provencher that he was heading back to Red River to pick up his things for reassignment. But instead of capitulating to Simpson and the bishop, Belcourt simply moved his mission just below the border to Pembina, where Norman Wolfred Kittson, an agent for Henry H. Sibley of St. Paul, had established an American trading post. Outside—but *just* outside—the jurisdiction of the HBC, Belcourt was still in a place where he could agitate among the Métis.

By the spring of 1849, as Simpson was introducing Eden Colvile to the trade, Chief Factor John Ballenden at Fort Garry had decided enough was enough and charged Métis hunter Pierre Guillaume Sayer and three other Métis men—McGillis, Laronde and Goullé—with illicit trafficking in furs, based on an exchange of fur for liquor with Norman Kittson at the Pembina post. For the HBC, the trial would be a first legal test of its monopoly on trade in North America. For the Métis, the trial put their emerging independence as a nation on the line.

Controversy about illicit trade had driven HBC officers, such as Assiniboia governor Alexander Christie, to take a number of small actions that combined to create a much bigger consequence than intended. After taking office in 1844, Christie had tried to limit such trade with threats to open mail and seize goods imported by anyone who was suspected of collusion with non-HBC personnel. Just before Christmas in his first year of office, he issued a proclamation that company ships would not even unload goods addressed to anyone in Rupert's Land, from any point of entry, unless the recipient had first signed a promise that he was in no way involved in illicit trade of any description. While this warning may have had some small effect at the time, the unintended consequence of Christie's actions was that it raised the ire of Red River settlers, who saw huge conflicts between their interests and those of their masters in the HBC.

Worries about safety and fairness in trade topped a long list of settlers' grievances. They wanted to live in peace with more control over their lives. So in addition to ferment in the Métis community, there was now also serious discontent in the growing parishes of Assiniboia. Settlers wanted an impartial governor and representatives on their governing council who would be elected, instead of being appointed by the London Committee of the HBC.

To quell at least a portion of this discontent, the London Committee retained the services of Major William Bletterman Caldwell, late of the British army, whom they commissioned to travel to Assiniboia to command a small body of Chelsea pensioners who were to keep order at Red River. But they also appointed Caldwell to replace Christie as governor of Assiniboia. Caldwell was the first governor not previously associated with the Hudson's Bay Company. Yet by 1849, after Caldwell had been in office for a year, the situation had not improved. The settlers were even more disgruntled than they had been when he had arrived, and the Métis were pushing harder than ever for self-determination.

In retrospect, if the Sayer trial had not happened when it did, something similar surely would have transpired. Had George Simpson been at Red River in the spring of 1849, though, history might have taken a different turn.

As it was, Caldwell made a colossally bad call. The trial was set for early May, before the buffalo hunt had begun and before the boat brigades had left for York Factory, which meant that Assiniboia was teeming with hundreds of restless Métis. And when Caldwell heard that a demonstration was planned for the day of the Sayer trial, he set the trial date to Sunday, May 17—Ascension Day, an important Catholic holiday—thinking that this might catch the Métis busy with other things.

They were not. The priest who had replaced Father Belcourt called an early mass that morning to make sure that the service would be finished before the trial began, and as part of the proceedings, a letter from Belcourt was read out that stirred the pot even more. By trial time, there were five hundred armed Métis under the leadership of Louis Riel (father of future rebel Louis Riel Jr.) both inside the Fort Garry courthouse and swirling angrily on the grounds outside. It was a testament to the leadership of Riel and "Chief of the Half-Breeds" James Sinclair (who, ironically, was Simpson's brother-in-law *à la façon du pays* through his sister, Betsy, who had borne the Governor's first child in Rupert's Land, and who was now happily married to Robert Miles) that the mob was restrained if still incensed about the charges. They wanted free trade but knew that the wheels of justice had to turn unfettered to confirm that right legally.

On the bench at the Quarterly Court of Assiniboia that sunny May morning were three magistrates who would listen to the arguments: Adam Thom, recorder of Rupert's Land; Major William Caldwell, governor of Assiniboia; and Cuthbert Grant, long-time Warden of the Plains and sheriff of Assiniboia. Grant's position of leadership in the Métis nation was fast being eroded by a new generation of nationalists for whom the HBC was their sworn enemy.

Adam Thom, as senior magistrate, fielded a jury of five French-speaking settlers and seven English-speaking settlers. The Métis, for the most part, spoke French. Pierre Sayer was represented by James Sinclair, aided by Louis Riel and his bristling crowd of onlookers. The prosecution laid out its case with facts on which there was no disagreement. One version of the proceedings had the prosecutor arguing that Sayer was trading with the permission of the company, which would have given the jury reason to acquit but, more important, would have defused a potentially explosive situation with the Métis. But this was somehow all beside the point. Free trade was the issue. Sinclair, for his part, argued that Sayer and the others were simply sharing goods among family members and were guilty of no crime. And that is where history took a strange turn.

On the recommendation of the jury, Judge Thom pronounced Pierre Sayer guilty of illicit trading, a verdict that upheld the HBC monopoly in the highest available court. But because of the circumstances—some members of the jury were sure that the Métis were convinced they had the ancestral right to free trade with the Americans—the jury recommended mercy in sentencing. Taking this into account, Adam Thom levied no fine or punishment on Pierre Sayer and dropped the charges against the other three men. On hearing this, the mob chose to respond to the implicit message in the sentencing rather than to the guilty verdict, and left the courtroom singing "*Le commerce est libre! La traite est libre!*" ("Free trade! Free trade!"), which, for all future purposes, meant that the HBC monopoly on trade had been unsuccessfully challenged in a court of law but had been successfully challenged by the will of the people.

Sir George arrived by canoe at Lower Fort Garry (also known as the Stone Fort) with Edward Hopkins and Eden Colvile on June 15 and must have known instantly that something drastic had happened in Assiniboia, though it would have taken some time, even for Simpson, to divine the full impact of the Sayer trial on life as he had shaped it at Red River. As always, one of the first things he did was to have an audience with Cuthbert Grant and some of the emerging Métis leaders, and from this he would have learned—though not in as many words—that Grant's currency had dropped suddenly as a result of the trial. In the fullness of time, Simpson would come to see the Sayer trial as the turning point in Grant's life, moving him, as an ally of the old regime, slowly into obscurity. Grant had been on the bench with Caldwell and Thom during the trial, which, in spite of efforts to conduct a full and fair examination of the facts, and notwithstanding the recorded verdict, had alienated him not only from the Métis but from the HBC as well.

In his meetings with the Métis, who had perennially turned to him for help with their circumstances at Red River, Simpson must also have realized that although the crux of the matter was free trade, the bigger issue at stake was self-determination. The Métis were calling for the administration of justice at Red River in the French language. Although one of the reasons Adam Thom had been appointed as recorder was his ability to speak French, which he had learned while working in Montreal, on the bench of the Quarterly Court of Assiniboia Thom would hear depositions only in English. For that and other reasons of misjudgement laid at the recorder's feet, the Métis wanted Simpson to remove Thom from his post. They also wanted total abolition of duty on American goods. And they wanted political representation on the Council of Assiniboia. With the company moving to separate matters of trade from matters of settlement, and with Thom and Caldwell both compromised and on their way out (Caldwell was in due course replaced by Eden Colvile as governor of Assiniboia), Simpson was technically powerless to act on this wish list. But over the next decade he would continue to push for Métis interests in the west.

The irony is that while, at this juncture in his life, Simpson chose to befriend and to support individuals of the Métis nation, he represented a company—and a society—that essentially did not recognize Native rights. Louis Riel Jr. would be hanged for treason, and it would take another century before Native peoples, including the Métis, were recognized as among Canada's founding peoples.

———

Eden Colvile carried on to the west from Red River, doing what Simpson could not, and leaving Sir George to pack his things after the week-long Council meeting at Norway House and make tracks back to Lachine. What kind of reception he received from his family his private correspondence does not reveal, but we do know that he maintained at least a physical relationship with his wife on return in the early autumn of 1849, because on June 14 of the following year, John Henry Pelly

Simpson—a son he dubbed "Moses," and his last with Frances before she died—was born while the Governor was back on the trail somewhere between Michipicoten and Norway House.

This had been the story of George Simpson's personal life. Except for the very occasional glimpses provided in surviving private personal correspondence, there is no direct evidence of any kind of emotional attachment to anyone or anything beyond himself and the HBC. He could muster illusions of warmth and friendship, could give his family endearing nicknames, but beyond that it appears that at his core the Governor was not sustained by matters of the heart. On July 20, 1847, his old friend J.G. McTavish died in Montreal of cholera. Had Simpson not been in a canoe on the north shore of Lake Superior heading from Fort William to Michipicoten Post, he might have attended the funeral and expressed his condolences personally to one of his young wife's best friends. As it was, Frances was there to comfort the widowed Mrs. McTavish on her husband's behalf. Two days after Christmas 1848, his uncle and father-in-law Geddes Simpson died at Stamford Hill in Middlesex. This was the man who gave him his start in business—and his daughter—and yet there is no record of even a ripple of emotion.

His wife, the delicate debutante he had whisked from her hearth at New Grove House, had been in steadily declining health since her first pregnancy at Red River. In those early years of their marriage, when Simpson was sufficiently worried about her well-being to alter his travel plans on behalf of the HBC, there are glimmers of emotional attachment, even love, for his young cousin—but in the end what mattered most to him was his business status and the legitimacy the marriage conferred on him.

The affection-starved Frances had struggled for breath from the moment she contracted tuberculosis in 1845, but by then she and Sir George were on totally different trajectories. Each one of her earlier pregnancies and deliveries had been difficult in its own way, and it appears that the birth of child number four was also a challenge. But still Sir George,

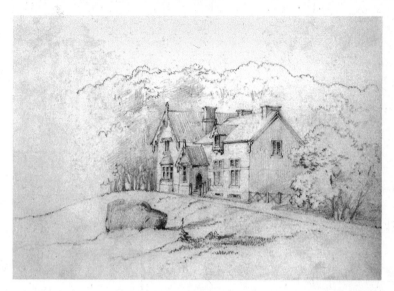

The first property George Simpson owned in North America was his summer home on Isle Dorval, in the St. Lawrence River, just upstream from the village of Lachine.

with his own infirmities, carried on indifferent, if not oblivious, to the frailties that surrounded him at Lachine. Simpson's apoplexy returned in early 1851, but again he rallied and pressed on. Sir John Henry Pelly died in London on August 13, 1852, after a long illness, leaving Andrew Colvile—finally—to assume the chair of the London Committee, becoming the eighteenth governor of the HBC and thereby bringing to fruition a design, of which George Simpson was an integral element, that had been sketched in Colvile's dreams more than forty years before. But by now, Colvile's interest in the fortunes of the HBC had waned, leaving his aging protégé to do more or less as he pleased in North America.

After years of gasping from progressive lung disease and, from the day they were wed, struggling to cohabit with George Simpson, Frances finally succumbed to tuberculosis on March 21, 1853. She was forty years old when she died, probably with Sir George at her side, or at least in the house. Daughter Frances was nineteen, Gussy was twelve, Margaret was nine and little John Henry Pelly Simpson was not quite three. In exhausting seasonal moves from their grandparents' house in England to Lachine and back, Frances had been a constant for her children, and her death must have been quite a blow for them. The younger three would have clung to the skirts of their older sister, who was just that much older, or to the embrace of their governess, Mary Barston. Or perhaps they would have turned to their aunt Isobel Finlayson, who had become a mother figure of sorts for them at Hudson's Bay House during their mother's long illness. As fate decreed it, Frances died when Sir George was in residence at Lachine, not in England or Washington or somewhere else. Whether his children turned to him at this darkest of times in their lives we can only guess. George Simpson was not incapable of warmth, when it pleased him.

Yet Simpson seemed insulated from the heartache of it all. We do not know how he responded to his young wife's passing, or what he wrote to his widowed mother-in-law about Frances's death. Frances was buried in the Protestant Mount Royal Cemetery in Montreal. History does not record anything of Simpson's response to her passing, except that he seems to have kept moving, always moving, in preparation for that year's travels to the interior.

Still extant, however, is his tribute to Governor Pelly. In a letter to HBC London secretary Archibald Barclay, written a month after Sir John's death, there is genuine feeling, but either by language or habit the sentiment is eclipsed by a formality that epitomizes Simpson's detachment from matters of the heart:

Lachine
6 September 1852

Sir

Since addressing you on the 4 instant, I have received your letter of the 20 ultimo, conveying the melancholy intelligence of the death on the 13 August of Sir John Henry Pelly. Although your letter of 6 ultimo had in some measure led me to anticipate this sad event, the announcement has nevertheless occasioned me deep sorrow. From Sir Henry's conspicuous position in the commercial world his death may be considered a public loss, and to the Hudson's Bay Company, from the deep interest he took in their affairs during an ordinary lifetime, it may be said to be irreparable.—I trust I may be permitted to add my individual testimony to the worth, and my personal regret at the loss of our late Governor, who for so many years had honoured me with his confidence, our public intercourse having ripened into feelings of warm regard, so that in him I lose, not only a highly respected official superior, but a kind and valued friend.

> I am, Sir
> Your obt Servant -
> [signed] G. Simpson[1]

If Simpson was tipped off-balance by these deaths of the early 1850s, he was certainly back on track by 1854. Strangely, after talking with Frances for years about building a house of their own at Lachine— Frances would certainly have known about (and perhaps dusted) the silver candelabrum from the officers of the trade that had come in 1839 with funds and encouragement to build a house called Beaver Lodge—it was only after she died that Simpson moved to purchase land on which to build. Having looked across the water from Hudson's Bay House at Lachine to a verdant little island in the St. Lawrence River, Simpson finally purchased Isle Dorval in 1854 and commissioned plans for a generously proportioned brick house to be set among mature shade trees and a rambling English garden. But supervision of this project had to be summarily handed off to Duncan Finlayson or another functionary at Lachine come spring because, like a bird drawn north in the lengthening days of April, Sir George was restless to head back out to Rupert's Land. By now, having invested heavily in New World transportation projects, he would leave Montreal in the comfort of a first-class coach on the train, headed on new steel rails for Toronto, Detroit, Chicago and the Sault, before settling back into his familiar place in the *Rob Roy* with Edward Hopkins, chief guide Morin and his old friends the Mohawk voyageurs.

Travelling with Sir George that year was a nineteen-year-old apprentice, Henry John Moberly, who was heading into the country on a five-year engagement to take up his first HBC posting in the Saskatchewan District. Moberly was not a journal keeper, like Lord Caledon or some of the others who had had the opportunity to experience the Governor firsthand, but in later life he sat down and told his story to writer William Bleasdell Cameron. The account shows that the old flair of Sir George could still impress.

Simpson had sent Moberly ahead from Lachine with his canoes. The Governor himself had rounded up a new judge to continue the never-ending process of tidying up the Red River settlement, and the two of them, with another officer headed west—perhaps to soften the rough edges of travel for the judge—had agreed to meet Moberly and the canoemen at Sault Ste. Marie. The train arrived late one evening, but to everyone's amazement, the Governor barked "*Lève! Lève!*" a few hours after they'd gone to sleep, and the whole entourage was on the water, headed into the darkness of Lake Superior at one-thirty in the morning. Moberly was deeply impressed with the voyageurs and with Simpson's style. Here is how he described leaving the Sault:

> I was now to learn how Sir George travelled. He had a picked crew
> of Iroquois canoemen from Caughnawaga, above Montreal, than
> whom there are no better in the world. They were dressed in red
> shirts and trousers of rough serge, with red L'Assompcion belts
> wrapped about their waists. Sir George and his secretary slept until
> seven o'clock [in the canoe] that first morning, the crew paddling
> silently and steadily, except when Sir George, still apparently asleep,
> raised his arm and slipped his fingers in the water. The steersman

no sooner noticed this than he put added force into his stroke, the others followed suit, and the canoe fairly leaped ahead.[2]

If we are to believe Moberly's recollections, "fairly leaped ahead" does not begin to describe the accomplishments of these voyageurs. "In four days," wrote Moberly, "we reached Fort William." The distance between Sault Ste. Marie and Fort William by water is over four hundred miles, which means that through wind, snow and rain these canoes averaged over 150 miles per day, not including the time the voyageurs spent stopping to eat and sleep and to check in at Michipicoten Post along the way. This pace and schedule apparently sat better with Moberly than with the new recorder headed for Red River. Moberly wrote, "The day we left Fort William the judge grumbled so much about being forced to travel in snow and rain without opportunity for sleep that Sir George was induced to leave him with two canoes en route for Red River, with permission to travel to suit himself."[3]

Along the way, to have some fun with his officers and with the tenderfoot coming into the country for the first time, Simpson took to introducing young Moberly as the new chief factor of Saskatchewan. Having seen Eden Colvile and other offspring of well-heeled London Committee members and HBC shareholders jump the promotion queue on the basis of social standing, this was nothing new to the officers, but Moberly thought it was delightful. "I was seated among the 'big bugs,' and to carry off the joke Sir George took wine with me before anyone else. That settled it, though I myself thought it was merely an act of courtesy toward a stranger."[4]

At Norway House, obviously somewhat in awe of his good fortune to be travelling with the boss, Moberly described Simpson meeting with the Northern Council. "Everything was discussed and arranged for the coming year for the Northern Department, which reached from the United States border along the Rockies to the Arctic Ocean and east to Hudson Bay and Fort William." But the observant Moberly went on to describe a side of Simpson that had never before emerged in written characterizations of the Governor:

An amusing incident, but one which for a time seemed likely to end in tragedy, occurred after breakfast [at Norway House]. M. de S., a French-Canadian, brave but excitable, in charge of Isle a la Crosse, sent a formal challenge to Mr. S., a member of one of the old Scotch families settled in Canada, a cool, self-possessed officer and a gentleman whose personal courage was undoubted. The latter was astonished and asked to be informed when and in what manner he had incurred the resentment of M. de S. The only reply he was able to elicit was: "I vill not be insulted by any man! I vill shoot him or he vill shoot me!"

At length Mr. S. said: "If my friend insists, I suppose I must oblige him."

A meeting was arranged for the following morning. Sir George, hearing of it, enquired of M. de S. what Mr. S. had done to insult him.

"He called me a 'miserable' at breakfast this morning," said the Frenchman, "and either I vill shoot him or he vill shoot me!"

"Why, so he did!" exclaimed Sir George. "Now you mention it, M. de S., I recall distinctly his using that expression. I won't interfere further."

Sir George called Mr. S. aside and voiced his surprise that that gentleman had, at the public mess, called his brother officer a miserable person.

Mr. S. heatedly denied the charge, but the Governor insisted that he had himself heard it. Mr. S. was amazed. Although he was quite positive he had made no such statement he could not convince others of his innocence.

Mr. S. and M. de S., it developed, slept in adjoining rooms, separated only by a thin board partition. M. de S. was a heavy snorer and rather touchy about it. Mr. S. had appeared late at breakfast that morning, and when Sir George remarked it, explained that "That confounded miserable kept me awake all night!"

The Frenchman at once took this as applying to himself and his snoring propensity, and became instantly and properly indignant. What

Mr. S. really referred to, however, was Victor Hugo's *Les Miserables*, in which he had become interested during the evening and continued reading until near daylight. Sir George had seen the joke at once and in a spirit of fun kept it up all day, divulging the secret, only in time to prevent real mischief, at dinner in the evening. As a result, the only shots fired were from the necks of Hudson's Bay dark brandy bottles.[5]

George Simpson was sixty-two years old and clearly of active mind and spirit as he joked with officers at Norway House. He was in his thirty-fourth year in the trade, and in all but three of those years, and against substantial physical odds, he had made his way to Council meetings by canoe. Those with him and around him bent to his every need, but there was toughness and durability in Simpson's constitution that still astounds. He seemed to be renewed and reinvigorated by his time on the trail and never more so than on his return from his 1854 trip to Rupert's Land, when, in the spirit of Hogmanays past, in a parlour dalliance early in 1855 he sired yet another child, this time with Mary Labonte, a servant at Hudson's Bay House at Lachine. And, in a now-familiar pattern, although this time not with an Aboriginal woman, Simpson appears to have convinced his manservant, James Murray, to marry this woman and to raise the child as their own. Frances Georgina Murray was born on October 17, 1855, and, like some of Simpson's other children born out of wedlock, was provided for in the Governor's will in a minor way.

Throughout his life, Simpson's appetite for sex was eclipsed only by his appetite for business, perhaps one tied to the other. Shortly after his tryst with Mary Labonte in January of 1855, he packed his cases yet again and headed to Washington to continue negotiations with the Americans over settlement of the outstanding Oregon issues. A letter to his mentor, now HBC governor, Andrew Colvile indicates that his animal spirits for business and his vigour for the subtleties and minutiae of negotiations were, like his entire constitution, undiminished by time:

Hudson's Bay House
Lachine
20 January 1855
A. Colvile Esquire

My dear Sir,

I left this morning for Washington on the 11. and arrived there on the evening of the 13 inst.

I had several interviews with Mr. [Sir John] Crampton [British minister to the United States], who was unfortunately confined to the house from the effects of a fall which prevented his accompanying me to Mr. [William Learned] Marcy's [American secretary of state]; he, therefore, gave me a note of introduction, with which I presented myself & was immediately admitted to an audience. My first visit was purely preliminary, as Mr. Marcy had not then time to discuss the question of the Company's negotiation, but he gave me to understand the Government had decided that $300,000 was the utmost they would offer both companies. I stated that under present circumstances, but more particularly in consequence of the hostility the Company experienced from all classes within the American Territory—the press, the Courts the Government officials and the public at large—they were more anxious than ever to come to an arrangement with the U/S Government it being almost impossible for them to maintain their footing in the country. I said further they were prepared to meet the Government as to the amount of compensation & suggested that the difference between the Company's demand of $1,000,000 & the offer of $300,000 should be halved & the amount fixed at $650,000. Mr. Marcy replied the Government would be firm in adhering to the basis of $300,000.[6]

But Simpson knew that the Americans would likely not move from $300,000, and with the passage of time were likely to pay even less for

HBC "rights" below the forty-ninth parallel. While he asked for Colvile's opinion, he advised him to accept the terms.

After yet another mad dash later that spring to Council meetings in the west, via train and canoe, Simpson was back in Lachine by the end of July, sitting for a portrait painted by Stephen Pearce that was commissioned as a gift by his senior officers in the trade. The Governor looks crabbed and tired in his portrait, his face showing every one of his sixty-four years and every mile of rough trail travel. But his body is erect, almost trim, as he stands at his Lachine desk, in long frock coat, starched wing collar and ample silk cravat, a gold chain and watch fob conspicuous in the buttonhole of his tailored waistcoat. And behind him, in a handsome, tall bookcase, are impressive leather-bound narratives of all the North American explorations that really matter: Hearne's *Journey*, Mackenzie's *Voyages*, Thomas Simpson's *Discoveries*, John Rae's *Expeditions to the Arctic Sea*, John Richardson's *Fauna of America* and, his pride and joy, a two-volume set with gold on polished leather, just like the others, entitled *Narrative of a Journey Round the World*.

But before the paint was dry, Simpson had left again, this time for England, conveniently one week prior to the birth of his eighth daughter.[7] He was back on a Liverpool packet ship on December 22 for his umpteenth North Atlantic crossing, returning to Lachine in January just in time to witness wedding preparations for his daughter Fanny (Frances). Life for the Governor must have been a blur, unless motion stemmed the tide of memories and regret that stasis could not.

Fanny had met and fallen in love with Angus Cameron, nephew of Chief Factor Angus Cameron, as a result of more than two decades of dealings between her father and the old Nor'Wester in posts from Lake of Two Mountains to Fort Timiskaming. Young Cameron had been a banker in Elgin, Scotland, but had come out to North America in 1848 and, with the help of Governor Simpson, who had taken the young Scot on as something of a protégé, had secured a job at the Bank of Montreal. His career was advancing nicely, with Sir George's help, but the smiles

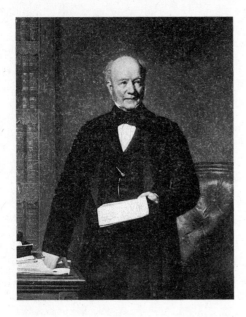

Stephen Pearce's portrait of Sir George, shown standing in his Lachine office next to his shelves of exploration books (including his own Round the World *volume).*

and assistance waned when Simpson learned of the bank apprentice's designs on Fanny. Indeed, just prior to his return to Lachine from London in December 1855, Simpson wrote to the old Nor'Wester Cameron of his concerns about his daughter falling for a suitor below her station: "As regard the projected union—your nephew Angus has stood very high in my regard, ever since I became acquainted with him; and as he seems to have made himself agreeable to my Daughter, I did not withhold my consent, altho his position in life was not such as (considering my circumstances) I might have looked for in a Son-in-Law: so that if the young people be of the same mind when I get back, as they appeared to be when I left Canada, their marriage may take place."[8]

Take place it did, at St. Stephen's Church in Lachine, with the Governor finally attending a ceremony to offer the hand of one of his daughters in marriage. And, when Fanny's first "trial" came along a year later, Sir George was by all accounts pleased enough with the arrival of the baby boy to stop in Toronto on his way west in 1857 to become godfather to namesake George Simpson Cameron. Alas, in an echo of

Simpson's own history, George Simpson Cameron, the little boy they called "Chieftain" in honour of his maternal grandfather, died suddenly before his second birthday.

—

In the middle of these family affairs, trouble was brewing in London that would sound the death knell for the HBC's monopoly in North America as well as for the reign of its long-time overseas governor. The Industrial Revolution, which had invigorated an increasingly influential middle class in Great Britain, had called into question many of the perquisites of the privileged upper classes. Influential people were questioning government-sponsored monopolies such as that held by the Hudson's Bay Company in North America. But even more damaging to the HBC were increasingly vocal critics in North America. Fallout from the Sayer trial had caught the ear of Whitehall Whigs, and in Canada people like George Brown, editor of the Toronto *Globe*, and William McDougall, editor of the *North American*, were openly attacking the Hudson's Bay Company's exploitive policies.

Just as American settlers in Oregon had begun to define themselves as part of a cultural whole, linking south to California and east to Washington and the New England states, so there were those in the Canadian government who were beginning to think of Canada in more expansive terms, "from sea to sea." Influential Canadian politician Philip VanKoughnet argued in a London newspaper: "The charter of the Hudson's Bay Company—no charter—no power could give to a few men exclusive control over half a continent. That vast a territory stretching from Lake Superior and the Hudson's Bay belonged to Canada—or must belong to it."[9]

Members of the British parliament knew that the HBC's operating licence was coming up for renewal. Driven by serious unrest in Canada and on the domestic front, Lord Palmerston, then prime minister, struck a select committee to "consider the state of those British Possessions in North America which are under the Administration of the Hudson's Bay Company, or over which they possess a License to Trade, and who are empowered to report their observations, together with minutes of evidence taken before them, to The House."[10]

George Simpson, naturally, was among about a dozen highly placed witnesses who were called to testify before the select committee. He left Lachine, in failing health, for London in January 1857 and was on the stand in an imposing hearing room at Westminster on February 16 and March 2. It seems evident from the transcript that from the moment the Governor sat down he did not respond well to this kind of interrogation. The Hudson's Bay Company was essentially on trial and, as its chief executive officer in North America, he was being called upon to account for its actions or inaction with respect to treatment of Aboriginal peoples, settlement, and prosecution of its various business concerns.

Simpson had grown used to being the intimidator, with money, power and influence on his side. Now the tables were turned, and it wasn't long before he started, uncharacteristically, to sweat: "[Chairman] I believe you hold an important situation in the administration of the territories of the Hudson's Bay Company? —I do. What is it? I have been Governor of their territories for many years. How long have you held that situation? —Thirty-seven years I have been their principal representative. As governor the whole time? —Yes; I have held the situation of governor the whole time. What is the nature of your authority in that capacity? —The supervision of the Company's affairs; the presiding at their councils in the country, and the principal direction of the whole interior management." And so on it went, for 1,423 questions.

The interrogation started to heat up when the topic turned to possibilities for settlement on company lands. Simpson was trying to stick to the argument that there were really no good lands for settlement on HBC territories, hoping that he might bluff the committee on lands they had never seen. But committee member Mr. Gordon led him into a trap:

> 772.[11] [Mr. Gordon] If I understand you rightly, you think that no portion of Rupert's Land is favourable for settlement, but that some portions might be settled? —Yes.

773. [picking up Simpson's book] In your very interesting work of a "Journey Round the World," I find at Page 45 of the first volume this description of the country between the Lake of the Woods and Rainy Lake: "From Fort Frances downwards, a stretch of nearly 100 miles, it is not interrupted by a single impediment, while yet the current is not strong enough materially to retard an ascending traveller. Nor are the banks less favourable to agriculture than the waters themselves to navigation, resembling, in some measure, those of the Thames near Richmond. From the very brink of the river there rises a gentle slope of greensward, crowned in many places with a plentiful growth of birch, poplar, beech, elm, and oak. Is it too much for the eye of philanthropy to discern through the vista of futurity this noble stream, connecting, as it does, the fertile shores of two spacious lakes, with crowded steamboats on its bosom and populous towns on its borders?" I suppose you consider that district favourable for population? —The right bank of the river is favourable, with good cultivation; that is to say the soil is favourable; the climate is not; the back country is a deep morass, and never can be drained, in my opinion.

774. Do you see any reason to alter the opinion which you have there expressed? —I do see that I overrated the importance of the country as a country for settlement.

775. [Chairman] It is too glowing a description, you think? —Exactly so.

What Simpson could not, or would not, tell his interrogators was that this description, published under his name by Mr. Colburn, had never been touched by his hand. It had been written by Edward Hopkins and twice embroidered: once by Archibald Barclay and once by a man known for his florid prose, Adam Thom. The Governor had been caught by the committee in a trap of his own making.

A hundred or so questions later, committee member Gordon used a similar tactic to explore Simpson's views about the HBC's stewardship of the settlers at Red River (which, after all, had been a company sponsored initiative). But to do this, after a few preliminary questions, he pulled out a book by one of Simpson's arch-enemies:

815. I suppose it was during the time you were Governor that a certain Mr. John McLean, who has published "Notes of a Twenty-five Years' Service in the Hudson's Bay Territory," was a servant of the Company? —Yes, he was so a part of the time.

816. I will read you an extract as taken from his book, and you can say how far it is correct. "A single Scotch farmer," says Mr. M'Clean, "could be found in the colony able alone to supply the greater part of the produce the Company require; there is one in fact who offered to do it; if a sure market were secured to the colonists of Red River they would speedily become the wealthiest yeomanry in the world; their barns and granaries are always full to overflowing; the Company purchase from six to eight bushel of wheat from each farmer, at the rate of 3s. per bushel, and the sum total of their yearly purchases from the whole settlement amounts to 600 cwts. flour, first and second qualities; 35 bushels rough barley; 10 half firkins butter, 28 lbs. each; 10 bushels Indian corn; 200 cwt. best kiln-dried flour; 60 firkins butter, 56 lbs. each; 240 lbs. cheese; 60 hams. Where he (the Red River farmer) finds a sure market for the remainder of his produce, Heaven only knows, I do not; this much, however, I do know, that the incomparable advantages this delightful country possesses are not only in a great measure lost to the inhabitants, but also the world, so long as it remains under the dominion of its fur-trading rulers." Do you agree in the comment of Mr. M'Clean there? —Certainly not.

817. In point of fact, do the Company purchase from the farmers settled in the neighbourhood of the Red River Settlement, all the corn the farmers are able to sell? —We are not able to let the quantity of corn to be held in depot that we require. I have written over and over again to the person in charge, to get all the grain he could for the purpose of being held at the depôt, and we can never get our quantity.

818. [Mr. Gordon] Will you allow me to remind you of one other sentence in your interesting work. It is at page 55 of volume I: "The soil of Red River Settlement is a black mould of considerable depth, which, when first tilled, produces extraordinary crops, as much, on some occasions, as 40 returns of wheat; and even after 20 successive years of cultivation, without the relief of manure or of fallow, or of green crop, it still yields from 15 to 25 bushels an acre. The wheat produced is plump and heavy; there are also large quantities of grain of all kinds, besides beef, mutton, pork, butter, cheese, and wool in abundance." Do you adhere to that statement? —I do.

819. And yet you think it unfavourable for cultivation? —Yes.[12]

The Emperor was cornered as the interrogation continued. On the second day of testimony, the select committee circled back to the land between Lake Superior and Lake Winnipeg, wondering about inconsistencies between what they had read and heard from other witnesses about settlement potential and about the treatment of Aboriginal peoples in this area and what they had heard from Simpson. Perhaps the most telling moment for the Governor came when committee member Mr. Roebuck read a passage from yet another book by a traveller who passed through this region. When it came time to answer a direct question about the author of this book, Simpson out and out lied:

1598. Did you know a book called "The Life of Thomas Simpson"? —I did.

1599. By whom was it written? —It was written by Mr. Thomas Simpson. [Simpson had to know that this was written by Thomas's brother Alexander.]

1600. And if that is an extract from Mr. Thomas Simpson's book, you say it is an exaggeration? —I do not know what part of the country he speaks of.

1601. Between Lake Superior and Lake Winnipeg? —There is a very thin population there.

1602. Who was Mr. Thomas Simpson? —Mr. Thomas Simpson was a distant relative of mine.

1603. Was not he a long time in the Company's service? —No.

For a man with George Simpson's passion for precision to characterize a first cousin as a "distant relative" is just odd, or evidence of a failing or seriously conflicted mind.

Reflecting back on this sad moment in the denouement of Simpson's career, an HBC London Committee member characterized Sir George's testimony before the select committee as a "wretched expedition."[13] He went on to say, "Simpson's mind was by that time beginning to give way. I had a high opinion at one time of his abilities but [after his testimony] I thought him deficient in sound judgement and latterly his nerves had quite given way."[14]

The Governor, too, knew that things were breaking up. He returned to Lachine and wilfully continued the alternating rhythm of life, west for Councils in the summer and home to Lachine for the winter. Parliament had renewed the licence, with the proviso that lands on Vancouver Island and other ground suitable for settlement be withdrawn from company control and put back into government hands, but the end of the monopoly was in sight. The end of the monopoly had been in sight, in fact, since the Sayer trial. Andrew Colvile, having finally achieved the pinnacle of power, stepped down after only four years, and Henry Hulse Berens took his place as governor. Privately and in confidence, Simpson wrote to the new HBC governor about his intention to resign before he was too much longer in the saddle: "It will occasion me regret to sever my connection. It is high time I rested from incessant labour. Moreover, I am unwilling to hold an appointment when I cannot discharge my duties to my own entire satisfaction. I shall therefore make way for some younger man, who I trust may serve the Company as zealously and conscientiously as I have done."[15]

Simpson's last horizon was in sight.

CHAPTER XIX

THE EMPEROR'S LIGHT
GOES OUT

B y the spring of 1857, when the Governor's small pedicured feet started to itch for his annual migration to Councils in Michipicoten and Norway House, at Lachine the gentle sounds of bark canoes being loaded by chirpy voyageurs had been all but drowned out by the whistles of steam trains heading to and from Toronto and Detroit on the newly completed Grand Trunk Railway. Better than anyone, Simpson knew that in the long term the railway meant settlement, which, as he had seen in Red River and Oregon Country, would eventually kill the fur trade in areas of his domain. But in the short term, both for the HBC and for his own entrepreneurial prospects, the railway meant new efficiencies for moving people and freight and other business opportunities.

While the company itself did not invest directly in these new forms of industrial capitalism (to its eventual peril), some members of the London Committee bought securities through Baring Brothers investment house in London in these emerging North American transportation ventures, and the shrewd and connected Simpson—ensconced in the middle of all this in Montreal—doubled and redoubled his personal fortunes through the buying and selling of stocks, bonds and debentures on banks, railways, canals, harbours, bridges, mines, telegraph and gas companies, and steamship companies. With Simpson's personal involvement in the Grand Trunk as an investor, it was only natural that as soon as possible after October 1856, when the last spike was driven into the last twenty-foot section of cast iron fifty-five pound,[1] brought by ship to Canada from Britain, the Governor would forgo his beloved seven-fathom canoe *Rob Roy* and its loyal crew for a well-sprung velvet-covered seat in a private car on the Grand Trunk Railway, with his servant James Murray, secretary Edward Hopkins and a cook and personal steward to see to his every need.

Because of inhospitable geography and the HBC's lack of interest in settlement anywhere other than Assiniboia and the west coast, the railway pushed west in the United States long before it did in Canada. In 1857, Simpson would have travelled west by train through Toronto to Windsor, but because there was as yet no bridge or tunnel on the Detroit River, and because the Grand Trunk had been built purposely at a larger gauge than US railroads to prevent American trains from running troops into Canada faster than had been possible in the War of 1812, the Governor and his entourage would have had to disembark from one train, cross the river by barge or ferry, and re-embark on the other side to continue their journey west through the state of Michigan to Chicago, Illinois, and on through Wisconsin to St. Paul, Minnesota. Rail would not reach the banks of the Mississippi River at St. Paul until the following year, so at some point west of Chicago on his inaugural train trip, Simpson would have had to move back to a horse-drawn conveyance. But here too, Simpson, as a business associate of strategic American politicians and an investor in American corporate interests, including the Michigan and Central Railroad Company, would have been given royal treatment.

For by this time in his life, although his allegiance to the HBC remained strong, his work as an independent entrepreneur had created its own social status. His wife was deceased and the day-to-day care of

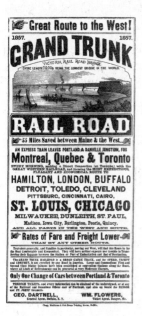

Simpson was quick to respond to changes in technology, putting westbound freight on the railway as soon as it was open for business. But the Emperor of the North knew, better than anyone, the value of the canoe as an icon.

his younger children was in the capable hands of the Finlaysons and the staff at Hudson's Bay House at Lachine. His aunt and mother-in-law were quick to take the children when they were home in London. And the affairs of the HBC were more or less running themselves on the backs of people who were sure their omniscient boss had magical powers. Simpson was free in these last working years to position himself among the New World gentry and to distance himself forever from his humble Ross-shire roots.

If one was to conjure an image of the self-made man in North America, then it could easily be that of the Governor trundling west on the brand-new Grand Trunk Railway, ensconced beneath an ornate clerestory of a private railcar beside the polished brass fittings and mahogany frame of a chattering stained-glass-detailed window. The beaver topper would have been neatly secured in its monogrammed leather carrying case, and the blue-lined tartan cape stowed. But, as a man of station, he would most certainly have retained the high-waisted pinstripes and tailored frock coat over the starched collar and cuffs affixed with studs to match golden cufflinks, hunting-horn fob, chain and chiming pocket watch, tucked into the stretched pocket of an outrageous red paisley silk vest.

A year later, in 1858, Simpson went west a second time by train, this time with an old acquaintance from the London Committee, Edward Ellice. In his correspondence of later years, Simpson often lamented the fact that there were fewer and fewer left of the HBC and NWC personnel who had lived through the amalgamation of 1821; there remained throughout the Governor's lifetime a sense of kinship and camaraderie among the old-time officers of the trade. But McTavish had died and so too had gone, either retired or deceased, many of the other gentlemen of the trade with whom Simpson had cut his managerial teeth. However, one who had stayed the course and done exceptionally well, though much more quietly and with much more family money and influence to begin than Sir George ever had, was Edward Ellice.

If there is one vignette that captures the essence of Sir George at the height of his career, it is his reunion and trip west with Ellice. Fate conspired with circumstance to bring these two old-timers together in the opulence of another private car on the Grand Trunk Railway in the spring of 1859. Simpson was sixty-six, Ellice seventy-five. Physically both were perhaps staying upright with burnished hardwood canes with fancy three-knob filigreed silver handles, their adjutants marking the way; but mentally, both had business minds hungry for economy and opportunity.

In 1818, two years before he had more or less single-handedly negotiated the amalgamation deal with Andrew Colvile, Edward "Bear"[2] Ellice, sole agent for the NWC in London, had been elected to the British House of Commons. With Nor'Westers William and Simon McGillivray, he had done well financially as a result of the amalgamation of the two companies (albeit, many argued, at the expense of the NWC, which effectively disappeared as a consequence of this deal), but Ellice brought to that windfall a fortune made by a father and four uncles who had also thrived as agents in the Montreal-based trade. From his father, Ellice had inherited the seigneury of Villechauve, also known as Beauharnois,

324 square miles on the south shore of the St. Lawrence River south of Lachine, which he was able to manage and develop through the 1830s and 1840s from his London home.

The personal connection between Ellice and Simpson, though not well documented in the historic record, was a direct consequence of the amalgamation of the two companies. On the signing of the deed poll, Ellice became a major shareholder of the HBC and was elected as a director of the new concern. And from that point on, as a member of the London Committee, using his access to the British cabinet, his parliamentary seat, his connections in the City of London, and his carefully honed liaisons with the press, Ellice became an unofficial advocate for the HBC. Although his name was rarely mentioned in print or correspondence, Ellice's quiet work in the margins was evident throughout all contestations of the HBC's monopoly, work that included, for example, the installation of his son, also Edward, a new parliamentarian, onto the select committee to which Sir George had had to testify in 1857.

In this role as a behind-the-scenes operative in London social and political circles, Ellice would have certainly crossed paths with Simpson on his trips to Fenchurch Street, but he more likely earned Simpson's respect and admiration as a man after his own heart, a possible additional role model for the Governor alongside their mutual friend Andrew Colvile.

In addition to his advocacy for the HBC, Ellice served as the go-to parliamentarian for any and all matters colonial between North America and the British government. As a businessman with major investments and interests in North America, Ellice had been a strong proponent of the uniting of the two Canadas. Further evidence of his influence on matters can be seen in his promotion of Lord Durham as a possible candidate with "large powers for the exercise of authority and conciliation"[3] to lead efforts to unify Upper and Lower Canada and to ensure that his son—the same son who later served on the select committee—was Durham's private secretary when Durham was dispatched to North

America. Ellice had also been involved at the highest levels, again unofficially, in negotiations with the Americans over matters of concern to the Crown and over the HBC's possessory rights in Columbia.

Drawn by Simpson's reports to the London Committee of the success of his 1857 train journey and of the smooth handling of a test shipment of forty tons of freight, Edward Ellice knew instinctively that this dramatic change of circumstance needed first-hand examination. Hence, in 1858, in conjunction with a second test shipment of HBC goods—this time totalling one hundred tons—Ellice decided to sail to North America for a grand rail adventure, the second of two trips (the first having been in 1836) he would take to North America in his lifetime. He would accompany the Governor and see again for himself these emerging nations and nascent business propositions in which he had a substantial personal and professional stake. One imagines the two old gentlemen—one Bayman, one would-be Nor'Wester—in their Victorian finery, Simpson more flamboyantly appointed in his haberdashery than the understated Ellice, sipping gin in their lounge chairs or against the ornate wrought iron railings of the verandah at the back of the train, one-upping each other with tales of the trade.

Where lesser business types might have looked at the ten-fold population growth between Chicago and St. Paul and thought, say, of starting a retail clothing store, a hardware store or a lumber operation, or perhaps an interconnected chain of stores or factories or an integrated manufacturing/transportation system of some kind, Ellice and Simpson confirmed as they made their way west on the train that what they really wanted to do was start a bank.

From their own pockets the old fur traders reckoned they could produce seed funding of $50,000 each. This, with enthusiastic testimonials about the phenomenal growth of western commerce, would raise additional contributions from friends and associates, perhaps reaching an initial capitalization of $250,000, which could be leveraged to twice that, depending on how the project proceeded. As an example of how straightforward Simpson was in his dealings, even at this lofty level

of private commerce, here is a letter he wrote to Minnesota governor
Alexander Ramsay to confirm proposed arrangements:

Hudson's Bay House
Lachine 3 November 1858

My dear sir,

During our recent visit to Saint Paul, the attention of my fellow
traveller, the Right Honble. Edward Ellice, and myself was drawn to
the apparent deficiency of banking capital and accommodation at
that growing place. It appeared to us that a good opening presented
itself for the profitable employment of capital and we have accordingly
come to the determination of ourselves establishing a Bank in Saint
Paul next year.

Mr. Ellice is to give $50,000 in the name of his son, Mr. Edward
Ellice Junr. (Member of Parliament); I have subscribed a like sum, and
a few of our friends have made up $50,000 more; —in all, $150,000 as
a beginning. We should increase our capital to $500,000 and further
as the business might require.

We are rather at a loss on what basis to establish our Bank; whether
under a Charter or as a private concern. There would be a good deal
of formality to go through in obtaining an Act of Incorporation &
probably some delay, both of which we should be glad to avoid. —If
chartered, our Bank would be under Government control, which,
besides restricting the rate of discount &c, might otherwise hamper
our operations; —the only return, I believe, being the right to circu-
late notes. —We are, on the whole, rather disposed to do business as
capitalists, —lending money on real and personal security and doing
general banking business, *without* circulating notes of our own.—

Is there in Minnesota any General Banking Law, limiting the
liability of partners in private banks? Suppose we had several, say 25
partners, how could we sue and be sued?; could we plead in the name
of the firm, or must the name of each individual partner be given? If

chartered, we might use the corporate name & be represented by our Cashier or President, —at least I presume such would be the case under your laws. —I should feel much obliged if you would favour us with your valuable opinion on this point and also with any hints for our guidance, which your experience might suggest.

Our Staff, in the first instance, would consist of a Cashier and Clerk, assisted by a local Board of Direction. The Agent of the Hudson's Bay Company at Saint Paul, who would be one of our Superior officers (I think I may say that measure is now decided on) would be one of our Directors. It would be gratifying to Mr. Ellice and myself if you would act as a member of the Board. The duties of the office would not be burdensome, indeed we should not propose the arrangement if likely to occupy much of your valuable time; but we think it important to the prestige and success of the Bank that your name should be associated with it. It might, perhaps, be agreeable to you to take an interest in it as a partner.

It would be desirable to secure as our legal advisor, the leading man in the profession at Saint Paul. Can you recommend any gentleman to us?

Mr. Ellice is about to sail to England, but I shall be in communication with that gentleman on this subject, and will acquaint him with your views, when you may find it convenient to favour me with them. —In the meantime, I shall consult with my friend Mr. Royal Phelps of New York—as I am anxious to have our arrangements completed in time to commence operations next Spring.—

Believe me, My dear sir,
Very faithfully yours,
G Simpson

Governor Ramsay
Saint Paul
Minnesota

P.S. I think it may be advisable that the intention to establish a Bank should be kept secret, until we are prepared to go into operation; I shall, therefore, feel obliged by your considering this letter confidential, for your private information only. —It would be advisable to look out for premises at once, and I should be glad to know if there are any you would recommend. The same premises might serve for the Hudson's Bay Company Agency & the Bank. For the latter, there would be required offices below & a dwelling house for the Cashier above. Fireproof vaults &c might be erected after we obtained possession; but the building itself must be of stone or brick, & situated in the best business part of town. If there be no premises that would suit us in the market, I should be obliged if you would ascertain if we could procure a lot on which to build. —I heartily recommend that these enquiries should be cautiously made, as if the object of them were known, parties having premisses or lots for sale would be disposed to advance their terms. G S[4]

Although the bank idea was never realized, it does stand as testament to Simpson's entrepreneurial spirit and capacity for moving in high circles—in this case, working with the new governor of the newly created state of Minnesota, the ranking official in the district.

Simpson was also interested in establishing steam transportation on the Red River. Rail could get freight to St. Paul, Minnesota—indeed, since the previous year, track had been laid down right to the banks of the mighty Mississippi. But there was still the matter of getting it up and down the north-south axis to Assiniboia. If only they could position powered ships on the Red River, thereby making a seamless and very economical steam connection between transatlantic shipping and the Red River settlement! Many credit Simpson as being "the driving force behind steam boating on the Red River."[5] About this time, the Governor purchased at least $6,000 of "Bonds of the County of Ramsay, State of Minnesota," dedicated, among other projects, to an incentive program to promote the placement of a steam vessel on the Red River. Exactly how the Governor advanced this cause or whether Edward Ellice was in on it is not clear, but the man who actually sweated to drag a steamship overland from the Mississippi to the Red River north of St. Paul—a St. Paul contractor and riverboat captain called Anson Northup—got a nasty surprise when he decided to play with the likes of Simpson and his cronies.

In the spring of 1858, a year after Simpson's initial meetings with city officials in St. Paul—and perhaps just after Simpson and Ellice passed through and conceived of their banking scheme—the St. Paul Chamber of Commerce posted a reward of $1,000 to the first person who could put a steamboat on the Red River. The unsuspecting Anson Northup took the bait, probably expecting that the first person with a steamship on the Red would have a captive shipping market for the increasing amount of freight travelling up and down the river to Assiniboia. He knew as well that the Hudson's Bay Company was always looking for efficiencies. But before Northup would take up the challenge, he went to the members of the St. Paul Chamber and renegotiated the prize from $1,000 to $2,000.

Northup purchased a paddle-wheeler called the *North Star* and, in the winter of 1858, took it as far up into the headwaters of the Mississippi as he could go—north of St. Paul, up rapids and over shoals to the Crow Wing River, where he eventually ground to a halt in shallow water. That winter, through the worst snow and cold that the American prairie could muster, Northup and a hardy crew dismantled the 90-foot-long *North Star* and dragged the bits—including an 11,000-pound boiler—150 miles from the Mississippi watershed over the divide to a point on the Red River about 10 miles north of the town of Moorhead, Minnesota. With dollar signs in his eyes, the ambitious entrepreneur renamed his reconstructed vessel after himself, and in the spring of 1859 the *Anson Northup*, with its namesake at the wheel, steamed its way from Fort Abercrombie in the Dakota Territory to Fort Garry in a scant four days, arriving triumphantly on June 10, 1859.

Although he had espoused great interest in this innovation, Simpson travelled west again on the train in 1859 but chose to travel by cart to

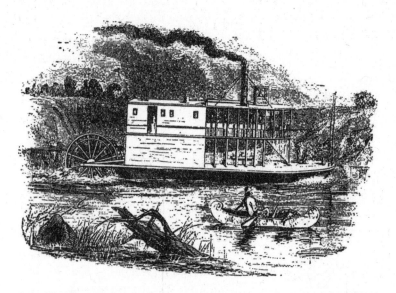

Anson Northup thought he had a captive market on the Red River with his steamer. Thanks to George Simpson, Northup lost his shirt, and his boat, to the competition, who renamed the vessel and gave the HBC a prearranged 50 per cent discount on freight rates to and from the railway.

Red River, arriving a week before the *Anson Northup* steamed up to the pier. Simpson might have been on the dock for her arrival but he had chosen not to travel with Northup on that maiden voyage. And that, to Northup, should have been ample warning that something nefarious was in the works.

Having invested much of his own time, money and energy in the project, perhaps blinded by the $2,000 prize, Northup got a terrible shock when he steamed back upriver to Fort Abercrombie later that year. To his dismay the contractor discovered that no one—including the HBC—was interested in doing business with him. While he had been lugging boilers over frozen ground, Governor Simpson had been in cahoots with the Burbank brothers of St. Paul, who had secretly agreed to give the HBC a 50 per cent discount on freight rates on the Red in return for the company's financial help in securing a vessel. There was absolutely nothing Anson Northup could do to capitalize on his investment. He was forced to sell his smoke-belching pride and joy to the Burbanks, who, with a purchase loan and a fat shipping contract in hand from the HBC, started immediately into the steam-shipping business on the Red River. The first order of business for the Burbanks was to rename the boat *Pioneer*, although they might more aptly have named it *Sir George Simpson* for his part in all of this.

———

George Simpson maintained an equally uncompromising grip on his core business concerns, knowing that with increasing criticism of the HBC's monopoly, he was obliged to carry out the obligations of the company's royal charter and to implement the terms of the deed poll to the letter, lest anyone be provided with ammunition to attack what was continuing, somewhat improbably, as a profitable business operation.[6] Because of his synoptic grasp of all things North American and his tremendous capacity for carrying a working knowledge of company history in his everyday dealings, Simpson must have known that the railway meant the end of York Factory as a depot for the HBC. He must have known that the technological tide that was washing wave after wave of settlers into the country south of the border would soon start doing the same in Rupert's Land and that those same forces would eventually erode any hope of the fur trade continuing in its traditional pattern. He must have known that the days of the HBC's cozy monopoly were numbered. But there was time yet to prosper. British colonial secretary Sir Edward Bulwer-Lytton[7] had led a charge to revoke the HBC's licence for operation in New Caledonia, Columbia and Oregon Country but had soon learned that the British government had neither stomach nor money for managing affairs that were being handled by the HBC. Simpson knew this as well and took advantage of the situation at every available opportunity, for corporate profits and for personal gain.

By now, democracy inside the HBC was a total illusion. Where once Councils might have actually been swayed by the vote of attending chief traders and chief factors, Simpson now just did as he pleased, whether they liked it or not, whether they even attended Council or not. In 1859, for example, he stepped from the train and, after a cart ride to Red River, settled back into a canoe for an old-style trip to Norway House. But spring that year was unusually late, and the brigades (along with the gentlemen who travelled with them, by Simpson's edict of long before) were delayed. His old friend and confidant Robert Miles explained Simpson's response to this delay in a private letter to a colleague in the trade: "Sir George and Hopkins I hear reached Montreal on the 16th July—the Western Brigades being detained by Ice at the Grand Rapids, he was awaiting at Norway House for them Seven days, consequently he did their business for them before hand & Settled their Council in one day— This is brisk work & must fully carry out the terms of the deed poll with respect to the business assigned therein to the Councillors—Bah!"[8]

One is inclined to forget, given the Governor's robust business activities in the late 1850s, that the man was nearly blind and still suffering from apoplexy. He was truly never happier nor healthier, it seemed, than when he was on the move, but there was no doubt his overall health was in steep decline. In February 1859, at Lachine, Simpson had a particularly severe attack and, having rallied after yet another round of intensive bleedings (there was still not much the medical profession could do for his condition), he wrote to Henry Hulse Berens in March to say that he was thinking about retirement—that is, he was not *actually* retiring, but he was thinking about steps the company might take in the event that he did retire. Wording was important. By now, Andrew Colvile had either lost interest in or fallen out of favour with the London Committee, and with him had gone the idea that his son Eden would be the heir apparent for Simpson's job. Eden Colvile had served his time at Red River but returned home after a devastating flood in 1852 to assume many of his father's business directorships, eventually taking a seat on the London Committee, and eventually becoming HBC governor.

The question of who might replace him as top man in North America was very much on Simpson's mind as he mustered strength to board the train yet again in May 1860 to make his way west to the Northern Council. This time, however, his iron will could not overcome his failing constitution. He had to admit that if he were to persist beyond St. Paul, he would almost certainly die.

The Emperor, finally, had had enough. He was forced to limp home on the train with Edward Hopkins at his side, his life more or less hanging in the balance. By June he was well enough to continue correspondence and wrote a private and confidential letter to Governor Berens:

> Mr. H. McKenzie has sent to the Secretary copies of a letter I have addressed to him from Prairie du Chien and Saint Paul, which will have prepared you for the announcement of my return hither after having proceeded far enough to prove beyond all doubt that my strength was unequal to the fatigues of the journey to Red River. My medical advisor strongly dissuaded me from making the attempt but I was so anxious to preside at the Council that I disregarded his warning. We were unfortunate at the offset; the weather was sultry, the railroad trains were crowded, the hours long and inconvenient and altogether it was trying to a person in good health and I felt the fatigue severely and day by day, the worst symptoms of my late attack returned. The stage beyond St. Paul is 250 miles to Georgetown, in wagons over a country without roads, inns or accommodation for travellers; had I attempted it I have little doubt that it would have proved fatal. It became therefore a question of life or death, and I thought it better to return than to leave my bones to bleach on the plains of Red River.[9]

Two months later, he considered his situation again. Though not ready to actually resign his post, he had been thinking more about who might succeed him. Again, he wrote to Berens:

> Mr. Colvile informs me, he has at my request, communicated with you on the subject of my withdrawal from active duty and the grant

of a retiring pension.— I have served the Company very actively for more than Forty years, and my wish is, to continue to do so while I have health and strength: but, my late illness admonishes me, that the time is coming when I must take more rest, and hence my reason for now opening this question.— The kind manner in which, Mr. Colvile reports, you and the Deputy Governor met the suggestion of a retiring pension, is very gratifying, as evidence that the Board appreciate my past services.— But to yourself individually my thanks are especially due as in this and other matters affecting my private interests I feel you have been influenced by personal regard, as much as a sense of official duty.—

I do not now address you for the purpose of formally tendering my resignation, but to offer some suggestions as to future arrangements connected therewith.— It is possible you may already be looking for a successor, and may find it difficult to satisfy yourself as to the qualifications of the candidates who suggest themselves to your mind.— You may remember that when I was at home in the Spring of 1857 attending the Parliamentary committee on Hudson's Bay Company affairs, I had communication with your lamented predecessor Captn Shepherd and yourself on the appointment of some one to act as Governor in the event of a sudden vacancy, and that Mr. W^m McTavish was furnished with a Commission as acting Governor under Date 29th of June 1857 of which a copy was sent me confidentially.— That appointment has not been made known, but the fact that McTavish still holds it, might be an objection to the appointment of a stranger over his head.— That difficulty I think might be obviated, by an appointment which would be generally acceptable of Mr. Dallas.— From what I have seen of that Gentleman's correspondence, and heard of his management on the West side, I think he would do justice to my office with the duties of which he has already some acquaintance as well as experience of the business of the interior. But, it is possible circumstances might prevent his acceptance, in that case, I think you would do better to look to the Service for a Governor than to send a Stranger into the Country at the risk of offending some of your most valuable officers.[10]

Alexander Grant Dallas was a successful man of business who had been elected to the London Committee of the HBC in 1856 and subsequently sent to sort things out on the west coast, where the Puget Sound Agricultural Company was in disarray and where the Committee was worried about Chief Factor James Douglas's ability to reconcile company business with matters of colonial concern in Victoria. But neither Dallas, nor anyone for that matter, while he might have had attributes necessary to "do justice to [Simpson's] office," could ever have hoped to outdo Simpson's amazing constitution or upstage his role in planning the drama that was the last act of his life.

The buzz in Montreal since the formation of the Grand Trunk Railway had been the commissioning of a bridge across the St. Lawrence River which, at seven thousand feet in length, was to be the longest in the world. The boon to business and to travellers was that this would connect trains in Canada to harbours on the coast of Maine, Massachusetts and New York that were open year round. George Simpson, of course, was intimately connected with the financing and politics of all things transportational in Montreal. And while he stood to gain financially from investments in concerns that would benefit from the bridge, he also saw in its completion an opportunity to do something else for which he had scraped and striven for his entire life—something extraordinary, something memorable, something that only he, George Simpson, could execute.

The structure, which some hailed as "the eighth wonder of the world," was to be named the Jubilee Bridge in honour of Queen Victoria (the bridge was in the end named the Victoria Bridge). Construction began in 1854 and, over the next five years—using 6 steamboats, 3,040 men, 4 locomotives, 72 barges, 144 horses and over $6.6 million—a parade of icebreaking piers was built up from the bottom of the St. Lawrence. Onto these sturdy legs were placed giant tubular sections of metal bridge made in England and shipped by boat to Canada. After a first train crossing in

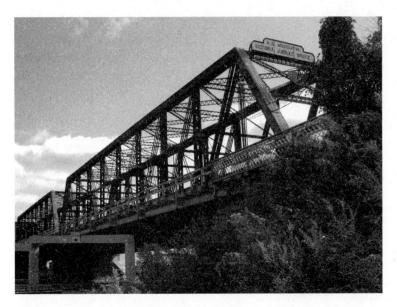

The Victoria Jubilee Bridge in downtown Montreal, as seen today.

December 1859, the Queen was invited to come to Canada to officially open the bridge named in her honour, but she declined. Instead she sent her eighteen-year-old son and heir, Albert Edward, the Prince of Wales (later Edward VII). Naturally, the Prince had to be royally entertained while he was in Montreal, before he headed further inland on his grand tour of the united Canadas, and somehow, using his considerable influence and skills of persuasion, Simpson managed to engineer the spectacle of his dreams. But this event would not happen in downtown Montreal, where it most certainly would be upstaged by the bridge. It would happen at Lachine, under the guise of having the future king to lunch at the dining table of Simpson's new house on Isle Dorval.

While this occasion might have been, in Sir George's imagination, one prelate welcoming another, in reality the event was shaped by the Governor's hunger to "arrive" at some position of ultimate social standing. Available Montreal lodgings were deemed unfit for the Prince of Wales and his entourage. The next best option was the home of Lieutenant

General Sir William Fenwick Williams, a Crimean War veteran now in command of the British garrison at Montreal. Williams having been displaced from his home during the Prince's visit, Simpson immediately offered him the use of his country home on Isle Dorval. This act of generosity gave the Governor the leverage he needed to advance the idea of an outing to Isle Dorval: he could entertain the Prince after he had completed the formalities at his mother's new bridge.

In mid-August 1860, in anticipation of this event, sailors from the British man-o'-war *Valorous*, which was anchored in Montreal harbour as part of the royal armada, rowed four of the warship's cutters up the Lachine Canal to position them for the planned crossing to Isle Dorval. That gesture was all quite public but, while the people of Lachine festooned their homes with flags and bunting and others hastily erected and decorated with ribbon and greenery no less than eight or nine triumphal arches on the road through Lachine leading past the town brewery, the Ottawa Hotel and Hudson's Bay House, George Simpson met quietly with his voyageur foreman from Caughnawaga with whom he had travelled so many days and so many miles over forty years in the trade. He was about to provide a very different and distinctively Canadian welcome.

August 29, the day of the big event, dawned rainy but the colours of the flags and the bunting were radiant against the dusty greens of late summer trees and the golden checkerboard of maturing corn and grain crops in orderly fields on the south shore of the river. From the main wharf next to the HBC warehouse at Lachine, well-wishers who gathered early to salute the Prince could see, through copses of mature trees across a half mile of open water, glimpses of ornate verge boards, chimneys and the louvered bay windows of Simpson's summer house. Had they looked closely, they might have seen the movement of flags and a number of people with red and white vessels, jostling just out of sight on the downstream end of the island.

By midmorning, the sky had cleared, the roads had dried and the cicadas were once again singing the sounds of summer on the verdant

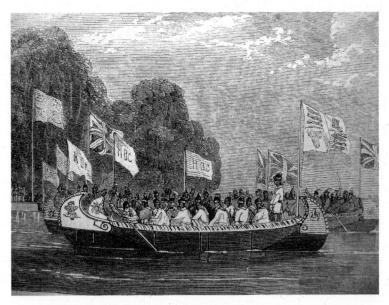

The pageant for Edward, the Prince of Wales, was a grand event that some thought may have precipitated the death of George Simpson.

shores of the St. Lawrence. Into this, with townsfolk cheering every inch of the nine-mile way between downtown Montreal and Lachine, drove the carriages of the Prince of Wales and his entourage, expecting a little cutter ride across the open water and a private reception at the home of the HBC governor.

No sooner had the Prince taken his seat in the royal cutter and the navy hands taken to the oars than out from behind Isle Dorval came a blaze of colour and sound. Ten thirty-five-foot *canots du maître*, each manned by ten or more Mohawk voyageurs with paddles flashing in unison at sixty strokes per minute, and with Union Jacks flying astern and HBC flags on pitch poles lashed into mast steps toward the front of each boat, surged around the corner. The paddlers wore new red flannel shirts and blue breeches. On their heads were blue and red hats festooned with feathers. The canoes were freshly painted a vivid red along the waterline with white detail under HBC insignias on prow and stern.

No sooner had they come into view than they were paddling abreast, ten magnificent big canoes in a line across, bearing down on the Prince's cutter, the voyageurs harmonizing at the top of their lungs to the rhythm of their strokes. The pageantry was all Simpson.

Approaching the Prince's cutter, still at speed, the line parted in the middle as if to let it pass. Instead, with the manoeuvrability of energetic paddlers glad to be pleasing their governor but even more delighted to be driving their craft without the usual five tons of freight, all ten canoes spun effortlessly, five on each side, and finished up in formation, with the Prince in the middle, then escorted the "royal barge" up to the dock at Isle Dorval. Meeting the wide-eyed and smiling young prince on the dock, elegantly attired and pulling himself up to his full five-foot-seven-inch height, was Sir George. "Welcome, your Highness, to my humble home," he said, as the riot of canoemen drifted back from the dock and the band of the Royal Canadian Rifles struck up a tune on the lawn.

Because this was a private function, no one was really sure in retrospect who was at the luncheon table that day. It was known that on one side of the host, General Williams, was the Prince and on the other was Governor Simpson. A best guess by a reporter from the Montreal *Morning Herald* put the guest list at about forty, including a generous sampling of the who's who of Montreal: the duke of Newcastle, Lord Lyons, the marquis of Chandos, the earl of Mulgrave (who, with the earl of Caledon, had accompanied Simpson to Red River), Lord Hinchinbrook, the bishop of Montreal, the bishop of Rupert's Land, General Bruce, Mr. Englehart, the Prince's equerry, Major Teasdale, the Hon. John Rose, Sir Allan MacNab, Sir E. Taché, Colonel Bradford, Colonel Rollo, Admiral Milne and a generous smattering of Royal Navy captains from the ships anchored down below. The *Herald* reporter added that "no ladies were invited, nor were any present, except three immediately connected with Sir George Simpson, viz, Mrs. [Frances Anne] Hopkins [the painter and second wife of Simpson's secretary, Edward Hopkins], and her sister Miss Beechey, and Mrs. McKenzie

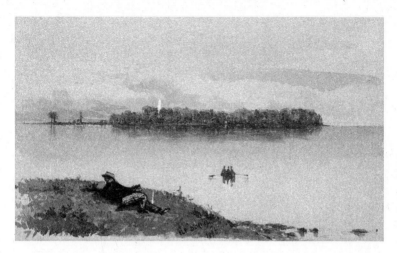

It was on Isle Dorval that Montreal politicians entertained the Prince of Wales just prior to Simpson's death in 1860. All that is left now among trees and cottages on smaller lots on the island is the well and foundation of this once grand country estate.

[wife of the HBC officer at Lachine who had taken over for Duncan Finlayson on his retirement a year or so earlier]."[11]

After lunch, the guests strolled along the herbaceous borders of the sumptuous English gardens Simpson had had constructed, while the band played quietly on the lawn. Later on in the afternoon, the Prince, who had been quite smitten with the canoe pageant—and had been reminded of it as the ten canoes and hundred-plus paddlers circled the island throughout the meal singing voyageur songs—requested that he might join the canoemen for the return journey. Forthwith, the HBC ensign on one canoe was replaced with the royal standard and, with similar formation paddling, the canoes made their way back to cheering crowds on the dock at Lachine, but not before taking a trip across two miles of open water to the south shore, where the paddlers' wives and families in the Mohawk village of Caughnawaga (today's Kahnawake) got a glimpse of their men escorting British royalty.

The event was a smashing success, with one small glitch. When they returned to Lachine, to Simpson's and the paddlers' utter horror, the last image the Prince had of the noble Mohawks, from the bow of the steamship *Kingston* before he rode through the Lachine rapids for a sunset pass under the Victoria Bridge, was described in an account of the event published in *The Illustrated London News*: "The Prince very kindly took his stand at the bow of the boat, thus giving the people assembled a capital opportunity of seeing him. Some amusement was caused by a stalwart red-man who appeared to have been drinking freely of whisky. He loudly proclaimed his intention of looking up on the face of his 'Great Father,' and, when he did get a sight of the little Prince, set up three or four lusty cheers upon his own account, waved his hat in the air and declared that he could now die in peace."[12]

The pageant was Simpson's last. After the canoe reception on Wednesday, he had three days to bask in the reflected glory and adulation of all concerned for having orchestrated the event. Friday's paper, which carried more details of the canoe reception, summed up coverage by saying, "We are enabled to state that the Prince and all who had the good fortune to be with him, entirely enjoyed the whole affair; which, from its peculiarities and successful management, will probably make a more lasting impression on His Royal Highness than anything else that has been, or will be, done to entertain him in this country. We consider the Hudson's Bay Company are entitled to the thanks of the Canadian public, for their liberality and spirit in getting up this unique excursion, which, besides gratifying our royal visitor, afforded a most agreeable holiday to several thousand persons, who were enabled to witness the scene from the shores of the noble St. Lawrence."[13] On Saturday, making his way back by carriage from yet another midday reception in Montreal, Simpson had another massive stroke. Six days later he was dead.

It fell to his long-time secretary, Edward Hopkins, to inform the London Committee:

Hudson's Bay House
Lachine 7 September 1860
Thomas Fraser Esquire
Secretary
Hon: Hudson's Bay company

Sir,

It is my mournful duty to have to report, for the information of the Governor & Committee, the death of our late respected Governor, Sir George Simpson. He experienced a severe attack of apoplexy on Saturday last, the 1st inst: and after six days of severe suffering, terminated his active and useful existence at half past ten o'clock this morning. I will not presume to dwell on my personal feelings at this sudden close of one and twenty years close official intercourse and personal friendship, nor on the deep distress this sad calamity has brought upon Sir George's family. Those feelings, I am assured, will be shared by the Board and by every member of the service over which our deceased Governor had so long and ably presided.—

During the earlier and later stages of his illness, Sir George Simpson was calm and collected and made all such arrangements as he deemed necessary in reference to the Company's and his own affairs. He particularly requested me to communicate to the Board that the charge of this establishment devolved upon me,—a charge which with the experience of nearly twenty years I trust to be enabled to conduct to the satisfaction of the Governor & Committee. Chief Factor H. McKenzie had been previously appointed to the charge of the Ottawa River business and was to have taken his departure for Fort William (Lac des Allumettes) yesterday, but, considerately, delayed leaving Lachine in order to attend upon Sir George during his illness. As Sir George's family are still here, we have, on consultation, so far ventured to deviate from the arrangements he had made, as to defer Mr. McKenzie's departure from hence until we are apprised of the pleasure of the Board in the matter, and learn from the Executors their wishes in reference to the family of the deceased. In so doing, we believe we have anticipated the desire of the Governor & Committee to consult the comfort and convenience of the family.—

You will excuse me for not entering on other topics in this letter, but I shall address you on the business of this establishment by next mail.

I may mention that I have lost no time in communicating the foregoing sad intelligence to Chief Factor W^m. Mactavish.

> I am
> Sir
> Your obedient Servant
> Edwd M. Hopkins[14]

Two weeks less a day after there had been such pomp and colour in and around Isle Dorval, George Simpson was buried in Mount Royal Cemetery beside his wife, in a ceremony befitting a king. A description in the Montreal evening newspaper gave a fulsome picture of the event:

The Funeral of Sir George Simpson.— In accordance with the arrangements we formerly announced, the last remains of the deceased Governor were brought by special train from the Hudson's Bay House at Lachine, to the terminus in Montreal yesterday afternoon. The body was accompanied by the relatives of the deceased, and friends of the family, and a goodly number of residents of Lachine. The Caughnawaga Indians escorted the melancholy cortege from the House to the landing where the train was in waiting; and as the coffin was placed in the car appropriated for its reception, the red men and their squaws sung a wild, and doleful but solemn dirge, in commemoration of the departure of "the great chief" above the sky, of one of their best friends. This tribute of regard and respect from the Indians was much felt; and though few could understand the burden of the chant they so piteously wailed forth—there was scarcely a dry

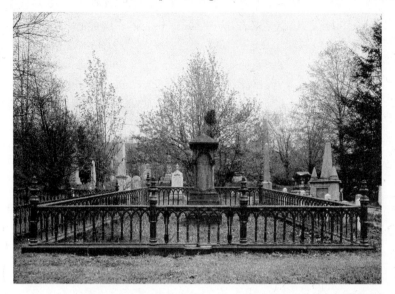

Simpson's original grave (since replaced) in Mount Royal Cemetery, Montreal, was a grand structure with iron fence and handsome stone that eventually disintegrated for want of upkeep.

eye among the assembled mourners. The Reverend John Flanagan, of Lachine, for many years the spiritual adviser and warm and attached friend of the deceased, in full canonicals, accompanied the mourners. At the Bonaventure Street Station several hundreds of our citizens were in attendance to receive the remains, and accompany them to the English Cathedral, where the funeral rites were to be performed. The pallbearers were Hon. G. Moffatt, Mr. T.B. Anderson, Mr. J. Miles, Mr. D. Davidson, Mr. J.B. Greenshields, and Mr. Hugh Taylor. The chief mourners were Mr. G.W. Simpson, nephew of the deceased; Mr. Cameron, of Toronto, his son-in-law; Mr. Hector M'Kenzie, of the Hudson's Bay Co.; Mr. Hopkins, Sir George's Secretary; and Mr. Clouston, H.B.C. Upwards of twenty carriages were in attendance— among others, those of the Cabinet Ministers, and that of General Sir W.F. Williams, Bart. His Lordship the [Anglican] Bishop also had his carriage in attendance. Arrived at the Cathedral the procession halted;

and the body having been removed from the hearse it was met at the
door by the venerable Dean [Bethune], and Mr. Flanagan. The latter
read the introductory sentences, commencing, "I am the Resurrection
and the Life saith the Lord;" which was followed immediately by the
solemn tones of the organ pealing forth Handel's Dead March—the
most magnificent requiem mortal ever composed, if, indeed, the great
sacred musician was not like the singer of old, inspired from on high
to make his great effort perfection. . . . The remainder of the beautiful
service of the Church of England for the burial of the dead was read
most impressively by the Dean; and the responses were given by the
congregation with an earnestness and distinctness which seemed
to prove that out of the fullness of the heart the mouths spoke. At
the conclusion of the service, the Organ again pealed forth its wail
of regret for the departed—the body was borne from the Church
and replaced in the hearse, which, followed by carriages bearing the
mourners, proceeded to Mount Royal Cemetery, where the deceased
was laid in the family vault. Requiescat in pace![15]

News of the Governor's passing travelled like quicksilver over the
moccasin telegraph as well as through the more conventional communication channels of the trade. It was fitting, perhaps, that the most apt
characterization of this seismic event in the history of the trade would
be in a letter[16] written by Chief Factor Dugald MacTavish, the nephew
of Simpson's only true friend in the trade, John George McTavish. He
wrote: "The Little Emperor's light has gone out."

AFTERWORD

The broad constellation of Sir George Simpson's toponymy—brooks, bays, lakes, capes, channels, streams, straits, villages, mountains, municipalities and, of course, Simpson Pass, west of Banff, Alberta—speaks to the man's geographic reach in North America, but his influence, particularly in Canada, went well beyond that. The very notion of a nation from sea to sea, linked by rivers flowing east to west, was one that George Simpson brought to life in the emerging public consciousness of nineteenth-century Canada. He was among those who pushed to expand the Hudson's Bay Company's operation westward over the Rockies, beyond the catchments of rivers flowing into Hudson Bay. But Simpson was almost alone in making sure that those lands in Columbia and New Caledonia were kept in British hands. As de facto agent for Westminster, Simpson negotiated effectively and strategically with the Russians and, through his various schemes—from "scorched earth" overtrapping policies in Columbia to strategic siting of company forts and skillful negotiation with politicians in Washington—he effectively countered the "fifty-four-forty or fight" campaign and carved out an empire separate and distinct from the United States of America.

Possessory rights were not settled between the American government and the HBC until a decade after Simpson's death, and land dealings with the Russians dragged on for years as well, but from 1820 onward one of the unsung champions of the idea of a cohesive cultural and economic whole from Atlantic to Pacific, divided from America in the west by the forty-ninth parallel, had to be George Simpson. And in many respects, Simpson's negotiations with the Russians and the Americans, as chief agent of the HBC in North America, became an exemplar for processes that confederated the provinces and that led, finally, to the sale, for £300,000, of Rupert's Land and the North-Western Territory of the HBC to the Government of Canada in 1870. As surely as these events took place, George Simpson should be counted among Canada's founding fathers.

To appreciate the Governor's legacy fully, one must also consider the darker consequences of his actions with regard to Aboriginal peoples. Simpson became well aware early on, through first-hand experience in the trade, that the HBC absolutely required the participation of the First Nations in the process. Entering the trade when he did, after nearly three decades of "war" between the North West Company and the HBC, he witnessed the effects of flagrant use of alcohol as an incentive for Indians to trade with one side or the other and the catastrophic effects on motivation for First Nations participants in the trade who learned very quickly to play one company against the other in order to realize maximum credit for the minimum number of furs delivered. At Fort Wedderburn and elsewhere in his travels early on in his career, Simpson had also seen the pernicious effects of dependence on Aboriginal peoples—shifts in expectations and diet, the possibility of disease that came with moving into a European-partnered trade economy from generations of self-sustaining, inter-tribal trade and reliance on a land-based economy. Because Simpson headed the HBC in North America through the heyday of its successes in the nineteenth century, there are historians prepared to place responsibility for this dependency on Simpson. For example, historian Robert Bone writes,

The fur trade dictated the nature of relations between Natives and Euro-Canadians. As the fur trade evolved, so did this relationship. At first each party needed the services of the other, they were more or less equal. With time, however, Indians became more and more dependent on the fur economy. With the industry's decline their dependency shifted to the federal and provincial governments . . . While his main objective was to increase the profits of the company, Simpson realized that such profits could only be achieved if the Indian way of life also prospered. He supported the concept of sup-plying Indians with food when country food—fish and game—was in short supply. Such a policy led the Indians into an ever-increasing and now systematized state of dependency . . . Not surprisingly, the economic dependency so effectively mastered by the Hudson's Bay Company under George Simpson was "inherited" by the Canadian Government.[1]

At the level of everyday interaction with the First Nations, George Simpson was, by all accounts, known and respected—loved, even—for his ability to listen, for his respect for Aboriginal people as operatives in the trade and for his sense of fair play. One need look no farther than his relationship with the Métis of Red River to see that he seemed to have more patience, more understanding and, as a consequence, much more currency with North Americans of Aboriginal and mixed blood. For their part, the Indians and Métis seemed moved by his oratory and by his response to their concerns as voiced at the many powwows and meetings he convened or conducted from one side of his domain to the other. Indeed, George Simpson had what appears in the historical record as a respect for Aboriginal people as business operatives. Simpson the Scottish pragmatist, Simpson the businessman did what he needed to do, said what he needed to say, traded as he needed to trade to keep the First Nations on side: this was just good business strategy. But despite the adulation that flowed back his way—Mohawk participation in his funeral is perhaps the most meaningful example of this—Simpson never

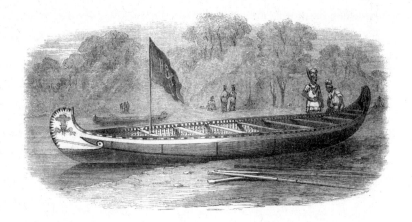

J.H. Pelly's successor in London as governor of the HBC, H.H. Berens, at Simpson's urging, directed that the canoe used by the Prince of Wales should be sent back to England as a gift to Queen Victoria, "a memento of the Prince's visit to her North American dominions."

considered non-whites anything like persons of equal standing. We must recall an early letter to his mentor, Andrew Colvile, from whom he had absorbed many of these racist attitudes, saying that "an enlightened Indian is good for nothing."[2]

Yet Simpson's unique political legacy cannot be denied. Had not a leader of his ilk come forward after the NWC-HBC amalgamation, the new concern may well have foundered in any one of the possible storms that raged during his career. There was the variable market for fur; there was the shift from beaver to other types of felt and fibre when large areas of Rupert's Land were trapped out; there were the wide-ranging problems with settlement and the internal challenges to the HBC's monopoly; there was the almost constant wrangling with other newcomers to the continent, such as the Russians and the Americans, as they sought to control what had up until that point been First Nations territory; there was the complex matter of dealing with the Aboriginal trappers, who procured the pelts in the first place; there was the matter of lethargy in a disgruntled workforce spread out in 110 little posts across an inhospitable land; there was the problem of transportation; there was the constant hemorrhage of waste and graft in a company system with absentee overseers—Simpson took all of these challenges in his stride and managed them with aplomb. And although the directors of the HBC did not move with the times into the age of steam, by investing in canals and railways, nor did they take advantage, after 1871, of leases on western land rich in resources of petroleum, the fuel of the second Industrial Revolution, Simpson did what he could to show them by example in the 1850s that there was money to be made in this kind of forward-thinking entrepreneurship.

Sir George Simpson certainly shaped Canadians' imaginative idea of their country. His sponsorship of Peter Warren Dease, Thomas Simpson and John Rae[3] was conflicted, but it resulted in the completion of the upper coastline on the map of North America, leaving those who came later to look north, instead of south, east or west, for glimmers of some historical essence of who we are. As a patron of the arts, George Simpson was directly responsible for advancing the work of two paint-ers—Paul Kane and Frances Anne Hopkins—who might otherwise not have travelled as they did throughout Canada, recording life on the land and rivers *a mari usque ad mare* during the denouement of the fur trade. Kane's paintings of Indian villages across the west and Hopkins's paint-ings of voyageurs and big bark canoes are defining Canadian images that are part of the canon of romantic works on which some significant part of the Canadian national identity was—perhaps still is—constructed.

And, of course, Canadians' continuing interest in canoe pageantry and their preoccupation with canoe iconography in advertising and popular culture can also be traced back to George Simpson, who, though one of his first decisions on the job was to replace canoes with the more efficient York boats on the major fur-trade routes, kept the bark canoe, dressed up with flashy voyageurs, piper and outrageous travel schedule, as his own unique image of New World corporate governance.

Whatever we may think of Sir George Simpson, his place in Canadian history is secure.

AUTHOR'S NOTE

My original impulse to explore more fully the life and times of Sir George Simpson had something to do with the fact that he holds, to this day, the record for the longest North American canoe trip ever completed in a single season—from Lachine to York Factory and thence from York Factory to the mouth of the Columbia River on the Pacific Ocean in the present-day state of Washington. This was no mean feat for a man who never picked up a paddle except to awaken or discipline his voyageurs. But beyond that remarkable achievement, as I have made my way around Canada by canoe over the last forty years, crossing the Governor's trail two or three times a season, I have come across more features with Simpson's name attached to them than are named for any other person. In fact, the Canadian Geographical Names Database lists 92 geographic features named Simpson, in contrast to Dease (19), McTavish (22), Rae (33), Cartier (35), Franklin (50), even Hudson (80)—most of those 92 are directly attributable to the peregrinations and achievements of Sir George.

I had also read Grant MacEwan's book *Fifty Mighty Men*, and had seen the claim that Simpson sired upward of seventy children between Montreal and the Pacific—hence earning him the ribald if apt title

"Father of the Fur Trade." And, like any semi-serious student of the history of that trade over the years, I had read and heard stories of Sir George—his legendary toughness; his skinny-dips in the darkness after four hours of sleep; his temper; his flair for pageantry, fancy clothes and beaver hats; his surprise entrances to trading posts with voyageurs in full regalia paddling in unison to the skirl of Colin Fraser's pipes. Since I was old enough to comprehend as a first-generation Canadian, sometime around Mrs. Barber's grade four class at Edward Johnson Public School in Guelph, Ontario, that this country has a history carved into the wilderness, Simpson has lived in my imagination as a larger-than-life character.

But history, in the main, has not been kind to George Simpson— probably for good reason. As Peter C. Newman wrote in *Caesars of the Wilderness*, "He was a bastard by birth and by persuasion."[1] Perhaps his anonymity in his home town of Dingwall, his omission from the list of famous people buried in Mount Royal Cemetery or his lack of inclusion in the long list of supporting Fathers of Confederation is in some strange way retribution for the shortcomings of his four decades of toil for the HBC in North America. Perhaps nowhere is there a more telling comment on Sir George's just deserts than in the inner sanctum of the Hudson's Bay Company Archives in Winnipeg.

The records are housed in a giant, climate-controlled, fireproofed cement vault built into and over the raked floor and stage of a retrofitted vintage theatre just north of the Manitoba legislative building in downtown Winnipeg. Typically, a researcher never gets beyond the reading room, which is absolutely fine because there is no nicer place to be when the afternoon sun streams in across Memorial Provincial Park through the massive west windows. Every hour on the hour, the reassuring ticking of the "Elsworth, London" grandfather clock toward the south end of the long, quiet space is punctuated by a crisp musical chime that, in its own way, like everything in the place, draws one gently, irrepressibly back in time. After registering, a researcher hunts through the finding aids, submits to the desk a written request for materials, noting title, cataloguing details and carrel number, and waits. In due course, depending on how busy the librarians are, requested items are retrieved from the vault by a staff member and hand-delivered to each work station.

One of my visits to the HBC Archives, in April 2004, happened to coincide with the tenth anniversary of the Hudson's Bay Company's gifting of this entire collection to the Province of Manitoba through the Hudson's Bay Company History Foundation. I attended the reception and, as part of that event, participated in a tour of the inner sanctum—the vault. We passed through the door that, to this point, I had associated only with the appearance and disappearance of neat librarians and small-wheeled trolleys. Down a hall and a set of stairs, through locked and air-sealed doors, all the while being watched by security cameras, we made our way. Finally, in a smallish sterile room that had the feel of an observation room or execution chamber—there were windows with closed blinds on just one side of the room—the guide explained the damaging effect of light, any kind of light, on artifacts, especially paper. "But," she continued, "to give you an idea of what's in the vault, we've reconstructed a diorama of Sir George Simpson's office, which I'll show you as soon as I flip the lights on and open the blinds."

The lights went on, the blinds opened and I couldn't contain my laughter. They had certainly recreated an office with Simpson's desk and chair, carved, as I recall, with *Alis nutrior* and Napoleon's falcon volant getting ready to fly the coop. There was a bookshelf of leather-bound post journals. Over there, in Simpson's own hand, was the famous Character Book, not far from the burnished brass and wood of the Albany packet box. And in the middle of all this was a cardboard cut-out of the man himself, a blow-up of the portrait by Stephen Pearce, standing beside the desk. But instead of having the likeness made life-sized, someone—an archivist with a wicked sense of humour—had reproduced it at only about three-quarter scale, making the Governor seem even smaller than he was in real life. No one else seemed to get the joke.

Throughout three years of intensive research and writing on this project, I'll have to admit that some days I was not a fan of Sir George, especially when it came to his treatment of women and his underlings, and particularly of his cousin Thomas. The more I learned about his exploits, the more enmity I seemed to harbour for the man. But it was in this same reading room that something of an epiphany occurred in this regard, an event that became a turning point in my research.

Typically, when a request is made for a particular old or valuable record, the trolley brings microfilm, which a researcher must then load into a reader and attempt to decipher as white writing on a black background. Reading microfilm is an acquired skill (and likely the reason why anyone who spends any time in such places wears glasses), and it is an effective way to make the materials available for wide distribution to as many researchers as possible around the world. But while one can get factual content and certain types of contextual information from microfilm, there is no direct connection between the writer and the reader of the material.

I had spent a great deal of time learning about Sir George from microfilm and had captured the best of this either by transcribing directly or, on occasion, by having copies made of relevant pages to take home with me to Ontario to have on hand for the actual writing process. But the more I stood in places across Canada where I knew Sir George had stood, and the more I pored over his journals and ledgers and correspondence, the more I hungered for a more direct, more intimate connection with the man himself. The microfilm, useful as it was, was still proxy to the real thing. I had seen his desk. I had laughed at his little likeness. I had cursed his insensitivity. I had marvelled at his expansive grasp of a vast amount of information that ebbed and flowed from an empire ten times the size of the Holy Roman Empire, about one-twelfth of the earth's land surface. I was learning the facts and the nuances that arise from comparison of the facts and from reading between the lines. But I needed more. I needed his actual handwriting. So, for the next request, instead of placing it in the appropriate receptacle on the main desk in the reading room, I handed it directly to the librarian, with a request to see the real thing. "Why?" she asked. "I'd like to touch something he touched. I'd like to behold the man himself through his writing." And from that moment on, the trolley brought white gloves, a Plexiglas book stand and leather-bound pages that felt and smelled every bit as good as their contents tasted. Simple as it may sound, seeing Simpson's writing brought to me the first tangible connection to the man behind the reputation.

It was impossible not to be moved by the fact that that one signature held sway for forty years over more people, with bigger budgets, more moving parts, more international connections, more overall complexity, than anything any of the other governors in British North America ever had to deal with—in a domain into which the Canadas could be placed, end to end, side by side, five or six times over. This was an astonishing achievement for one man.

———

Readers will notice a variety of spellings, grammar and usage in quotations from archival documents. Where necessary, I have amended the text in small ways for clarity.

ACKNOWLEDGEMENTS

Many thanks are due to my spouse, Gail Simmons, and daughters, Molly and Laurel, who know better than anyone that writing is solitary in the doing but, in the living, a gloriously collaborative if occasionally ticklish caper; and also to my long-time publisher and editor, Phyllis Bruce, friend and ally in the writing process. This book would not have happened without you.

Thanks also to my trusty nephew/travel agent/tour guide/hotelier/researcher Graham Singh in London, England; Sir William Lyon at the private office of De Beers Brack in Liverpool; John Porter at the Kendal Mountain Film Festival; Matthew Ellis and family at Glebe Croft in Lazonby; Robin Ashcroft at Rheged; Miles Davis and Deb Cooke at Knockbain Farm, overlooking Sir George's birthplace on Cromarty Firth, and Ian and Pat McLeod at the Dingwall Museum; Roddie Macpherson in Avoch; Selina Lawrie and family at Bellevue, near Beauly; Dr. David Munro, director and secretary of the Royal Scottish Geographical Society in Glasgow; Sarah Haddon at the Glen House Estate near Innerleithen; Marc Croft at the Public Records Office of Northern Ireland in Belfast; and my extended family across the UK, particularly the McPhersons and the Sugdens, for their wonderful welcome and hospitality, especially Uncle Colin McPherson for his company and connections on the road from Inverness to Orkney and countless places in between.

On this side of the Atlantic, many thanks are due to Shandé Kegan on Dorval Island; David Pelly in Ottawa; Pamela Wachna at the Market Gallery in Toronto; Dale Lahey in Guelph; Barbara Huck and Peter St. John, Matthew Lawrence and Sonya Jantz, Anne Morton and the ever-helpful staff at the HBC Archives, and Cameron White, all in Winnipeg; David Finch in Calgary; the staff of the Archives of British Columbia in Victoria. And closer to home, many thanks to Kathy Harding in suburban Inverary; Pamela Manders and staff at the Queen's University Special Collections Library; Bob Moore and Tom Caine at the Smiths Falls Railway Museum in eastern Ontario; and most especially the editorial, production and publicity staff at HarperCollins, with whom it was—and is—a joy to work. Your various contributions to this project have made all the difference.

Finally, I acknowledge the support of the Canada Council for the Arts, which last year invested $20.1 million in writing and publishing throughout Canada.

APPENDIX I

SIR GEORGE'S FAMILY TREE

Although he was likely not as fecund as historian and politician Grant MacEwan would have us believe ("70 children between Lachine and Victoria"), George Simpson was an active philanderer who—at least so far as the historic record is able to show—sired eleven (probably thirteen, and very likely more) children with at least eight women, only one of whom was his wife. Some of these children did well; others died early or did not thrive—but whatever success they did achieve had little to do with their father.

His first child, Maria Louisa Simpson, born in England in 1815, was the best looked after of all his natural children. Simpson provided a £500 dowry when she married, and when she and her first husband moved to Northumberland County in the eastern part of what is now the province of Ontario in Canada, Simpson appears to have helped them become "landed" through the purchase of property on their behalf. Simpson left Maria £100 in his final will. Thanks to the detailed genealogical work of Dale Lahey, we know that Maria Louisa produced the second-longest chain of Simpson descendants (111 in 2003), including renowned Canadian broadcaster Shelagh Rogers.

His second daughter, Isabella, appears to have been disowned by her father when she married Inverness lawyer John Cook Gordon, because Gordon was possibly mulatto. She died young, at only twenty-five, probably in childbirth. Likewise it was an early and tragic death for Simpson's other Maria, begotten with Betsy Sinclair in Rupert's Land. At only sixteen, after "Maria of Rupert's Land" had been sent to Norway

House, she met and married a young British botanist and died with him in a canoeing accident at Little Dalles Rapid on the Columbia River during their honeymoon journey to the west.

The governor's three natural sons from Rupert's Land, James Keith Simpson (b. 1823 of "Mrs. Keith"), George Stewart Simpson (b. 1827 of Peggy Taylor) and John Mackenzie Simpson (b. 1829 of Peggy Taylor), all of whom found modest success in the fur trade, were mentioned in a will Sir George drafted in 1841, prior to his journey around the world, but were absent from his final will and testament. Lahey reports a line of 76 descendants from George Stewart ("Geordie") in British Columbia and California and a thriving clan of John Mackenzie ("Johnny") Simpsonites in Manitoba, numbering 347, including the Simpson genealogist himself.

Of the remaining two natural daughters, Ann Simpson (b. 1828 of "Ann Foster") and Frances Georgina Murray (b. 1855 of Mary Labonte), and any other offspring born out of wedlock in the Caribbean before he joined the HBC and, after 1820, on the west coast, in Sitka or in Siberia or Russia (of whom, given the Governor's libidinous excesses, there must, in all probability, have been at least one or two), we as yet know nothing. They were not part of the Governor's affairs in life and were certainly not mentioned in his will.

For his first child born in wedlock, George Geddes (b. 1831), whose death Simpson appears to have genuinely grieved—in spite of having without remorse dumped Peggy Taylor and her two healthy boys before running off to England to marry his eighteen-year-old cousin Frances—Simpson seemed to have a special place in his heart. Having a "son and heir" of the right colour seemed to matter to Simpson. He remembered each of his three daughters of wedlock with a £15,000 bequest from his estate, but the remainder of his considerable fortune (see Appendix II) he left to John Henry Pelly Simpson (b. 1850), who seems to have warmed the place in the Governor's heart made cold by the untimely death of his first-born son and heir. Of his children born in wedlock, it is Margaret Mackenzie Simpson (b. 1843) who had the longest line of descendants. In 2003 they were mostly in Scotland. Christopher Ronald Ross Haddon (who moved from Scotland to Australia in 1982) is the current keeper of the silver canoe given to Sir George by the earl of Caledon in 1842.

George Simpson's descendants, according to Dale Lahey, "have distinguished themselves in the fields of the fur trade, politics, medicine, agriculture, business and industry, radio and television, and the military"[1]—a happy consequence of his liaisons with women in the UK and Rupert's Land.

SIR GEORGE'S FAMILY TREE

Rev. Thomas Simpson of Avoch
- m. Isobel Mackenzie —— William Simpson (mother died 2 days later)
- m. different Isobel Mackenzie —— George Simpson (1792–1860)

William Simpson — w. Unknown Woman — George Simpson (1792–1860)

Children of William Simpson:
- George (b. 1759)
- John (b. 1761)
- Alexander (b. 1763)
- Jean (b. 1764)
- Thomas (b. 1766)
- Mary (b. 1768)
- Roderick (b. 1770)
- Duncan (b. 1771)
- Geddes (b. 1775)

George Simpson (1792–1860):

w. Unknown British Woman 1 — Maria Louisa Simpson (1815–1891)
- m. Donald Mactavish (1796–1849) — 6 children who begat at least 111 descendants in Ontario
- m. Donald Campbell (1808–1892) — 1 child

w. Unknown British Woman 2 — Isabella Simpson (1817–1842)
- m. John Cook Gordon (1803–1853) — 2 children

w. Betsy Sinclair in Rupert's Land — Maria Simpson (1817–1838)
- m. Robert Wallace (d. 1838) — died together in canoe accident; no descendants

w. "Mrs Keith" in Rupert's Land — James Keith Simpson (1823–1901)
- m. Catherine Moignon (1831–after 1901) — 2 children

w. Ann Foster? in Rupert's Land — Ann Simpson (b. 1828) — no descendants

w. Margaret Taylor in Rupert's Land
- George Stewart Simpson (1827–1894) m. Isabella Yale (1840–1927) — 5 children who begat at least 76 descendants in British Columbia and California
- John Mackenzie Simpson (1829–1900) m. Amelia Fidler (1839–1900) — 10 children who begat at least 347 descendants in Manitoba

m. Frances Ramsay Simpson
- George Geddes Simpson (1831–1832) — 3 children
- Frances Webster Simpson (1833–1881) m. Angus Cameron (1823–1864) — 1 child, died in infancy; m. Edward F. Hodder (1836–after 1881) — no descendants
- Augusta d'Este Simpson (1841–1888) — 1 child
- Margaret Mackenzie Simpson (1843–1871) m. Alexander D. Gordon (1830–1863) — 3 children who begat at least 40 descendants in Scotland; m. James Butler-Hughes (1825–1871) — no descendants
- John Henry Pelly Simpson (1850–1898) — no descendants

w. Mary Labonte in Lachine — Frances Georgina Murray (1855–1913)

Adapted from Lahey, *Fed by Their Wings.*

APPENDIX II

INVENTORY OF ESTATE OF LATE SIR G. SIMPSON

Bank Stock, Bonds and Other Stocks and Securities

500 shares	Bank of Montreal	$100,000
200 shares	City Bank of Montreal	$16,000
55 shares	Bank of British North America	$13,383
124 shares	Commercial Bank of Canada	$12,400
270 shares	La Banque du Peuple	$13,500
164 shares	Bank of Toronto	$16,400
100 shares	Ontario Bank	$1,600
40 shares	Bank of Upper Canada	$2,000
774 shares	Montreal Telegraph Company	$30,960
40 4/10 shares	Montreal and Champlain Railroad Company	$1,332
110 shares	New City Gas Company	$4,400
600 shares	Montreal Mining Compoany	$1,800
100 shares	Michigan and Central Railroad Company	$5,000
26 1/5 shares	Richelieu Navigation Company	$2,620
2,000 shares	Huron Copper Bay Company	$900
56 1/3 old shares	Ottawa River Steamers	
56 1/3 new shares	Ottawa River Steamers (combined value)	$10,000
8 debentures or bonds	Montreal Harbour Loan	$12,166.67
17 debentures or bonds	Montreal Harbour Debentures for the deepening of Lake St. Pete	$20,000
3 debentures	Montreal and New York Railroad Company Loan, Province of Canada	$6,000
4 debentures or bonds	Signed by William Molson, Johnston Thomson and Thomas Ryan, Esquires, Trustees, headed "Province of Canada"	$4,000
10 debentures or bonds	New York Central Railroad Company Sinking Fund	$10,000
8 debentures or bonds	Consumer's Gas Company of Toronto	$8,000
6 debentures or bonds	County of Ramsay, State of Minnesota	$6,000
part interest	County of Ramsay, State of Minnesota	$250
Total value		**$298,711.67**

Executors: Duncan Finlayson, David Davidson, James Blackwood Greenshields
Signed by them in the presence of Notaries Isaac James Gibb and R. [Beanfield]
December 1860.
Source: HBCA "Sir George Simpson" Search File

NOTES

PROLOGUE

1. George Simpson, *Narrative of a Journey Round the World, During the Years 1841 and 1842*, 2 vols. (London: H. Colburn, 1847), Vol. II, 249–50, 257.
2. Robert Sahr at Oregon State University, using Consumer Price Index conversion factors to determine the value of American dollars from 1665 to 2012, estimates that a US dollar around the time of Simpson's round-the-world trip would be worth about $20.14 of today's US dollars. Using an estimate of 3.26 roubles to the dollar, consistent with the period 1840–1860, this would mean a rouble in Simpson's day would have been worth about $6.17 today.
3. Simpson, Vol. II, *Narrative of a Journey Round the World*, 258.
4. Ibid., 259.
5. Edward Hopkins married Frances Anne Beechey (later Hopkins), the famous fur trade artist.
6. Simpson, Vol. II, *Narrative of a Journey Round the World*, 261–62.
7. Ibid., 261.
8. Ibid., 286–87.
9. Ibid., 306.
10. Ibid., 306.
11. Ibid., 307.
12. Ibid., 271.
13. Ibid., 368.
14. Ibid., 393.

CHAPTER 1: DINGWALL

1. A.S. Morton, *Sir George Simpson: Overseas Governor of the Hudson's Bay Company* (Toronto: J.M. Dent, 1944); John W. Chalmers, *Fur Trade Governor: George Simpson, 1820–1860* (Edmonton: Institute of Applied Art, 1960); John S. Galbraith, *The Little Emperor: Governor Simpson of the Hudson's Bay Company* (Toronto: Macmillan, 1976). In a 2006 paper, Simpson family genealogist Dale Lahey convincingly fixes Simpson's birth date for the first time ("How Old Was Sir George Simpson? An Exercise in the Genealogical Proof Standard," *Families*, February 2006, 42–59). Using the established "genealogical proof standard," he marks Sir George's birth year as 1792. For the purposes of this book, Simpson's birth date—though still not known absolutely—will be considered 1792.

2. D.T. Lahey, *Fed by Their Wings: The Descendants of Sir George Simpson* (Guelph, ON: Datel Publishing, 2003), x. It is interesting to note that in spite of the absence of a birth record or much other evidence indicating birth out of wedlock, the otherwise very careful descendant who researched and wrote this first Simpson family genealogy reports that Sir George was "son of George Simpson and Mrs. George (Simpson)," giving the impression that the governor was conceived in a matrimonial bed. Lahey, in congruence with other writers on Simpson's early years, makes no accommodation for a natural mother in young George's life, allowing that "he was raised in a household consisting of his father, his aunts Jean and Mary, and his grandmother, Isobel Mackenzie, the relict of the Reverend Thomas Simpson of Avoch" (1).

3. Rev. Hector Bethune, "Parish of Dingwall, Presbytery of Dingwall, Synod of Ross," in *The New Statistical Account of Scotland 1845* (Edinburgh: Blackwood, 1845), 224.

4. Not including one son with his first wife, Bell, who died in childbirth in 1757, Thomas had nine children, with his second wife, Isobel. George (Sir George's father) was the oldest, born in 1759, followed by John (1761), Alexander (1763), Jean (1764), Thomas (1766), Mary (1768), Roderick (1770, who died at three months), Duncan (1771) and Geddes (1775). Which older children were living at home when Thomas died in 1786 we can only guess; the youngest two boys would still likely have been in school. We do know with reasonable certainty that the two girls in the family, Jean and Mary, were with Isobel when she moved to Dingwall.

5. Andrew Blaikie's work is of particular relevance here; see Andrew Blaikie, "Scottish Illegitimacy: Social Adjustment or Moral Economy," *Journal of Interdisciplinary History* 39 (1998): 221–41, and A. Blaikie, E. Garrett, and

R. Davies, "Migration, Living Strategies and Illegitimate Childbearing: A Comparison of Two Scottish Settlements, 1871–1881," in *Illegitimacy in Britain, 1700–1920,* ed. Alysa Levene, Thomas Nutt, and Samantha Williams (Houndmills, Hampshire, UK: Palgrave Macmillan, 2005), 141–67.

6. In point of fact, there are some who claim that MacBethad mac Findláech, also known as Macbeth, the last Celtic king of Scotland, was born in a castle near the present-day town of Dingwall. The place, in summer at least, is an unlikely setting for that play—it is not sufficiently foreboding.

7. Now a charity shop.

8. Shrove Tuesday, the day before Ash Wednesday and the beginning of Lent, has been in many cultures a time of revelry and spring celebration, marking the return of the sun in the northern hemisphere, but it is also a chance to indulge before the privations of Lent.

9. From Norman Macrae, *The Romance of a Royal Burgh: Dingwall's Story of a Thousand Years* (1923; Dingwall, Scotland: Dingwall Museum Trust, 1974), 177–79.

10. Bethune, "Parish of Dingwall," 223–24.

CHAPTER II: LONDON

1. A replica of which is currently on display at the London Maritime Museum.

2. Robert Wedderburn, *The Horrors of Slavery; exemplified in the life and history of the Rev. Robert Wedderburn . . .* (London, 1824), 4–5.

3. *Bell's Life* (London), February 29, 1824.

4. Ibid.

5. T.G. Burnard, *Mastery, Tyranny, and Desire: Thomas Thistlewood and His Slaves in the Anglo-Jamaican World* (Chapel Hill: University of North Carolina Press, 2004).

6. Lahey, *Fed by Their Wings,* 18.

7. Thomas Douglas Selkirk, *Observations on the present state of the highlands of Scotland, with a view of the causes and probable consequences of emigration* (Edinburgh, 1806).

CHAPTER III: ABOARD THE JAMES MONROE

1. Murial R. Cree, "Three Simpson Letters: 1815–1820," *The British Columbia Historical Quarterly* 1 (1937): 119.

2. As distinct from the longer, coarser guard hairs, which were of little value for felting.

CHAPTER IV: TO RUPERT'S LAND

1. Alan Seaburg, in the *Dictionary of Unitarian and Universalist Biography* (www.uua.org/uuhs/duub/index.html), a project of the Unitarian Universalist Historical Society. Seaburg draws heavily on a 1971 biography of Thomas Perkins by Carl Seaburg and Stanley Patterson, *Merchant Prince of Boston: Colonel T.H. Perkins, 1764–1854* (Cambridge, MA: Harvard University Press, 1971).

2. Nicholas Garry, *The Diary of Nicholas Garry: A Detailed Narrative of His Travels in the Northwest Territories of British North America in 1821; Originally Composed, Edited and Annotated from His Grandfather's Original MS. by Mr. Francis N.A. Garry in 1900* (1900; Toronto: Canadiana House, 1973), 25.

3. Ibid., 30–31.

4. Ibid., 39.

5. Cree, "Three Simpson Letters," 121. This is the same letter as that quoted above.

6. HBC to William Williams, February 26, 1820, Letter Book 619, HBCA [Hudson's Bay Company Archives] A/6/19/, fos. 89d–90, 162–67.

CHAPTER V: FORT WEDDERBURN

1. As quoted by Jennifer S.H. Brown in Clarke's entry in *The Dictionary of Canadian Biography*, online edition.

2. From a letter to Robert McVicar, post manager at Fort Resolution, September 26, 1820 (George Simpson, *Journal of Occurrences in the Athabasca Department by George Simpson, 1820 and 1821, and Report,* edited by E.E. Rich [Toronto: Champlain Society for the Hudson's Bay Record Society, 1938], 57).

3. Ibid., 71.

4. Ibid., 55–56.

5. The writer who coined the term "smoothing" with reference to Simpson was University of Toronto professor of history Chester Martin, who wrote the excellent introduction to Simpson's *Journal of Occurrences,* lvii.

6. Simpson, *Journal of Occurrences,* 63.

7. Ibid., 62.

8. Ibid., 66.

9. Ibid., 86–87.

10. Ibid., 101.

11. Ibid., 102.

12. The de Meuron Regiment, originally raised in Switzerland in 1781, served the Dutch East India Company until it went bankrupt in 1795, at which time various of these soldiers entered British service. Some of them ended up in Assiniboia, attempting to keep peace between the Selkirk settlers and the Métis. On occasions such as this, it was apparent that at least some of the de Meurons caused as much insurrection as they quelled.

13. Betsy's youngest brother, James, was born in 1811 and her oldest brother, William, was born in 1794, which meant that when she was with twenty-eight-year-old Simpson in 1820 she would have been no older than sixteen.

14. Simpson, *Journal of Occurrences*, 261.

15. Ibid., 290.

16. Ibid., 366.

17. Ibid., 349.

CHAPTER VI: NORTHERN GOVERNOR

1. The amalgamation of these two companies is a study in its own right, covered fully elsewhere. In skeletal form, the amalgamation agreement that was negotiated by Edward Ellice and Simon McGillivray Sr. on behalf of the North West Company with Andrew Colvile and others as representatives of the HBC London Committee presumed that both interests would find equal shares of capital needed for trade and that annual profits would be divided into one hundred shares: twenty for HBC proprietors; twenty to the NWC wintering partners and their agents; forty for personnel conducting the trade in North America; five to Lord Selkirk's heirs; five to Simon McGillivray and Edward Ellice in compensation for the loss of their London agency, which was tied to NWC trade; and ten kept in reserve. The deed poll, a separate document, was signed on the same day as the amalgamation agreement, March 26, 1821, and, similarly, would be in force for twenty-one years. The deed poll, among other things, detailed how the forty shares for personnel actually involved in the trade would be allocated. Rich's excellent history of the HBC details the deed poll's thirty-six clauses (E.E. Rich, *The History of the Hudson's Bay Company*, vol. 2, *1763–1870* [London: The Hudson's Bay Record Society, 1959], 407).

2. R. Harvey Fleming, ed., *Minutes of Council, Northern Department of Rupert Land, 1821–31* (Toronto: Champlain Society, 1940), 9–10.

3. Garry, *Diary*, 101–2.

4. Ibid., 96.

5. There appeared to be tacit agreement on both sides of the Atlantic that William Williams's time with the firm was winding down, partly because of

his advancing age, but also because of his involvement in some of the most heated arrests and controversies of the war with the NWC. However, he had been a loyal servant of the HBC, and to preserve this fact (and his dignity), the company chose to award him a salary in his new position of £1,200—20 per cent higher than Simpson's starting annual pay; and, more significant if not symbolic, the London Committee dated Williams's letter of commission one day prior to Simpson's, thereby making him, on paper at least, the senior HBC operative in North America at the time.

6. Growing public support for Adam Smith's *Wealth of Nations*, as well as for Benthamite thinking about notions of democracy, was in many respects contrary to the British government's move to strengthen and enlarge the HBC's monopoly in North America. The government knew that fighting in the fur trade was a liability, especially as it affected their Aboriginal partners, and that with the HBC representing government interests and acting as the unofficial British "agent" in British North America, granting an enlarged legal monopoly was not so much a move to support a monopoly as it was an effort to keep affairs across the Atlantic running without further embarrassment to the politicians at Westminster.

7. Letter to Andrew Colvile, in Fleming, ed., *Minutes of Council*, 390–91.

8. Ibid., 394–95.

9. Ibid., 396.

10. Ibid., 399.

CHAPTER VII: MANAGEMENT BY WALKING AROUND

1. Letter to McTavish, January 25, 1822, HBCA B239/c/1.

2. From a letter written at Fort Garry, May 20, 1822, in Morton, *Sir George Simpson*, 80–81.

3. Private letter to McTavish, June 4, 1822, at Red River Settlement, in Fleming, ed., *Minutes of Council*, 410–12.

4. Fred Stenson, *The Trade* (Vancouver: Douglas & McIntyre, 2000), 98.

5. John Tod, quoted in Morton, *Sir George Simpson*, 58–60.

6. Fleming, ed., *Minutes of Council*, 20–21.

7. Ibid., 24.

8. Ibid., 27. It is interesting to note that in addition to the major tightening of record keeping that Simpson introduced, the deed poll also made changes to accounting that facilitated assessment of business success, including the shift of year end for balancing the books for any given year from September 30 to

May 31, a change that allowed a better assessment to be made at Council time (in the summer) of how the company was doing financially.

9. Fleming, ed., *Minutes of Council*, 27.

10. Colin Robertson, *Colin Robertson's Correspondence Book, September 1817–1822*, ed. E.E. Rich (Toronto: Champlain Society, 1939), cxv.

11. It is interesting to note that Simpson was well aware that junior men in the trade could easily spend their entire annual salary purchasing goods from the company and that when this happened, their motivation to continue doing a good job declined. To avoid this he suggested, in another dispatch to the London Committee written in his first months as governor, that employees be allowed to borrow on account only up to two-thirds of their salary, the remainder being kept on account to ensure continued motivation and good behaviour.

12. Robertson, *Correspondence Book*, 387–88.

13. Ibid., 388.

14. Ibid., 388.

15. HBCA B.181/a/4.

16. Selkirk Correspondence, supposedly in a letter from Lord Selkirk to Lady Selkirk, September 8, 1836, as cited in a note in Fleming, ed., *Minutes of Council*, lxxii. The trouble with the reference is that the 4th earl of Selkirk had been dead for sixteen years by the time this letter was written. The "Lord Selkirk" reference here might be to his son, the 5th earl—but it's not clear that he had a son. He and his wife, Jean Wedderburn (Andrew Colvile's sister), had three children.

17. Simpson, letter to Andrew Colvile from York Factory, September 8, 1823, in George Simpson, *Fur Trade and Empire: George Simpson's Journal Entitled Remarks Connected with the Fur Trade in Course of a Voyage from York Factory to Fort George and Back to York Factory 1824–25, with Related Documents*, ed. Frederick Merk, rev. ed. (Cambridge, MA: Belknap, 1968), 201–2.

CHAPTER VIII: COLUMBIA

1. Simpson, *Fur Trade and Empire*, 5.

2. Ibid., 348.

3. Although Simpson quietly capitulated on this great scheme of his to use the Nelson River, the decision to try is an excellent example of his fearlessness to challenge conventional thinking. He may have learned from this bad decision to trust the knowledge of his voyageurs and Indian guides, who, in many cases, had generations of experience on the land.

4. Simpson, *Fur Trade and Empire*, 10.

5. Ibid., 12. It took Simpson until the Council of 1825 to make good on this promise, but, like an elephant, he never forgot. In the minutes of that meeting he wrote the following: "John Clarke, C.F. having contravened the 139th Resolve of Council of 1823 (directing Gentlemen in charge of Districts accompany their loaded craft inwards) by preceding his Brigade last season from York Factory to Norway House without any good cause being assigned to justify the same and a loss of pieces having been incurred by the Lesser Slave Lake Brigade which might have been avoided had the said John Clarke accompanied said Brigade it is 77. That all expenses connected with the loss in question be charged to the private account of the said John Clarke" (Fleming, ed., *Minutes of Council*, 117).

6. Simpson, *Fur Trade and Empire*, 23.

7. Although Simpson considered the river they were on at this point the upper Athabasca, it was really the Whirlpool River, a mountain tributary of the main Athabasca River.

8. This name was not given to this particular peak until 1827.

9. Simpson, *Fur Trade and Empire*, 30.

10. David Thompson found the pass after much hardship and very slim rations in late December 1810, arriving at the forks of the Canoe River and the Columbia on January 18, 1811.

11. Simpson, *Fur Trade and Empire*, 38. It's worth noting here that Simpson's movement through the Athabasca Pass and his experience with these clinker-built canoes might indeed have had an effect on the evolution of canoe design back in "Canada." The early decades of Simpson's tenure in North America were also the time when demand for recreational canoes was starting to build. At some point, in the Peterborough area, there was a design shift away from basic dugout and bark canoe construction to all-wood canoes made of strips of wood affixed to ribs—a design that was more like the clinker-built craft of the Columbia River Valley than anything anyone had seen by the 1820s east of the Rockies. On his trip through the Athabasca Pass, and based on his experience west of the Rockies, David Thompson made detailed journal notes on these all-wood canoes. Likewise, although Simpson had not Thompson's eye for technical detail, word of these unusual canoes would have travelled back with members of his party and may (although proof of this has yet to be unearthed) have played a direct role in a revolution in canoe design in eastern Canada.

12. Simpson, *Fur Trade and Empire*, 38.

13. W. Kaye Lamb, who wrote Fraser's entry in *The Dictionary of Canadian Biography*, online edition.

14. Simpson, *Fur Trade and Empire*, 39.

15. Ibid., 39.

CHAPTER IX: VICEREGAL CEO

1. Simpson, *Fur Trade and Empire*, 84–85.
2. Frederick Merk, in Simpson, *Fur Trade and Empire*, lvi.
3. In the sweeping terms of the original royal charter for the HBC, there are more rights given than duties or responsibilities assigned. Such was the legal tenor of the time. The actual clause that becomes the basis of the future expectation of stewardship of Aboriginal people reads as follows: "Do grant unto the said Governor and Company . . . shall for ever hereafter have, use, enjoy, not only the whole, entire, and only Trade and Traffick, and the whole, entire, and only Liberty, Use, and Priviledge, of Trading and Trafficking to and from the Territory . . . but also the whole and entire Trade and Traffick to and from all Havens, Bay, Creeks [etc.] . . . and to and with all the Natives and People, inhabiting, or which shall inhabit within the Territories, Limits and Places aforesaid." From the outset, however, unlike the French, the HBC sought to keep contacts between its servants and the Native peoples to an absolute minimum necessary for trade. At many posts, Indians were not even welcome in the trading room. But in practice, connections between the HBC and Aboriginal people—men as guides, women as workers and sexual partners—were an everyday and necessary part of life for the HBC.

   It became apparent, almost from the outset of the HBC's operations in North America, that these activities profoundly affected the lives of the Native peoples that were HBC trading partners, especially during the "war" with the NWC for control of the North American fur trade. But in most instances, as far as the London Committee was concerned, the less detail it heard about this matter, the better. It was only when questions about what the HBC was and should have been doing with and to Aboriginal people under the auspices of the charter arose at different times during its history, especially in conjunction with the issue of settlement and during hearings into the company's monopoly, that the expectation of care for Aboriginal people became a company-invoked lever to prop up the argument that it was taking its charter responsibilities seriously (and was therefore entitled to keep operating under the charter). There was no doubt that there were often significant gaps between the intent of the charter, as written, and the actions and intents of HBC operatives, including George Simpson, in the field. This disconnect is treated substantially in a variety of sources, including R. Douglas Francis, Richard Jones, and Donald B. Smith, eds., *Origins: Canadian History to Confederation* (Toronto: Holt, Rinehart & Winston, 1988), and, from an Aboriginal historian's point of view, in Olive Patricia Dickason, *Canada's First Nations: A History of Founding Peoples from Earliest Times* (Toronto: McClelland & Stewart, 1992).

4. These comments come from a letter to Colvile dated May 20, 1822. The letter is among the Selkirk Papers in the Canadian National Archives (Selkirk Papers 7587) and is mentioned in E.E. Rich's introduction to Simpson's Athabasca Journal (Simpson, *Journal of Occurrences*, xl).

5. Simpson, *Fur Trade and Empire*, 96.

6. Ibid., 96.

7. Ibid., 99.

8. Ibid., 101.

9. Ibid., 138.

10. Ibid., 142.

11. Ibid., 143.

12. Ibid., 144.

13. Ibid., 150.

14. Ibid., 163.

15. Simpson, *Journey Round the World*, 76–78.

CHAPTER X: A MAN ON THE GROUND

1. Charles Dickens, *Little Dorrit*, chapter 3.

2. Although existing engravings always show the handsome symmetrical four-storey building on the south side of Fenchurch Street, just east of the intersection with Gracechurch Street, with its matching twin-pillared doorways separated by an arched and wrought-iron gated courtyard entrance, as numbers 3 and 4 Fenchurch Street, detailed city maps of the time show that this facade was actually assigned numbers 3 and 5. The structure corresponding to number 4 Fenchurch Street is an expansive U-shaped building, possibly including a warehouse, surrounding a courtyard that can be accessed only through the archway in the main building.

3. The title "governor" is confusing to the extent that it was used in different instances to refer to the members of the London Committee who, in modern parlance, would be considered directors of the company. And although George Simpson was titled "northern governor" or "overseas governor," this was often truncated to simply "governor," the same honorific used to describe the head of the London Committee.

4. G. Spraakman and A. Wilkie, "The Development of Management Accounting at the Hudson's Bay Company, 1670–1820," *Accounting History* 5 (2000): 3.

5. The HBC was still in a losing financial position when Simpson entered service. In 1821, the company reported a loss of £30,000. But by the next year, Simpson was able to generate a 4 per cent dividend for shareholders. By 1825,

the dividend had risen to 10 per cent, and it reached 20 per cent in the late 1820s and as high as 25 per cent in the mid-1830s. The dividend never fell below 10 per cent for the rest of Simpson's time in office.

6. Spraakman and Wilkie, "Development of Management Accounting," 7–8.

7. Fleming, ed., *Minutes of Council*, 122.

8. This refers to a £500 bonus and a £200 raise, boosting Simpson's annual salary to £1,200 per annum.

CHAPTER XI: "THE CHIEF WHOSE DOG SINGS"

1. Why this particular tartan was chosen may have had less to do with any familial connection to the Stuarts than with its flamboyant look.

2. Peter C. Newman coined the phrase "birchbark Napoleon" in his 1987 book *Caesars of the Wilderness*, vol. 2 of *Company of Adventurers* (Markham, ON: Penguin), a phrase that, as much as any, has stuck to Simpson in public consciousness.

3. A. Colvile to Governor Simpson, March 11, 1824, in Simpson, *Fur Trade and Empire*, 206.

4. Cited in Sylvia Van Kirk's groundbreaking 1972 article "Women and the Fur Trade," *The Beaver*, Winter 1972, 13.

5. The dinner bill from a Beaver Club dinner in September 1808, at which thirty-one members and guests dined, is as follows: 32 dinners, £12; 29 bottles of madeira wine, £6; 19 bottles of port, £5; 14 bottles of porter ale, £2 6s.; 12 quarts of ale, £8; 7 suppers, £8 9s.; brandy and gin, £2 6s.; cigars, pipes and tobacco, £5; 3 wine glasses broken, £3 9s.—a princely sum for one meal at that time.

6. HBC to J. Rae, Stromness, January 17, 1827, HBCA Letter Book 658, p. 161.

7. HBC to J. Rae, Stromness, February 14, 1827, Letter Book 658, p. 167.

8. HBC to J. Rae, May 4, 1827, Letter Book 658, p. 193.

9. HBC to George Simpson Sr., May 10, 1827, Letter Book 658, p. 195.

10. September 15, 1827, HBCA B.239/c/1, fol. 332.

11. When John Henry Pelly moved up to the governor's chair in 1822, this left vacant the deputy governor's position, which was filled by Andrew Colvile, who would become chair on Pelly's death in 1852.

12. Rich, *History*, 2: 457–58.

13. Simpson genealogist Dale Lahey, while concluding that the woman is Ann Foster, admits that if the case is "judged by the minimal requirements of determining paternity outlined by Stevenson, we must conclude that the entry lacks the 'greater weight of evidence' [Stevenson, Noel, *Genealogical Evidence*

(Walnut Creek, CA: Aegean Park Press, 1989), 2–7] and reserve judgement until corroborating evidence comes to light" (*Fed by Their Wings*, 56).

14. Lahey, *Fed by Their Wings*, 55.

15. March 20, 1828, HBCA, D5/3, fos. 168–69.

16. Archibald McDonald, *Peace River: A Canoe Voyage from Hudson's Bay to Pacific by Sir George Simpson in 1828—Journal of the Late Chief Factor Archibald McDonald (Hon. Hudson's Bay Company), Who Accompanied Him*, ed. Malcolm McLeod (1872; Edmonton: M.G. Hurtig, 1971), 32.

17. McDonald, *Peace River*, 4.

18. Ibid., 18.

19. Ibid., 22.

20. Ibid., 22.

21. Colin Fraser, who added the colour and pomp to Simpson's second Columbia journey, did not work out all that well as a contributor in other ways to the expedition, as the Governor had hoped he would. On the way home, Simpson wrote to McTavish and confided that "the Piper cannot find sufficient Wind to fill his bag," and later that "Colin breaks in by degrees I rub him against the grain as frequently as worth, he is a piper and nothing but a piper" (B.239/C/1). Having come all this way to pipe for the illustrious governor, he found himself assigned to York Factory as a steward in the officers' mess, after which Simpson appears not to have travelled with him, although the record of this one memorable trip with Colin Fraser has lingered on, giving the impression that the relationship between Simpson and Fraser was much longer and stronger than it actually was.

22. McDonald, *Peace River*, xxvii–xxviii.

23. Ibid., 24.

CHAPTER XII: ITCHING TO MARRY

1. McDonald, *Peace River*, 46–47.

2. Simpson was interested in the Fraser as a navigable waterway, so he instructed the majority of his crew to travel down that river; however, he was also interested in options for travel and the movement of goods, so he, with McDonald and Hamlyn (using the horses and guide services that were part of the HBC infrastructure in the New Caledonia District), crossed from the Fraser Valley to the Thompson River on horseback and continued on the Fraser by canoe, hooking up with the main party at the confluence of the Thompson and the Fraser. Not surprisingly, Simpson arrived there nine days ahead of the group that had come directly down the Fraser, but

he is still credited with orchestrating the first European descent of this wild western Canadian river.

3. McDonald, *Peace River*, 27.

4. HBCA B.239/c/2, fos. 8–11d.

5. So named for the darker colour of their skin, the offspring of French traders and Aboriginal women who now populate the Métis nation were in the parlance of the trade referred to as *bois brûlés*, or "burnt-wood," people.

6. Alexander Simpson, *The Life and Travels of Thomas Simpson, the Arctic Discoverer* (London: Richard Bentley, 1845), 47.

7. Average life expectancy in North America in 1805 was about thirty-six years. By 1830 the situation had improved slightly, but still only about one-third of North Americans could expect to reach sixty years of age.

8. William Todd to George Simpson, 1849, HBCA D.5/25, fol. 390d.

9. George Simpson to J.G. McTavish in Campbelltown, London, December 5 and December 26, 1829, HBCA B.135/c/2.

10. Ibid.

11. George Simpson to J.G. McTavish, Bellevue, January 8, 1830, HBCA B.135/c/2.

12. George Simpson to J.G. McTavish, 73 Great Tower Street, London, January 26, 1830, HBCA B.135/c/2.

13. George Simpson to J.G. McTavish, London, February 13, 1830, HBCA B.135/c/2.

14. As cited in Van Kirk, "Women in the Fur Trade," 14.

15. HBCA George Simpson search file, transcribed from original record April 27, 1960.

16. George Simpson Sr. was the eldest of nine children born to Rev. Thomas Simpson and his second wife, Isobel Mackenzie. Besides Geddes, who was the youngest, born in 1775, the only other sibling in the wedding party could have been "W. Simpson," who might have been William Simpson, the only child of Rev. Thomas and his first wife, Bell, who died two days after William was born in 1757. Had George Sr. been present at the wedding, he most certainly would have been in the wedding party and would have signed the register as a witness to his son's marriage. That he was not there, and that communication with George Sr. regarding the procurement of a piper was done through the HBC London office, speaks to—but does not in any way authenticate—some level of estrangement between father and son.

17. HBCA D.6/4, fol. 29.

18. All quotations that follow are from Frances's journal: HBCA D.6/4, fol. 4.

19. The cook from New Grove House, who had come with them to provide sustenance to Frances and her new husband, would have had to adapt her culinary

skills to campfire and post kitchen cooking, but this was probably less of a shift from the hearths of London than one might imagine. Nevertheless, the life that went with it must have been a bit of a shock.

20. Excellent context for the roles and relationships of women in the fur trade can be found in Sylvia Van Kirk, *Many Tender Ties: Women in Fur-Trade Society, 1670–1870* (Winnipeg: Watson & Dwyer, 1980).

21. A. Simpson, *Life and Travels of Thomas Simpson*, 66.

CHAPTER XIII: DARK DAYS IN RED RIVER

1. There was probably never any doubt in Simpson's mind that the place to reside, were he to stay in North America, was Montreal, but it may have been because of the friendship with McTavish and his new wife, or to show Frances a slice of fur trade life on the frontier, that he chose to live in Red River immediately following his marriage.

2. HBCA B.135/c/2, fos. 54–54d.

3. Ibid., fol. 57.

4. Ibid., fol. 56d.

5. Ibid., fol. 58.

6. Ibid., fos. 63–63d.

7. Excerpt from William Sinclair, letter to Frances Ermatinger, August 15, 1830, A B 40 Er 62.3, Ermatinger Papers, British Columbia Provincial Archives.

8. HBCA B.135/c/2, fos. 66–67.

9. McTavish had a marriage *à la façon du pays* with another Aboriginal woman before Nancy McKenzie, and had two children with her. It was relatively common practice, when a country wife was summarily left to her own devices or "turned off" by a trader, for his children to be killed or abandoned, and this is likely what happened to McTavish's first offspring in Rupert's Land.

10. HBCA B.135/c/2, fos. 68d–69.

11. Ibid., fol. 71d.

12. Ibid., fol. 78.

13. Ibid., fol. 72.

14. Ibid., fol. 76d.

15. Ibid., fol. 88.

16. Ibid., fol. 84.

17. Ibid., fos. 84–84d.

18. McTavish wrote around this time, "I had thought of getting away in one or two outfits but I am so miserably poor that I am afraid of coming to want if adrift in the world—I have been thoughtless in money matters having hopes

of getting some windfall which would have made up matters, disappointed in this I of course must now do for the best, and all I can to economise for the future" (McTavish, letter to James Hargrave, Moose Factory, December 18, 1833, in James Hargrave, *The Hargrave Correspondence, 1821–1843*, ed. G.P. de T. Glazebrook [Toronto: Champlain Society, 1938], 124).

19. Thomas Simpson, letter to Alexander Simpson, in A. Simpson, *Life and Travels of Thomas Simpson*, 80.
20. Simpson to McTavish, HBCA B. 135/c/2, fol. 96d.
21. HBCA B. 135/c/2, fol. 86d.
22. HBCA A.12/10, fol. 64.
23. The story of Sir George's handwritten "Character Book" and how it came to be decoded was included in a digest of miscellaneous news and information under the heading of "The HBC Packet" in the June 1935 issue of *The Beaver*. For many years, the value of the Character Book was limited because Simpson had identified his subordinates by number only. However, in 1935, archivist Leveson Gower found among Sir George's papers a single sheet linking numbers with names that turned out to be the key. The book itself was finally transcribed and published as George Simpson, "The Character Book of Governor George Simpson, 1832," in *Hudson's Bay Miscellany 1670–1870*, ed. Glyndwr Williams (Winnipeg: Hudson's Bay Record Society, 1975).
24. Simpson, "Character Book," 177.
25. Ibid., 182.
26. Ibid., 169.
27. Ibid., 171–72.
28. Ibid., 175.
29. Ibid., 179–80.
30. Ibid., 171.

CHAPTER XIV: MERCHANT EMPEROR

1. This characterization of Simpson, referring to his almost superhuman capabilities for travel and supervision, was put forward in a letter written by HBC London Committee secretary Archibald Barclay, as quoted in Morton, *Sir George Simpson*, 278.
2. A. Simpson, *Life and Travels of Thomas Simpson*, 100–3.
3. Galbraith, in F.G. Halpenny, ed., *Dictionary of Canadian Biography* (Toronto: University of Toronto Press, 1966), 8: 815.
4. Derek Hayes, *Historical Atlas of Canada* (Vancouver: Douglas & McIntyre, 2002), 180.

5. William R. Swagerty, "The Leviathan of the North: American Perceptions of the Hudson's Bay Company, 1816–1846," *Oregon Historical Quarterly* 104, no. 4 (2003), http://www.historycooperative.org/journals/ohq/104.4/swagerty.html, 26.

6. Alice M. Johnson, "Simpson in Russia," *The Beaver*, Autumn 1960, Outfit 291, 7.

7. "Snapes" could have been an alcoholic beverage, possibly schnapps, or Simpson might have been more poetic in his writing. "Snape" is actually a ship-building term describing the bevel on the end of a large timber; it may be related to the British Navy term "splice the main brace," which is actually a term for a hefty tot of rum.

8. Johnson, "Simpson in Russia," 10–11.

9. Ibid., 11.

10. Ibid., 58.

11. One of the most intriguing elements of this deal was that these two companies were powerful enough to protect their peaceful joint interests in the Pacific northwest from future disagreements between their governments, including during the Crimean War of 1854–55. See also Reginald Saw, "Treaty with the Russians," *The Beaver*, December 1948, 30–33.

CHAPTER XV: GEORGE SIMPSON, MURDERER?

1. "Presentation to the Governor," *The Beaver*, June 1943, 49.

2. The candelabrum is currently in the collection of the Manitoba Museum in Winnipeg.

3. John McLean, *Notes of a Twenty-Five Years' Service in the Hudson's Bay Territory*, ed. William Stewart Wallace (Toronto: Champlain Society, 1932), 387.

4. Ibid., 333.

5. Ibid., 334.

6. This note may be found written on page xxii.

7. Simpson, "Character Book," 227–28.

8. A. Simpson, *Life and Travels of Thomas Simpson*, 52.

9. Ibid., 78.

10. Ibid., 84.

11. Ibid., 337.

12. The situation as characterized by Thomas's brother Alexander; ibid., 338.

13. A. Simpson, *Life and Travels of Thomas Simpson*, 340. Dease's father was Dr. John B. Dease, an army captain and deputy superintendent of the Canadian Indian Department, and his mother, Jane French, was of Caughnawaga (Kahnawake) Mohawk descent.

14. Beating his own remarkable record of 1,377 miles on snowshoes in 61 days, set when he snowshoed from Red River to Fort Chipewyan to meet up with Peter Warren Dease in January 1837.

15. The most unequivocal indictment of Simpson for this is by Marjory Harper, *Thomas Simpson: Dingwall's Arctic Explorer* (Dingwall Museum, Local Studies No. 2 [Dingwall, Scotland: Ross & Cromarty, n.d.], 9). It could be true, given that Thomas's letter to the Committee was written in mid-October 1839 and, even though it had to travel across the country in the winter mail packet and across the Atlantic by ship, it could have been received in London as early as February. The Committee's response was not written until June, which, given their calls for dispatch in continuing the explorations in the letter itself, is perhaps evidence of intervention to slow down their reply.

16. Harper, *Thomas Simpson*, 5.

17. A. Simpson, *Life and Travels of Thomas Simpson*, 357.

18. Alex McArthur, *A Prairie Tragedy: The Fate of Thomas Simpson* (Winnipeg: G.C. Mortimore, 1887), 11.

19. Among them, Douglas MacKay and W. Kaye Lamb, "More Light on Thomas Simpson," *The Beaver*, September 1938, 26–31; Vilhjalmur Stefansson, *Unsolved Mysteries of the Arctic* (New York: Macmillan, 1942); Harper, *Thomas Simpson*; and, as late as 1998, University of Manitoba historian J.M. Bumstead, writing in the *Winnipeg Real Estate News* ("The Strange Death of Thomas Simpson," *Winnipeg Real Estate News*, July 3, 1998, 3).

20. Harper, *Thomas Simpson*, 9.

21. Stefansson, *Unsolved Mysteries*, 182.

22. Ibid., 184.

23. Ibid., 188.

24. Harper, *Thomas Simpson*, 10.

25. What might be a naive misunderstanding about terminology could have led to the public claim by his brother that Thomas Simpson was the discoverer of the Northwest Passage. Simpson and Dease's first "discovery" was to chart, in the western Arctic, the unknown coastline between Return Reef (the limit of John Franklin's mapping) and Point Barrow (the eastern limit of known lands explored from the Pacific). Simpson and Dease went west from the mouth of the Mackenzie River and made this connection, which Thomas sometimes referred to as the "northwest passage" across the top of North America. In subsequent expeditions, they turned their attentions to the uncharted gap on the map between Turnagain Point and the Gulf of Boothia, which Simpson sometimes referred to as the "northeast passage." Within the geography of North America, making a distinction between the "northwest"

and "northeast" sections of the sea route across the top of the continent is completely understandable, and, to be sure, completing the map of the northern coast of North America was a significant achievement; however, Simpson and Dease (because Sir George thwarted his cousin's last journey, which would almost certainly have finished his mapping of unknown lands to the east of the Mackenzie River) did not make the connection in the "northeast," leaving Thomas with the claim of discovering the "northwest passage." Because, in a larger global context, the sea route across the top of North America was referred to as the "Northwest Passage," one could understand how a person, like Thomas Simpson's brother Alexander, who did not know the geography all that well could be confused about the scope of Thomas Simpson's claim.

26. Chester Martin, introduction to Simpson, *Journal of Occurrences,* lvi.

CHAPTER XVI: AROUND THE WORLD

1. McLean, *Twenty-Five Years',* 387–88.
2. The steam packet was a week to ten days faster than a conventional clipper ship in this crossing of the Atlantic, which must have pleased the Governor no end.
3. Lord Caledon's journal is held at the Public Records Office of Northern Ireland in Belfast, microfilm reference 496/1, D2433/B/8/33.
4. Ibid., D2433/B/8/33.
5. In Caledon's account it certainly sounds as if they opened a keg of rum that was *always* carried by Simpson to keep the voyageurs going, to have a toast or two with the disgruntled Indians at this location ("the nut was cracked"). Simpson's account, written years after the fact, may have been skewed for political reasons to give the impression that this was a dry consultation.
6. Simpson, *Round the World,* 43–44.
7. This is the first time a connection has been made between the contents of Lord Caledon's journal and the circumstances of George Simpson's connection to the Métis community of Red River. It is a link that could be explored in much more detail.
8. Stefansson, *Unsolved Mysteries,* 191.
9. Caledon, journal, Public Records Office of Northern Ireland, D2433/B/8/33.
10. The silver canoe is owned by Simpson descendant Christopher Haddon, who lives in Mount Macedon, Victoria, Australia. This artifact was on loan at the Canadian Canoe Museum in Peterborough, Ontario, in 2007.
11. Chalmers, *Fur Trade Governor,* 130.

12. Simpson renamed this lake "Peeche" after his guide on this first crossing.

13. The piece of the tree with Simpson's initials on it is now in the Whyte Museum of the Canadian Rockies in Banff, Alberta. It was not until one hundred years later that Simpson's first crossing of this pass was recognized with the placing of a historical monument. In an article about this event in *Saturday Night* magazine, author Charlotte Gordon was rhapsodic in her celebration of the governor as almost a founding father of Canada: "The recognition of Sir George Simpson is not only of national but of international significance in that his broad kingdom was of such regal extent. That a memorial to him should be in an Alpine setting, by deep-hearted rivers, with snow-crested domes as a background, is fitting for this energetic governor, who with broad vision helped to make firm the foundations of our Dominion" ("Memorial to Sir George Simpson: Famous Hudson's Bay Company Governor of a Century Ago to Be Honored," *Toronto Saturday Night,* August 18, 1928, 4–5).

14. Galbraith, *The Little Emperor,* 77.

15. Simpson, "Character Book," entry No. 10, 176.

16. Galbraith, *The Little Emperor,* 77.

17. In due course, Simpson dispatched James Douglas to site and built this installation at the present-day harbour and town of Victoria on the southern tip of Vancouver Island, strategically below the forty-ninth parallel. The presence of this post was sufficient, when the Oregon Treaty was finally signed and extended the border to the coast along the forty-ninth parallel, to allow the whole of Vancouver Island to remain in British hands. James Douglas took up this post and, in doing so, became a founding father of the province of British Columbia.

18. Simpson, *Round the World,* 167.

19. James McCook, "Sir George Simpson in the Hawaiian Islands," *The Beaver,* Winter 1976, 48.

20. HBCA D.6/1, fos. 24–25.

21. HBCA D.4/60, fol. 131.

22. John McLoughlin, *The Letters of John McLoughlin from Fort Vancouver to the Governor and Committee . . . 1825–39,* ed. E.E. Rich (Toronto, 1841–44), 166.

23. Ibid., 171. It is also important to mention that however ruthless Simpson was in dealing with McLoughlin's charges against him with respect to John Jr. and William Rae, when McLoughlin finally retired, after three years of trying to clear his son's name, Simpson supported the Committee in awarding him a very generous pension.

24. Simpson, *Round the World,* 72.

25. Written and edited by a cast including Edward Hopkins, HBC secretary Archibald Barclay and Simpson's hand-picked scribe in Red River, Adam Thom; and published by Henry Colburn in London and Lea and Blanchard in the United States.

26. Charles R. Dod, *The Peerage, Baronetage, and Knightage of Great Britain and Ireland for 1854* (London: Whittaker and Co., 1854), 478.

CHAPTER XVII: Presiding at Lachine

1. On the survey attached to the deed of sale when Chief Factor James Keith purchased this property from its original owner, William Gordon, this street is referred to simply as Road to Montreal.

2. Clifford P. Wilson, "Sir George Simpson at Lachine," *The Beaver*, June 1934, 39.

3. "Fed by their wings" was used for the title of Simpson descendant Dale Lahey's book. This last translation may be found in Baron Modar Neznanich's compilation at www.byzantios.net/modar/motto.htm.

4. Galbraith, *The Little Emperor,* 175. Simpson was not beyond straight-ahead bribes, as evidenced by a gift of "10,000 golden reasons" offered to cabinet member Francis Hincks for his help in obtaining government contracts for a shipping line for which the Governor was a director and major investor.

5. One of the American claims that justified this action was that the HBC was a "Colonial Government" and not a trading company.

6. Simpson thought that with the right British forces in place, it would be possible to fight locally with the Americans only in the west, to settle the border issue. Historians, given the history of conflict between the Americans and the British from the Revolutionary War to the War of 1812 and the various skirmishes in between, agree that the view that this war would not involve forces right across North America was highly simplistic.

7. Rich, *History,* 2: 740.

8. Archibald Barclay to George Simpson, January 3, 1844.

9. HBCA D.5/15, fos. 590–91.

10. Alice M. Johnson, "Edward and Frances Hopkins of Montreal," *The Beaver,* Autumn 1971, Outfit 302(2), 4.

11. Chief Factor John Stuart, letter to Donald Smith, in Galbraith's article "The Little Emperor," *The Beaver,* Winter 1960, Outfit 291, Vol. 40(3), 22.

12. John Henry Lefroy to Lieutenant C. Younghusband, April 25, 1843, in John Henry Lefroy, *In Search of the Magnetic North: A Soldier-Surveyor's Letter from the North-West, 1843–1844,* ed. George F.G. Stanley (Toronto: Macmillan, 1955), 6.

13. Quoted in Margaret Arnett Macleod, introduction to Letitia Hargrave, *Letters of Letitia Hargrave*, ed. Margaret Arnett Macleod (Toronto: Champlain Society, 1947), xciv.
14. W.L. Morton, "Donald A. Smith and Governor George Simpson," *The Beaver*, Autumn 1978, 4.
15. Ibid., 7.
16. George Simpson to Donald Smith, as cited in Morton, "Donald A. Smith," 7.
17. George Simpson to John McLean, June 22, 1843. In McLean, *Notes of a Twenty-Five Years' Service*, 307.

CHAPTER XVIII: DENOUEMENT

1. HBCA D4/73/146d.
2. Henry John Moberly, with William Bleadsdell Cameron, *When Fur Was King* (Toronto: J.M. Dent, 1929), 5–6.
3. Ibid., 12.
4. Ibid., 8.
5. Ibid., 15–17.
6. Frank E. Ross, "Sir George Simpson and the Department of State," *British Columbia Historical Quarterly* 2, no.2 (1938): 132.
7. Although it has never been proven with any particularly compelling evidence, a number of historians suspect that Sir George may have sired a second child with Mary Labonte, sometime between the birth of Frances Georgina Murray in 1855 and Simpson's death in 1860. The birth would have fit the libidinous pattern he had established throughout his working life.
8. Sir George to Angus Cameron, December 1955, in Lahey, *Fed by Their Wings*, 78.
9. *Canadian News* (London), October 15, 1856, in Galbraith, *The Little Emperor*, 194.
10. From the preface of Great Britain, Parliament, *Report from the Select Committee on the State of British Possessions in North America which are under the Administration of the Hudson's Bay Company with Minutes of Evidence Appendix and Index* (London: British Parliamentary Papers, 1857), iii.
11. Simpson's testimony began with the 702nd question asked by the select committee and continued until they finished at question number 2,125. These numbers are used to mark position in the transcript.
12. Great Britain, *Report from the Select Committee*, 50.
13. Characterization by the 6th earl of Selkirk of Simpson's defence of the HBC at the select committee hearings in London, in Galbraith, *The Little Emperor*, 197.

14. Selkirk to Bryce, January 29, 1882, Bryce Papers MG14 C15, Public Archives of Manitoba.
15. Simpson to Berens, private and confidential, March 22, 1859, HBCA D4/84a.

CHAPTER XIX: THE EMPEROR'S LIGHT GOES OUT

1. Rail is categorized by weight per yard. For fifty-five-pound rail, one yard of cast iron rail, in these early days of the Grand Trunk, weighed fifty-five pounds. Modern tracks, made of rolled steel, weigh more than twice that.
2. This moniker has variously been attributed to Ellice's days as the NWC's agent in Montreal or Toronto, referring to his handling of furs, but more likely it has to do with acumen with money and securities, especially in times when stock markets were in decline.
3. James M. Colthart on Edward Ellice, *Dictionary of Canadian Biography*, online edition.
4. Grace Lee Nute, "Simpson as Banker," *The Beaver*, Outfit 286, Spring 1956, 51–52.
5. "Steamboats on the Red River 1859–1871" (Institute for Regional Studies, North Dakota State University), www.fargo-history.com/transportation/steamboats.htm.
6. It was improbable given the changes in manufacturing and transportation technology, the rise of silk in the hat market and the vagaries of fur as a fashion accoutrement. After dividends to shareholders had risen from single digits in the early years to as high as 25 per cent in the mid-1830s, profits fell off during Simpson's reign, but he was able to maintain at least a 10 per cent annual dividend for the rest of his career with the HBC. Given changes in manufacturing and business through the mid-nineteenth century, this was a remarkable achievement.
7. Edward Bulwer-Lytton was the politician–cum–famously florid playwright and novelist who coined such phrases as "It was a dark and stormy night" and "pursuit of the almighty dollar."
8. From a letter in the Ermatinger-Tod papers in Library and Archives Canada, as quoted in Harold Innis, *The Fur Trade in Canada* (Toronto: University of Toronto Press, 1956), 321.
9. Simpson to H.H. Berens, Private and Confidential, dated Lachine, June 1, 1860, HBCA D.4/84a, fos. 57d–58.
10. Simpson to H.H. Berens, dated Lachine, July 31, 1860, HBCA D.4/84a, fos. 11–12.
11. "The Canoe Race," *The Morning Herald*, August 31, 1860.
12. *The Illustrated London News*, October 13, 1860.

13. "The Canoe Race."
14. HBCA Simpson Search File, J/16/3/29.
15. *The Evening Pilot* (Montreal), September 12, 1860.
16. As cited in Clifford P. Wilson, "The Emperor's Last Days," *The Beaver*, December 1934, 51.

AFTERWORD

1. Robert M. Bone, *The Geography of the Canadian North* (Toronto: Oxford University Press, 1992), 45, 52.
2. Simpson to Colvile, September 8, 1821, Selkirk Papers, PAC 7374.
3. Understanding this element of Simpson's leadership style, in the end, might help change history's view of the Governor's role in his cousin Thomas Simpson's death. Circumstantial evidence definitely points to pathological jealousy of his cousin's achievements. Indeed, as Ken McGoogan explains in *Fatal Passage: The True Story of John Rae, the Arctic Adventurer Who Discovered the Fate of Franklin* (Toronto: HarperCollins, 2001), Simpson was jealous of John Rae's exploration accomplishments as well. And while one can imagine Simpson saying out loud in the company of some of his Métis friends in Red River that the world might be a better place with Thomas dead, a more likely scenario explaining young Thomas's untimely end might well be that he died at the hand of a Simpson acolyte hoping to curry favour with the boss.

AUTHOR'S NOTE

1. Newman, *Caesars of the Wilderness*, 290.

APPENDIX I

1. Lahey, *Fed by Their Wings*, vii.

Bibliography

Beebe, Lucius. *Mansions on Rails: The Folklore of the Private Railway Car.* Berkeley, CA: Howell-North, 1959.

Bethune, Rev. Hector. "Parish of Dingwall, Presbytery of Dingwall, Synod of Ross." In *The New Statistical Account of Scotland 1845,* 210–35. Edinburgh: Blackwood, 1845.

Black, George F. *The Surnames of Scotland: Their Origin, Meaning, and History.* Edinburgh: Birlinn, 1946.

Blaikie, Andrew. "Scottish Illegitimacy: Social Adjustment or Moral Economy." *Journal of Interdisciplinary History* 39 (1998): 221–41.

Blaikie, A., E. Garrett, and R. Davies. "Migration, Living Strategies and Illegitimate Childbearing: A Comparison of Two Scottish Settings, 1871–1881." In *Illegitimacy in Britain, 1700–1920,* edited by Alysa Levene, Thomas Nutt, and Samantha Williams, 141–67. Houndmills, Hampshire, UK: Palgrave Macmillan, 2005.

Bone, Robert M. *The Geography of the Canadian North.* Toronto: Oxford University Press, 1992.

Brown, Jennifer S.H. "Linguistic Solitudes and Changing Social Categories." In *Old Trails and New Directions: Papers of the Third North American Fur Trade Conference,* edited by Carol M. Judd and Arthur J. Ray, 147–59. Toronto: University of Toronto Press, 1978.

——. *Strangers in Blood: Fur Trade Company Families in Indian Country.* Vancouver: University of British Columbia Press, 1980.

Bryce, Rev. G. *Mackenzie, Selkirk, Simpson.* Toronto: Morang & Co., 1910.

Bibliography

Bumstead, J.M. "The Strange Death of Thomas Simpson." *Winnipeg Real Estate News,* July 3, 1998, 3.

Burley, Edith I. *Servants of the Honourable Company: Work, Discipline, and Conflict in the Hudson's Bay Company, 1770–1870.* Toronto: Oxford University Press, 1997.

Burnard, T.G. *Mastery, Tyranny, and Desire: Thomas Thistlewood and His Slaves in the Anglo-Jamaican World.* Chapel Hill: University of North Carolina Press, 2004.

Chalmers, John W. *Fur Trade Governor: George Simpson, 1820–1860.* Edmonton: Institute of Applied Art, 1960.

Cline, Gloria Griffin. *Peter Skene Ogden and the Hudson's Bay Company.* Norman: University of Oklahoma Press, 1974.

Cotter, H.M.S. "The Birchbark Canoe: An Important Factor in H.B.C. Transport from Earliest Times." *The Beaver,* June 1922, 5–8.

Cox, Ross. *The Columbia River.* Edited by Edgar I. Stewart and Jane R. Stewart. 1832; Norman: University of Oklahoma Press, 1957.

Cree, Murial R. "Three Simpson Letters: 1815–1820." *British Columbia Historical Quarterly* 1 (1937): 115–19.

Cyriax, R.J. 1957. "A Note Concerning Thomas Simpson." Hudson's Bay Company Archives, Thomas Simpson search file.

Dickason, Olive Patricia. *Canada's First Nations: A History of Founding Peoples from Earliest Times.* Toronto: McClelland & Stewart, 1992.

Dod, Charles R. *The Peerage, Baronetage, and Knightage of Great Britain and Ireland for 1854.* London: Whittaker and Co., 1854.

Doolittle, I.G. *The City of London and Its Livery Companies.* London: Gavin, 1982.

Fleming, R. Harvey, ed. *Minutes of Council, Northern Department of Rupert Land, 1821–31.* Toronto: Champlain Society, 1940.

Flinn, Michael, ed. *Scottish Population History from the 17th Century to the 1930s.* Cambridge, UK: Cambridge University Press, 1977.

Franchère, Gabriel. *A Voyage to the Northwest Coast of America.* Edited by Milo Milton Quaife. Chicago: Lakeside Classics, 1954. Originally published in French in 1820.

Francis, Daniel. *The Imaginary Indian: The Image of the Indian in Canadian Culture.* Vancouver: Arsenal Pulp, 1992.

Francis, R. Douglas, Richard Jones, and Donald B. Smith, eds. *Origins: Canadian History to Confederation.* Toronto: Holt, Rinehart & Winston, 1988.

Fraser, Simon. *The Letters and Journals of Simon Fraser, 1806–1808.* Edited by W. Kaye Lamb. Toronto: Macmillan, 1960.

Bibliography

Galbraith, John S. "The Little Emperor." *The Beaver*, Winter 1960, Outfit 291, Vol. 40 (3), 22.

——. *The Little Emperor: Governor Simpson of the Hudson's Bay Company.* Toronto: Macmillan, 1976.

Garry, Nicholas. *The Diary of Nicholas Garry: A Detailed Narrative of His Travels in the Northwest Territories of British North America in 1821; Originally Composed, Edited and Annotated from His Grandfather's Original MS. by Mr. Francis N.A. Garry in 1900.* 1900; Toronto: Canadiana House, 1973.

Gordon, Charlotte. "Memorial to Sir George Simpson: Famous Hudson's Bay Company Governor of a Century Ago to Be Honored." *Toronto Saturday Night,* August 18, 1928, 4–5.

Great Britain. Parliament. *Report from the Select Committee on the State of British Possessions in North America which are under the Administration of the Hudson's Bay Company with Minutes of Evidence Appendix and Index.* London: British Parliamentary Papers, 1857.

Halpenny, F.G., ed. *Dictionary of Canadian Biography.* Volume 8. Toronto: University of Toronto Press, 1966.

Hargrave, James. *The Hargrave Correspondence, 1821–1843.* Edited by G.P. de T. Glazebrook. Toronto: Champlain Society, 1938.

Hargrave, Letitia. *Letters of Letitia Hargrave.* Edited by Margaret Arnett Macleod. Toronto: Champlain Society, 1947.

Harmon, Daniel Williams. *Sixteen Years in the Indian Country: The Journal of Daniel Williams Harmon, 1800–1816.* Edited by W. Kaye Lamb. Toronto: Macmillan, 1957.

Harper, M. *Thomas Simpson: Dingwall's Arctic Explorer.* Dingwall Museum, Local Studies No. 2. Dingwall, Scotland: Ross & Cromarty, n.d.

Hayes, Derek. *Historical Atlas of Canada.* Vancouver: Douglas & McIntyre, 2002.

Herman, Arthur. *How the Scots Invented the Modern World.* New York: Random House, 2001.

Innis, Harold. *The Fur Trade in Canada.* Toronto: University of Toronto Press, 1956.

Ireland, Willard E. "McLoughlin's Letters 1839–1944" [Review of Hudson's Bay Record Society, Vol. 6]. *The Beaver,* 1944, Outfit 275, Vol. 24(2), 45–46.

Johnson, Alice M. "Edward and Frances Hopkins of Montreal." *The Beaver,* 1971, Outfit 302, Vol. 51(2), 4–17.

——. "Simpson in Russia." *The Beaver,* 1960, 4–12, 58.

Lahey, D.T. *Fed by Their Wings: The Descendants of Sir George Simpson.* Guelph, ON: Datel Publishing, 2003.

——. "How Old Was Sir George Simpson? An Exercise in the Genealogical Proof Standard." *Families,* February 2006, 42–59.

Laing, Alexander. *American Sail: A Pictorial History*. New York: Dutton, 1961.

——, ed. *Saskatchewan Journals and Correspondence: Edmonton House 1795–1800, Chesterfield House 1800–1802*. London: Hudson's Bay Record Society, 1967.

Lefroy, John Henry. *In Search of the Magnetic North: A Soldier-Surveyor's Letter from the North-West, 1843–1844*. Edited by George F.G. Stanley. Toronto: Macmillan, 1955.

Levene, Alysa, Thomas Nutt, and Samantha Williams, eds. *Illegitimacy in Britain, 1700–1920*. Houndmills, Hampshire, UK: Palgrave Macmillan, 2005.

MacDonald, D.D. *A History of Dingwall Academy*. Inverness, Scotland: printed for the author, 1989.

MacEwan, Grant. *Fifty Mighty Men*. Saskatoon: Modern Press, 1958.

MacKay, Douglas, and W. Kaye Lamb. "More Light on Thomas Simpson." *The Beaver*, September 1938, 26–31.

Mackenzie, Alexander. *The Journals and Letters of Sir Alexander Mackenzie*. Edited by W. Kaye Lamb. Cambridge, UK: Cambridge University Press, 1970.

Maclean, Charles. *The Fringe of Gold: The Fishing Villages of Scotland's East Coast, Orkney & Shetland*. Edinburgh: Canongate Books, 1985.

Macrae, Norman. *The Romance of a Royal Burgh: Dingwall's Story of a Thousand Years*. 1923; Dingwall, Scotland: Dingwall Museum Trust, 1974.

McArthur, Alex. *A Prairie Tragedy: The Fate of Thomas Simpson*. Winnipeg: G.C. Mortimore, 1887.

McCook, James. "Sir George Simpson in the Hawaiian Islands." *The Beaver*, Winter 1976, 48.

McDonald, Archibald. *Peace River: A Canoe Voyage from Hudson's Bay to Pacific by Sir George Simpson in 1828—Journal of the Late Chief Factor Archibald McDonald (Hon. Hudson's Bay Company), Who Accompanied Him*. Edited, with notes, by Malcolm McLeod. 1872; Edmonton: M.G. Hurtig, 1971.

McGoogan, Ken. *Fatal Passage: The True Story of John Rae, the Arctic Adventurer Who Discovered the Fate of Franklin*. Toronto: HarperCollins, 2001.

McKay, John. *The Hudson's Bay Company's 1835 Steam Ship "Beaver."* St. Catharines, ON: Vanwell, 2001.

McLean, John. *Notes of a Twenty-Five Years' Service in the Hudson's Bay Territory*. Edited by William Stewart Wallace. Toronto: Champlain Society, 1932.

McLoughlin, John. *The Letters of John McLoughlin from Fort Vancouver to the Governor and Committee . . . 1825–39*. Edited by E.E. Rich. Toronto, 1841–44.

Moberly, Henry John, with William Bleasdell Cameron. *When Fur Was King*. Toronto: J.M. Dent, 1929.

Bibliography

Morse, Eric. *Canoe Routes of the Voyageurs: The Geography and Logistics of the Canadian Fur Trade. Canadian Geographical Journal,* 1961; Quetico Foundation of Ontario and the Minnesota Historical Society, 1962.

Morton, A.S. *Sir George Simpson: Overseas Governor of the Hudson's Bay Company.* Toronto: J.M. Dent, 1944.

Morton, W.L. "Donald A. Smith and Governor George Simpson." *The Beaver,* Autumn 1978, 4–9.

Newman, Peter C. *Caesars of the Wilderness,* Volume 2, *Company of Adventurers.* Markham, ON: Penguin, 1987.

"Presentation to the Governor." *The Beaver,* June 1943, 49.

Ray, Arthur J. *I Have Lived Here Since the World Began.* Toronto: Lester/Key Porter, 1996.

——. *Indians in the Fur Trade: Their Role as Trappers, Hunters and Middlemen in the Lands Southwest of Hudson Bay, 1660–1870.* Toronto: University of Toronto Press, 1974.

Rich, E.E. *The History of the Hudson's Bay Company,* Volume 1, *1670–1763.* Hudson's Bay Record Society 22. London: Hudson's Bay Record Society, 1958.

——. *The History of the Hudson's Bay Company,* Volume 2, *1763–1870.* Hudson's Bay Record Society 22. London: Hudson's Bay Record Society, 1959.

——. *Montreal and the Fur Trade.* Montreal: McGill University Press, 1966.

Robertson, Colin. *Colin Robertson's Correspondence Book, September 1817–1822.* Edited by E.E. Rich. Toronto: Champlain Society, 1939.

Rose, Rev. Daniel. "Parish of Dingwall (County of Ross)." In *Statistical Account of Scotland 1791,* 353–72. Edinburgh, 1791.

Ross, Frank E. "Sir George Simpson at the Department of State." *British Columbia Historical Quarterly* 2, no. 2 (1938): 131–35.

Royal Burgh of Dingwall. "Minutes of 18th Century Council Meetings" [1780–1784]. Dingwall Museum Trust Document 2548. Dingwall, Scotland.

Rutherford, Edward. *London.* New York: Ballantine, 1997.

Saw, Reginald. "Treaty with the Russians." *The Beaver,* December 1948, 30–33.

Seaburg, Carl, and Stanley Patterson. *Merchant Prince of Boston: Colonel T.H. Perkins, 1764–1854.* Cambridge, MA: Harvard University Press, 1971.

Selkirk, Thomas Douglas. *Observations on the present state of the highlands of Scotland: With a view of the causes and probable consequences of emigration.* Edinburgh, 1806. CIHM Microfiche 49523.

Simpson, Alexander. *The Life and Travels of Thomas Simpson, the Arctic Discoverer.* London: Richard Bentley, 1845.

Simpson, George. "Blue Bell." *The Beaver,* Autumn 1971, 58.

Simpson, George. "The Character Book of Governor George Simpson, 1832." In *Hudson's Bay Miscellany 1670–1870,* edited by Glyndwr Williams. Publications of the Hudson's Bay Record Society 30. Winnipeg: Hudson's Bay Record Society, 1975.

——. *Fur Trade and Empire: George Simpson's Journal Entitled Remarks Connected with the Fur Trade in Course of a Voyage from York Factory to Fort George and Back to York Factory 1824–25, with Related Documents.* Edited by Frederick Merk. Revised edition. Cambridge, MA: Belknap, 1968.

——. *Journal of Occurrences in the Athabasca Department by George Simpson, 1820 and 1821, and Report.* Edited by E.E. Rich. Toronto: Champlain Society, for the Hudson's Bay Record Society, 1938.

——. *Narrative of a Journey Round the World, during the Years 1841 and 1842.* 2 vols. London: H. Colburn, 1847.

——. *Part of Dispatch from George Simpson EsqR, Governor of Ruperts Land, to the Governor and Committee of the Hudson's Bay Company London, March 1, 1829: Continued and Completed March 24 and June 5, 1829.* Edited by E.E. Rich. HBC Series 10. Toronto: Champlain Society, 1947.

Spraakman, G., and A. Wilkie. "The Development of Management Accounting at the Hudson's Bay Company, 1670–1820." *Accounting History* 5 (2000): 59–84.

——. "Transaction Cost Economics as a Predictor of Management Accounting Practices at the Hudson's Bay Company." *Accounting History* 3 (1998): 69–101.

Stefansson, Vilhjalmur. *Unsolved Mysteries of the Arctic.* New York: Macmillan, 1942.

Stenson, Fred. *The Trade.* Vancouver: Douglas & McIntyre, 2000.

Swagerty, William R. "The Leviathan of the North: American Perceptions of the Hudson's Bay Company, 1816–1846." *Oregon Historical Quarterly* 104, no. 4 (2003): 478–517, http://www.historycooperative.org/journals/ohq/104.4/swagerty.html.

Thompson, David. *David Thompson's Narrative, 1784–1812.* Edited by Richard Glover. Toronto: Champlain Society, 1962.

Van Kirk, Sylvia. *Many Tender Ties: Women in Fur-Trade Society, 1670–1870.* Winnipeg: Watson & Dwyer, 1980.

——. "Women and the Fur Trade." *The Beaver,* Winter 1972, 4–21.

Verne, Jules. *The English at the North Pole.* London: G. Routledge, 1864.

——. *The Tour of the World in Eighty Days.* Boston: J.R. Osgood, 1873.

Wedderburn, Robert. *The Horrors of Slavery; exemplified in the life and history of the Rev. Robert Wedderburn . . .* London, 1824.

Williamson, Oliver. *The Economic Institutions of Capitalism.* New York: Collier Macmillan, 1985.

Bibliography

Wilson, Clifford P. "The Emperor at Lachine." *The Beaver,* September 1935, 18–22.

——. "The Emperor's Last Days." *The Beaver,* December 1934, 49–51.

——. "Sir George Simpson at Lachine." *The Beaver,* June 1934, 36–39.

Illustration Credits

Images not otherwise credited are from the author's collection.

Original maps by Dawn Huck:
60, 84, 134, opposite 340 (fold-out map).

Courtesy of Clipartreview.com:
Pages 5, 12, 30, 46, 66, 68, 71, 122, 133, 147, 171, 188, 208, 230, 291, 330, 362, 395, 403.

Courtesy of Glenbow Museum Archives:
Pages 137 (NA-1041-8); 174 (NA-3490-26); 279 (NA-3421-3); 314 (NA-1406-35).

Courtesy of Sara Haddon:
Pages iv, 2 (painter unknown, possibly Paul Kane or Stephen Pearce).

Courtesy of the Hudson's Bay Company Archive / Manitoba Provincial Archives:
Pages 58, 95, 128, 160, 209, 210, 232, 237 (painted by L.L. Fitzgerald, based on a photo of a Cyrus C. Cuneo painting commissioned by the Canadian Pacific Railway), 253, 271, 284, 314, 386 (painted by Stephen Pearce), 417.

Courtesy of *Illustrated London News*:
Pages 42, 411, 422.

INDEX

Two indexes are printed in the pages that follow. The first is an abridged index of marker events listed by their *date of occurrence*. The second and longer index is a standard *alphabetic index of subjects and concepts*. Page citations appearing in ***bold italics*** denote ***illustrations*** in this book.

EVENT INDEX BY DATE

Event Index by Date

Subject Index

Aberdeen (city), 28
Aberdeen (Lord Aberdeen), 359–60
Aberdeen University, 39, 44, 202, 237, 246, 325
aboriginal people. *See* First Nations people; *See also specific exemplars* [e.g. Cree (people)]
Act for Regulating the Fur Trade, 138
Addington, Lord Henry, 225
Adirondack Mountains, 83
Alaska, 5, 13, 179
Albany, (N.Y.), 82–83
alcohol. *See* liquor
Alexander (ship), 1, 3–4, 347, 350
Alexander I (Czar), 179, 298, 300
Aleutian Islands, 1
Aleuts (people), 298
Algonquin (people), 92
Allumette Island, 92
American Fur Company, 93, 297
Anderson, Alexander Caulfield, 311
Anderson, Dr. James, 311
Anderson, T.B., 417
Anglo-American Treaty (1846, re Pacific border), 360–61
Ashley, Gen. William H., 297
Assiniboia. *See also* Red River Colony; Selkirk settlement (Winnipeg), 74–75, 96, 109, 128, 136, 148, 175, 245, 279, 293, 296, 322, 332, 339, 369–75, 394, 401–2
    attacks upon the residents of, 59
    recruitment of settlers for, 58–59, 132
Assiniboine River, 58, 74, 136, 169, 176, 257, 273
Astor, John Jacob, 76, 81–82, 178, 188, 257, 297
Athabasca (district). *See also* Lake Athabasca, 59, 75–76, 96, 102–11, 113, 121, 123–27, 129, 137–38, 140, 143, 152–54, 158–59, 161, 163, 166, 169, 172, 175, 183, 281
Athabasca Pass, 173–76, 195–96, 198–99, 236, 245
Athabasca River, 110, 172–75, 183, 198
Avoch (Scot.), 25–27, 30–31, 44, 73

Back, George, 108, 118–20
Baines, Captain, 78, 80
Ballenden, John, 371
Bank of British North America, 356
Baranof Island, 342, 347
Barclay, Dr. Archibald, 362–63, 378, 389
Baring Brothers (investment firm), 393
Barston, Mary (Simpson governess), 378
Bathurst (Lord Bathurst), 61, 78, 81, 93–95, 100, 225
bear pelts, 214

bears, encounters with and tales of, 14, 175
Beauharnois, 356, 396
Beauly Firth, 214, 249, 289
Beaver (ship), 341–43
Beaver Club (Montreal), 231–32, 294, 356
"Beaver Lodge" (proposed Simpson residence), 307, 379
beaver pelts
    as a monetary unit, 214
    demand for, 71, 99, 138, 159, 179, 182, 300
Beaver River, 173, 183, 198
beavers, increasing scarcity of, 71, 113, 138, 160, 214, 308, 422
Beef-Steak Club (Montreal), 294–95
Belcourt, George A., 371, 373
Bella Bella, 342
Bella Coola, 299
Bellevue House (Scotland), *249*, 254
Belle Vue Point, 187
Ben Wyvis, 31–32
Berens, Henry Hulse, 297, 392, 405–6, 422
Berens, Herman, 210–11
Berens, Joseph, Jr., 210–11
Berens, Joseph, Sr., 210
Berens House, 110–11, *134*, 137
Berens River, 137
Bering Sea, 3, 315
Bernard, Jean Baptiste (chief guide), 240, 259, 275
Bethune, Rev. Hector, 37, 430
Bird, George, 199–200, 319, 322
Bird, John, 319–20, 337
births, out of wedlock. *See also* Simpson, Sir George, children born out of wedlock to, 20, 25, 28–29, 50, 52, 252
Black, Samuel, 104, 106–7
Black Ball Line, 66–69, 77, 256, 285
Blackburn, Isabella, 51
Black Isle (Scot.), 25–26, 30, 177, 202
Blackwater (Scot.), 31
Blackwood, William, 231
blankets
    as items of survival and comfort, 91, 160, 240, 272
    as items of trade, 91, 106, 169, 214–15
Boat Encampment, *134*, 136, 173, 175–76, 186, 195
bois brûlé. See Métis (people)
Bonaparte, Napoleon, 36, 48, 66–67, 170, 228, 353–54, 426
Bone, Robert, 420
Boothia Peninsula, 316

Subject Index

Subject Index

Subject Index

479

Subject Index